Your Life Your Choice
Let the Healing Begin
A JOURNEY OF DIS-EASE TO EASE

Healing Holistically of
Pancreatic Cancer

Your Life Your Choice
Let the Healing Begin
A JOURNEY OF DIS-EASE TO EASE

Healing Holistically of
Pancreatic Cancer

By Kelly Lang and Amy Lang

ISBN: 978-1-66785-417-5
ISBN eBook: 978-1-66785-418-2

DEDICATION
Kelly Lang

I'd like to dedicate this book to my Papa God.
He's my best friend, my biggest love,
and truest companion I could ever have.

Papa God loves each and every one of us,
and without Him as the Lord of my life
I would not be who I am today.

Thank God for saving a wretch like me
who is completely undeserving,
yet loved with a vengeance by her
Papa God that to this day still blows my mind.

Thank You, Papa God, for loving not just me,
but every single person on this gigantic earth.
Thank You for not saving me once, but twice now.
And thank You for the continuous love
You give with no strings attached.

May we all try to do that more—
love with a heart blown wide open with
no restraints, like Papa God loves.

INTRODUCTION
Kelly Lang

At 18 years old I became ill in health. It took a total of seven years to reverse my health situation. This is my story of overcoming illness via all-natural modalities, food as medicine, and with the help of practitioners and therapists to heal my ill body. It's taken a lot of hard work and dedication, but without others to walk alongside of me on this journey, life probably would be very different for me—or wouldn't be at all.

During all the years when I was sick, I had journaled on a daily basis, which helped me immensely in the healing process. I first thought I'd write a book. So, I did a lot more writing, which turned out to be for my own benefit. I chose not to publish those writings AS a book at the time. A few years later, after I healed, I started sharing my story in honest, open truth about my health, my life, my emotions, my thoughts, and even my prayers during the span of illness. I had my journals and writings to look back on as I blogged. I simply shared my life and my health story. There was a sincere interest in my story by my readers, which encouraged me to put my story into a physical book and an Ebook as well.

My story is raw and personal. That's about as real as it gets, right? My health has come full circle. As a woman who has nearly lost her life because of her ill health, I can't say how thankful I am to have my health back, restored tenfold! I'm very excited you chose to take this healing journey with me! With that being said, I cordially invite you to embark with me in "Your Life Your Choice Let the Healing Begin A JOURNEY OF DIS-EASE TO EASE Healing Holistically of Pancreatic Cancer".

May this story be a blessing to all who read it. May you see God's hand at work in the spoken and unspoken in my story.

PREFACE
Amy Lang

As I actively partook in life with Kelly, my daughter, in our home during her health journey from dis-ease to ease, there were days of great discomfort and pain. But also, there were important days of celebrating the small significant shifts as they began to happen... and many, many days of wonders to keep us encouraged. Kelly's my living miracle. I believe her story matters and can make a difference in this unpredictable world.

Journeys are meant to teach us many things: about ourselves, about others, and about life. Our journeys are also used to grow our faith and individual character. Most often I find the later to be true.

I was asked to share my thoughts and memories of her health journey when Kelly began the process of sharing her story in writing. Willingly, I wrote.

"ADVERSITY is like a strong wind. It tears at us and pulls everything off until what's left is what we really are"
-Arthur Golden

Within the bookends are stories of hope and healing, conversations had between Kelly and her family, her friends, with her Papa God, and conversations with her alternative health practitioners--whose names, business names, and locations have been changed. As we dug deep to find help for Kelly, starting at age 18 years old, there were people who came alongside to assist in bringing her to a higher level of healing what needed to be healed and detoxing what needed to be eliminated from her ill body. Kelly's health story is told uncensored, with boldness, and in detail of real happenings I witnessed daily. Her personal health experiences, all of which she practiced naturally and overcame illness with years of diligence, commitment to self, and with much respect for herself, is truly amazing! The road she chose to heal herself is in fact a road less traveled, and even much less talked about in mainstream health services and in the media. All-natural approaches to dis-ease are not new ideas--they are ancient, and most are proven cures in many cases. We hope you will enjoy our journey and our stories! And most importantly, we want you to enjoy your life because it's really your choice to how you live each and every day. Each choice you make matters—you only get one life here to live!

BEFORE READING THIS BOOK

Always check who the author is at the chapter's beginning for clarity as to who is writing, since Kelly and Amy are two different writers contributing to the same book. Putting Kelly's and Amy's writings together makes Kelly's story more complete, but it can make reading much more confusing if the reader doesn't note an author change at the beginning of a chapter.

The names and locations of all friends, of all healthcare individuals, and of all businesses besides Kelly's business and her families' names have been changed for confidentiality purposes. Although the conversations are factual, the people and their businesses are made up names... unless there is a reference and footnote to either for looking up more information on topic of discussion.

1

When Your Life Flashes Before Your Eyes in a Flood Gate of Memories...

Kelly

When your life flashes before your eyes in a flood gate of memories... This happens during the time of year between the months of August thru October, because they hold a lot of memories. Let me explain why.

For seven years, starting in August 2010, I was sick, having severe left-side pain that ripped into my gut. I choose all-natural routes of healing to cure whatever was going on deep inside my body, starting at that time in August. For the first five years I got by, struggling at times. But it finally came to the point where I needed serious help.

At year number five my health was at a critical point. I was malnourished, weak, pale, and having symptoms that were pages long. I was also depressed. Year number five was a turning point in my health. I got to the core issue, which exposed pancreatic cancer that I was starting to detox out of my body. I worked with multiple naturopathic therapists, chiropractors and doctors, and also did a gut healing program online, all before logging on with a brilliant clinician based in the United States who was a vital key to turning my health around.

It took a total of seven years to reverse my health. During all the years when I was sick, I had journaled on a daily basis, which helped me immensely in the healing process. I first thought I'd write a book. So, I did a lot more writing, which turned out to be for my own benefit. I chose not to publish those writings

AS a book at the time. A few years later, after I healed, I started sharing my story in honest, open truth about my health, my life, my emotions, and my thoughts. I had my journals and writings to look back on.

My story is raw and personal. That's about as real as it gets, right? My health has come full circle. As a woman who has nearly lost her life because of her ill health, I can't say how thankful I am to have my health back, restored tenfold!

When I received my test results with a clean bill of pancreas health in September of 2016, it was not a surprise to me. I had already known in my heart of hearts that I was free of cancer—free of dis-ease and ready to move on with my life and my choices. So naturally when the dog days of August arrive each year, my life flashes before me in a flood gate of memories of starting this healing journey, August of 2010 through October 2016, and I smile really big knowing all the progress that was made in gaining back my health in all-natural ways.

2

My Ill Health Journey Begins

Kelly

My left side hurts.

May/June 2010. I'd just graduated from high school. Life happened fast, and now I was 18 years old with no idea of what I wanted to do for a life work. Being uncertain about my future, thankfully that was okay with my family. Since I didn't know what I wanted to do, I decided washing windows with my dad was a good fit, which I'd done during the summers' past. I liked physical work, and washing windows was a very physically active job! *This will give me time to figure out what I might want to do with my future,* I thought.

"The best view comes after the hardest climb." -Unknown

July 2010. Our family was in the process of helping put together a benefit for a family friend who had cancer. It wasn't until mid-July that I said out loud, "Mom, my left side hurts." She looked at me immediately with concern shown in her eyes.

"Where does it hurt? Point to where it hurts, Kelly." She inquired, searching my eyes in all seriousness. I shared with her the painful physical symptoms of gas, bloating, headaches, and a dull ache that was very severe at times, and diarrhea. We talked at length, deciding it was time to pay a visit to the medical doctor.

A week-and-a-half later, I attempted to not squirm in my chair while in the waiting room at the medical clinic with Mom next to me. My abdomen hurt and my head was pounding. My hands were clammy. It was time. A physicians' assistant called my name. On the other side of the waiting-room

3

door, she had me stand next to the measuring tape to get my height, 5′ 6″, then she motioned me to the scale and I stepped on it. She wrote down 157 pounds. I was the heaviest I'd ever been. My weight didn't matter to me, as long as I felt well and healthy. And that's why I was there at the medical center. I didn't feel well OR healthy. I felt bloated, inflamed, and on fire.

Sitting down inside the examination room, getting asked many questions and telling her my symptoms, she jotted down notes in my file. She exited the room and the doctor came in and repeated her questions. Common procedure. I told the doctor, "I recently quit eating dairy and that seems to help some, but it doesn't make all my symptoms go away."

Mom spoke too, saying, "Kelly is the kid that never complains about pain. The fact that she has shared it is an obvious concern to us. Kelly came to me telling me about her pain. She could pinpoint it, but can't reach into it."

The doctor palpated my abdomen. At the end of being poked and prodded, she said, "I'm sure it's just some IBS (irritable bowel syndrome). But let's do some testing to make sure it's nothing else in the meantime."

At that point in my life, I hadn't had much patience. *IBS? Are you kidding me?* Immediately feeling defensive, I calmed myself down and Mom gave me that *I know you're ticked off but don't be a jerk* look. I attempted to throw the doctor's observation aside and focus on the conversation. My mind reeled.

I agreed to having blood drawn, give a urine sample, a test for West Nile disease and a few other diseases. "You should get your results via a phone call in a few days from my assistant," the doctor had told us. I'd nodded my okay, completed the tasks asked for before leaving the clinic, then Mom and I walked outside into the fresh air, at last!

My stewing silence lasted about ten steps or less, until I was far enough from the building before blurting out, "Are you kidding me? IBS? That has NOTHING to do with my left side pain." I was angry, steaming and starting to boil over. I had a headache bigger than what I went into the appointment with, my left side hurt, and yes… you could say I was a hot mess. I attempted to hold in my emotions, thoughts, and words that I wanted to say more of, and tried to be tough. I was on the verge of tears. By the time we got to the car,

4

hot tears were trickling down my face as I angrily swat at them. And so, my journey begins…

3

I Will NOT Be a Lab Rat

Kelly

My phone rang. Then my mind whirled as I looked at the caller ID number that came up on my cell phone. It was time to find out about my test results from the local medical clinic. *I wonder what they found wrong with me?* I thought inwardly.

"Hello?" I answered.

"Hi Kelly. It's Salena from the clinic. Well, I have both good and bad news for you. I'll start with the bad news", she stated. "Bad news is; we don't know WHAT'S causing your discomfort." There was a brief pause before offering, "The good news is that all your test results came back 'normal'. It's good that they came back normal, but that doesn't help with understanding why you don't feel good."

I stood looking out the window inside of our home, shaking my head in disbelief. *All these tests and not a single lead on what is going on inside of me? Why am I having these symptoms and in such pain and discomfort then?* I shook my head in order to clear my thoughts and listen to her as she'd started talking again.

"It must be a bad case of IBS. If it doesn't quit within the next 2-3 weeks give the clinic a call and we'll do further tests." She then guided our phone call to an end. Again, my mind reeled.

Mom had stood close by, listening to the conversation as my irritation had continued to grow. Sadness filled her eyes as I looked into them. My eyes and heart were filled with hurt, anger, resentment, disbelief, and questions, everything Mom could see inside of me. I locked in my emotions, clenching my jaw, desperately trying to cut off my feelings. Silence was short-lived before Mom gently questioned, "Kelly?"

The dam broke loose and words inside of me came spilling out, "Mom, I DO NOT want to be a lab rat! There is something much deeper than 'IBS' going on here. Something is really wrong, but I don't know what. I'm mad at the doctor... and the assistant. It's like they didn't even hear me with what I all shared with them. I wouldn't have gone in if I didn't feel this bad. I feel like they don't even believe me." Again, I stated, "I WILL NOT be a lab rat." I was fuming mad, all the while holding back hot tears. *Tears are weakness. I'm not weak. I won't give in to crying. Control yourself*, I thought.

Mom knew me well enough that she wasn't going to argue with me. Arguing wasn't going to help the situation. Right now, what the situation needed was for me to calm down. Mom slyly helped calm me... and we began a brief question and answer session.

"Okay. You don't want to be a lab rat. Let me make sure I understand what you are saying in that statement. Please explain that." She'd probed.

"I don't want to be looked at as 'a number' instead of a human being. I don't want to do a bunch of tests like they do on rats that ultimately lead to exactly what just happened--testing with no results, insights, or answers. And, I don't want to take medications –drugs, if that's what they recommend to help with the pain. My gut already hurts, so I'm not going to add drugs into the mix and be worse off than now." I paused before adding, "I just don't feel like this... um, well... feels 'RIGHT'." I paused again before finishing my explanation, "Something is really wrong, Mom... but I don't know WHAT."

Tears attempted to spill over onto my face, some breaking free resulting in me irritatingly grabbing for them. *Dang it.* I tried encouraging the log that now filled my throat to flow in the direction downward, instead of pouring my feelings out. We stood in silence for almost a minute.

"I hear what you are saying." Mom said shaking her head. "I understand where you are coming from. If this matters, I'm telling you that I do believe what you have shared with me about the physical pain you are feeling, Kelly. I know you. I hear you. And I stand behind you in whatever decision that you ultimately make in finding answers to your health problems." Tears were gently streaming down her face as she spoke fluently.

She believes me! I never doubted that though, I thought. *How is it that she makes crying look beautiful? I look like a sobbing, angry, hot mess when I cry. No crying for me!*

"Kelly, if you don't want to be a lab rat, what do you want to do in order to get some answers for your symptoms and left-side pain?" She ever so gently asked. I was speechless. How could I answer a question that I had so little information on to even begin an answer?

Truth was, Mom was dead right in asking the question. I was 18 years old, an adult, and I didn't fully know what "other" options I had. *I have to make my own choices because I am legally an adult now. Mom and Dad will help and guide me in my choices IF I want help and direction,* I thought to myself. I was really sick for the first time in my life, and I had no idea as to what the answer to her question was. I shook my head back and forth. "Kelly?" She lovingly tried me again.

"I don't know, Mom. I don't know." I stammered. "All I know is that I don't want to be a lab rat, and that this system of testing, labeling, and drugging isn't right for me. I really don't know what to say other than that right now." *I don't know Mama, I don't know...*

4

Stories Brewing

Amy

When I see arms flailing and legs moving fast from outside our kitchen window, there's a story brewing! This morning, as Kelly joined her cat, Goofy, for their daily morning adventure outside, I thought while watching, *what the heck?*

Then, explosive shouts of "NO! NO! NO!" penetrated the exterior wall, shattering through the overhead oven hood via the vent from where the action was taking place! My heart went faint with thoughts of *another stray cat, or maybe a visiting dog from the next-door lake area boat launch.* Kelly's vocal reaction drove my thoughts towards the worst. I dropped everything and ran to the garage, opening the service door. I saw, half ways across the road, my grown-up brown-eyed girl running FULL speed. I know full well she is in last place in the race ahead of her. I dash to the bedroom to wake my husband from his sleep, telling him of the immediate happening.

When I looked out the window minutes later, half ways back across the street, Goofy is leading her owner home. There's a story alright, but it will have to wait to be told until the two pals come in from their morning adventures!

And THIS mornings' adventure sparked memories of times past--raising our two children, Troy and Kelly, bringing to my mind choices leading to the good, the bad, and the uncertainties of life, love, and parenting. How many times did I REACT immediately to the adventures at hand in these areas, with possible outcomes being un-thought about? Too many to count. There's much to be said about choices: ours, others, and our children's. We each have daily opportunities to impact our own and other's lives positively, negatively, or otherwise because of our choices.

So, this morning, as I watched scenes of a brewing story in, "Adventures with Goofy and Friends" up close and personal, I saw my girl REACT immediately to help her pal who was in a bad situation. She didn't hesitate! She reacted with virtually no pause (paws, for effect!) and entered into the fight. *Hmm, this is feeling familiar*, I thought from my parental view.

It turned out that when Goofy was moved off of a stray cat, by Kelly when they were outside of my kitchen window view, the stray cat ran and Goofy was at its tail following! And so followed Kelly, beating foot to keep up through the neighborhood to rescue her furry friend Goofy. What a sight! The best and funniest part left unseen by myself, but maybe not unseen to unknown others, was when Kelly's arms and torso were moving faster than her legs. The top-weight won out, spilling herself onto a neighboring yard! She was unharmed by the fall physically, so the image in mind of the spill made me laugh out loud as she retold the story!

Eventually, the stray cat got away and Goofy was captured, redirected, and brought back home. THAT'S love. Real, genuine, unspoken LOVE. Love does. And this morning, love DID. Love was in action without a moments' hesitation.

As parents, the relationships we have with our kids are ever changing with the seasons of age, and with each situation. When Kelly came to me telling of her health symptoms, I immediately reacted inside, wanting to help in any way possible. She was 18 years old. She was an adult who could and would make her choices for the life she would choose to live. I knew that this would have to be her choice on how she was going to adapt to a Western-world medical system that is GREAT at so many aspects of healthcare, but in my opinion lacks in treating the whole person dealing with chronic illness. I knew my girl. I knew her well enough to know that prescription drugs would not be a part of her daily lifestyle.

My girl was going to have to make a choice on how she was going to get answers for what was going on inside her body, and I was going to be there to walk alongside of her no matter what. Because honestly, like Kelly with her pal Goofy, I would run after and support my brown-eyed girl wherever her health journey led her. And I did.

Kelly has a telling story to share of this difficult season of her life. I watched her live this one out, up close and personal for seven years. Every day WAS a journal page while she chose to let the healing begin in alternative ways of caring for herself. I watched her grow mentally, spiritually, emotionally, and change physically often. It was painful and sometimes overwhelming to adapt to her choices. It was also rewarding, joyous, and often times extremely peaceful in our home while on this journey with her. We became closer through than we two had ever been, and that is a gift that I wouldn't exchange for the world.

Since Kelly allowed me to walk next to her, help her in any and every way possible on this healing journey, it only seems natural for her to ask me to sporadically add my thoughts and memories. So, with that said, you'll be hearing from "Mom" now and then.

5

You Have to Start Somewhere

Kelly
I don't know Mama, I don't know…

My mind still didn't know what to think or what I should do next, until something just sort-of happened. A few days later Mom was talking with a friend, and somewhere in the conversation she'd shared about the pain in my left side.

Later that week, our friend was informed about a reflexologist who had helped someone whom our friend knew, someone who'd also had digestive issues. Remembering what Mom had told herself about me, the friend passed along some information to us, suggesting, "Maybe this will help Kelly?"

It was a place to start, right? Mom and I discussed it and agreed that the reflexologist was a good place to start.

At this time in my life, I really didn't know what the statement "Food as Medicine" meant. I was naive, truly still in the dark, about the importance of GOOD FOOD. That being said, I HAD already completely given up all dairy products. Yes, that was hard to give up, especially right away. So, what did I eat at this time in my life? I consumed a typical (SAD) Standard American Diet consisting of breads and grains, hormone filled meats, lots of homemade cookies and sugary items, chips, pizza, and other prepackaged snack foods. However, our family grew produce in a garden that was non-GMO, so our vegetables were clean. I mostly drank store boughten bottled flavored water, well water, and soda pop.

Sadly, I'd been fooled that if a food product is packaged and sold in a retail location then it is OKAY for us to eat. I've learned since then. It is just not true. Ingredient labels are required by law, but they are tricky. I now read labels on all products before buying anything.

Growing up I thought our family ate well. Mom made the majority of our meals--mostly home cooking with store boughten groceries and seasonal fresh produce or stored canned food from our garden. And the other meals that she didn't cook? Well, there were daily hot school lunches, meals out including fast-food restaurants, and family gatherings that always included snacks or meals. In the soon coming months ahead, I was in for an eye-opener on the subject of "food AS Medicine" that would change my life forever.

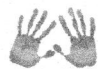

A few days later, after our friend had shared information on reflexology, I sat in the recliner at the Reflexologist's office with my feet outstretched and exposed. She asked me, "Have you had reflexology done on you before?"

"No." I replied.

"The feet are a map of your whole body. All your organs, your spine, sinuses… everything in your whole body is displayed on your feet! I'm also going to push on some points that might make you uncomfortable or even hurt a bit," she told me. *Can't hurt that bad*, I thought.

"Okay," I said.

Thus far, I hadn't told the reflexologist about the pain in my left side. Because we'd researched what reflexology was before going to the appointment, I had a good idea of what was going to happen. Honestly, I figured she would be able to find my painful areas based upon my feet being a diagram of the body. I was putting her to the test.

As she worked on my feet, she told me my pancreas and stomach appeared to be having problems. My eyebrows shot up in amazement. *Are you for real?* I thought, while giving Mom one of those looks. *Did she really just say that?* "Have you been having any abdominal pain or digestive problems lately?" She asked.

13

Surprised by how she knew something I didn't tell her, I spoke up. "I've been having a lot of left-side pain in the last month or so. The pain is dull and achy, but sometimes it gets so severe it takes my breath away. The symptoms I have are headaches, nausea at times, cold hands and feet, gas, bloating, and diarrhea multiple times every day followed by a couple days of regular bowel movements." My voice trailed off before I finished, quietly saying, "I went to the medical doctor. That wasn't very helpful."

The reflexologist said she knew of an acupuncturist, "Maybe she might be able to help with your left-side pain and digestive issues."

She gave us the contact information, and each a hug before leaving her home-based office, saying, "I hope you find out what's going on, Kelly, and that you get some answers."

Tears threatened to surface… a log forming in my throat. I swallowed it and said, "Thank you."

I shook my head as Mom and I walked out into the crisp afternoon air, while thinking, *a person that I've only known for an hour, but yet she knows that something IS going on inside of me that's problematic. I wonder if this acupuncturist person she mentioned might be able to give me some insights and answers?*

6

The Choice to Choose

Kelly

As Mom and I drove home from the reflexology appointment that late summer afternoon in August, Mom shared with me about a doctor she'd gone to that is licensed in acupuncture, chiropractic, and holistic medicine. She'd gone to her, Dr. Ann, for about ten months back in 2003 when she herself wasn't well in health. Mom said, "Dr. Ann helped change my health, and my life, for the better!"

I learned more about Mom's prior health journey that day on the drive home. Dr. Ann had used a variety of holistic methods of natural healing to reverse, and therefore improve, Mom's health. Some choices Mom made were to change her diet--eating organic produce, eliminating dairy, grains, and other specific foods, taking all-natural supplements, doing enemas and colonics, and practicing calming exercises, like simply deep breathing and palates. And yes, breathing IS important! Mom had her work cut out for her every day: implementing these changes all the while raising two kids, not feeling well, and running a household. In the ten months' time, Mom said she could think clearer, had improvements in her digestion, her energy had returned, and she felt better in her overall health.

Even from my 11-year-old perspective at the time of Mom's changes, I knew something was different with my her. Since we, my brother and I, were the kids and she was the parent, we had to eat some nasty tasting foods, which brought thoughts of *what is Mom feeding us? Who eats liver? I hate that we can't have our regular morning cereal. Troy's older! He should have to eat more than me!* Mom's new meal planning had changed our family's eating habits. Since she did the grocery shopping and cooking, Troy and I, and sometimes Dad too, had to eat some of her "interesting" concoctions. Unfortunately, we didn't cheer her on in her efforts to benefit our health, but we DID eat what was put in front of us.

"Kelly, I'm sharing this with you because the acupuncturist that we were just told about probably does more than just acupuncture." Acupuncture is a Traditional Chinese Medicine that most often uses food as medicine, all-natural supplements, and other helps to complement each other to bettering the patient. "If you choose to go and have an appointment with her, I'm willing to guess that she will probably be using some of the same helps that I did."

I was 18 years old and one head-strong, self-willed girl. I was like this as a kid too, strong-willed. Mom and I had butted heads a LOT, because I was so strong-willed. When we didn't see eye-to-eye, well, it was often times disastrous. I wasn't a good listener and didn't like being told what to do. But, more recently in the last five plus years, with both mom's and my hard work to change our ways, we're on a better path that's strengthened our relationship. It's hard to humble yourself, but we both had to, and let me just say… it was a process for both of us!

As I sat, clenching my jaw in the passenger seat on that drive home from the reflexologist appointment, my head pounded. *Supplements don't sound that hard, or BAD. Cleaning up my diet though, uh...* I had to ask what this would entail. "So, what do you think she'd say to me about my diet if I went there? Do you think that I'd have to 'clean it up'?" I inquired, slightly irritated. I didn't really want to hear Mom's answer, but I did want to know more of WHAT I might be getting myself into if I chose to see her.

"You'll probably be told to eliminate grains, refined and processed sugar, dairy…" which I'd already quit eating, "and probably some other more specific foods like tomatoes and potatoes."

Inwardly I groaned. Outwardly, I squirmed while making fascial expressions that boldly stated, *"I'm not a fan!"* *So, what am I going to be able to eat if I DO go see her*, I thought?

16

Days of severe pain, more pain than the month before, led the way up to the day of my acupuncture appointment. At home still, as I sat down to eat lunch, I thought about how my life could drastically be changing in just a couple of hours. *Am I really going to have to drastically change my diet?* Deep in my heart I knew the answer, but I didn't want to believe my thoughts. I finished my lunch, looked at the few cupcakes left in a container on the counter and thought, *I probably won't be able to eat these for a while, so I better enjoy it now.* Little did I know, then, that those would be the last cupcakes that I would ever eat again.

Now, looking back, remembering events, holidays, family gatherings and celebrations... each one had included food. Gatherings of most any kind really do revolve around food. I remember baking weekly, or more often twice a week with Mom and my brother, and making all kinds of Christmas cookies with my dad, Darren, too as the festive season came each year.

I remember Halloween tricks-or-treating, coming home and dumping out our multiple ice cream pails filled with candy. Troy and I would sort all the candy out on the living room floor. We'd eat candy for months after.

When I think about all the food choices made back then, I realize that I was CHOOSING what I was being exposed to, and that exposure was often to junk food. It was my life. And it was also my choice, kind of, as a child.

But my **CHOICE** as an adult is what this young woman's story you are reading is about. Choice--my choice to be made well, at ease again, or for maybe the first time ever in my life.

7

Moving Forward

Kelly

It was the end of August, 2010. I completed the paperwork in the waiting area, then was invited in to one of two therapy rooms. The acupuncturist, Mom, and I all sat down. The acupuncturist asked me many questions. Some questions included, "Where is the pain? When did the pain first start? How long does the pain last? What degree would your rate the pain? Is the pain better, or worse, at certain times throughout the day? Do you have headaches? Are your hands and feet cold? Do you crave certain foods? Have you had lots of stress in your life lately? Are your periods regular? Do you get any pain with your periods? How are your bowel movements; hard, soft, runny, etc.? What does your daily diet look like? Do you have any known food allergies?"

I answered the questions as best I could, and Mom would add into the conversation when she had some insights to share, including my health history growing up as a baby into a teenager. "As a baby, Kelly was very gassy. Her diapers were often pretty nasty and always loose; not your 'normal' smelly diapers. My husband always said, 'They were explosive!' As Kelly grew, she was often times gassy. As parents, we figured that would change as she got older. But, it didn't. Kelly took an 'allergy test' when she was 11 years old because she was having headaches and sinus congestion. Through that test we found out she had seasonal allergies and allergies to cats (we had two indoor cats at the time), dust, mold, and pollen. She was never tested for food allergies, though." Mom stated. The acupuncturist listened intently, taking notes.

"As parents, we were aware of how gassy Kelly was. She never complained about any pain or really complained about anything. We honestly thought her gas was due to stress in her life--stress coming in many different forms." Mom shared.

I stated, my hands folded across my abdomen, "In addition to gas, I would have abdominal pain--cramps, and headaches. I figured they were due to holding in the gas most of the time, waiting until I was alone to pass it."

"At 16 years old, Kelly was gassy daily." Mom stated.

I added, "The abdominal cramps and headaches were present quite often. Again, I wasn't one to complain about pain or say that I really didn't feel good. No one knew my stomach hurt until it really hurt bad, and then I would tell Mom, 'My stomach hurts'. I learned that passing the gas brought relief, so that was helpful."

The acupuncturist asked a few pointed questions and we moved forward with the appointment. "I would like to do some muscle testing so I can listen to your body, Kelly. Through this testing, the body can tell me a lot about what's going on inside by how it reacts to different bottles filled with specific ingredients when I place those individually in your hand. The various bottles contain foods, chemicals, vitamins, and mineral supplements, toxins, etc. I can also listen to the body by accessing the different meridians and their points. The meridians are a form of Chinese medicine," she shared.

"Okay." I said as I got up onto her examination table and laid on my back. I hadn't told her about my appointment with the reflexologist yet. It was time to see if the acupuncturist would find what the reflexologist found.

Through the course of questions, palpating, and listening to my body's reaction during muscle testing, she came to several conclusions. 1) I had several food allergies and intolerances. 2) My pancreas was VERY stressed and was having a hard time trying to do its function--making enzymes. Therefore, 3) my stomach was having problems digesting foods. 4) My liver was not functioning as optimally as it should, and 5) my adrenal glands were stressed, which was causing them to continually work overtime. *No wonder I'm feeling so bad!*

Upon hearing what she had found, she wrote a list of foods for me to take out of my diet. They included: ALL nuts, wheat, dairy, white rice, gluten, legumes, and all processed sugar.

As the appointment concluded, Mom and I asked a few more questions and then I was sent home with supplements to help: 1) The pancreas do its job. 2) My stomach to digest food properly. 3) And to aid my stressed organs to function better. I was then rescheduled to see the her again in two weeks.

I said to Mom on the drive home, "So I can't eat ANY of the foods that have any ingredients listed here," while pointing to the sheet of paper with the list of "foods to avoid" written on it?

"Yep," she said.

I had SO many thoughts… one of them being, *WHAT am I going to eat?*

8

Grateful Each Day

Amy

Life should never be taken for granted. How many times have I hit the floor running upon awakening in the morning and kept going, never being grateful for the moments in a day? What would happen if I didn't awaken, or one of my loved ones didn't wake from their sleep? Hard questions, for sure. But I've thought about those questions. Maybe you have too?

I take for granted a day, an hour, and minutes of time more often than not. But sometimes, just some times, a thought preludes a memory of a day gone past, provoking vivid memories, and then my heart is sprinkled full with a whole lot of gratitude!

If you're like me, you sometimes have to remind yourself to be grateful, even for the challenging happenings going on in your life. That may be foreign to some of you reading this--being grateful for something that is upsetting, difficult, hard, tragic, energy zapping, or brings a painful loss in your life. Why on earth would you or I be grateful for those kinds of things? Well, because those are the kinds of challenges that give us opportunities to build our faith, trust, and character, to shedding old skin for new growth layered beneath!

I know how it can sound, but with all my heart I tell you that I've been there on BOTH sides of being grateful for "the good things" and also "the hard things" in more recent years. I've learned to be grateful for the challenges I face that are not easy to embrace. I like to think I've come a long-ways. Because, well, I really have come a longways. And, I've seen others close to me who, too, have come to this kind of grateful for "the worst" to bring about the best changes in themselves. It's a choice, and that's what Kelly's story is about! Choice.

How does one choose to be grateful for physical pain in their life, for daily physical pain? THAT I cannot answer. But I've witnessed Kelly change to that kind of thinking and living--during and through her worst-of-worst times. I remember some of those really bad days; prayers said alone or with my husband, with my son, with friends, and Kelly too, asking for God to help us see His hand working in Kelly's circumstances, for Kelly to believe, trust, and see what He wanted to do in and through her painful days that led into years.

As a family of four, our lives were lived 24-hours a day, from our children's births into their teens and beyond, until now. Darren, my husband, often away in the cities working, or at home on weekends playing with us, or catching up on house chores inside and out, doing office work, and living life. Troy, our son, growing up in his sandbox, being on the lake, then in his late teens working daily for another man's dreams while building his own business on the weekends, ultimately going out on his own working for himself. And Kelly, who was often home with me helping in all ways, and during the summers in her later teens working part-time with her dad in the cities until she knew her life work to do, then pursuing that new dream of hers. Seems there were not, and are still not, enough hours in a day to get done the tasks during the gift of a 24-hour day. We all needed some rest, and often times we did take the time for getting rest and family play.

Our bodies need rest, but they also need so much more than rest. Clean water, nutrients, minerals, sunshine, warmth, positivity, other people; we need all these and so much more. Whether we have or lack any of these needs, we wear our health on our sleeve. Being human is a lot of work!

I, too, like many people, I am a work in progress to getting needed rest and becoming the best me in the challenges I have daily. I'm thankful for having good relationships with our adult children, which didn't come easily with the challenges of parenting. I learned to humble myself when in error, and asked for their forgiveness. I'm thankful for the work my husband does to provide

22

for us when the kids were growing up and starting their businesses too. Our seasons changed. We experienced health changes that challenged us individually. For Kelly, she eventually overcame her illness--more to come in this story, and gained many beautiful characteristics that even a seasoned, elder person may not attain to; patience, kindness, goodness, faithfulness and the like. All of these qualities stemmed from her health challenges then budded as she grew IN her painful illness, and bloomed big during her newest season of good health these last years. How awesome is THAT, I ask you, to see a delightful flower bloom out from her pain?

I hope to not take for granted a day of good health, feeling well and doing the tasks that each day brings. I hope not to take for granted my family--Darren's, Kelly's, Troy's, or anyone's beautiful characteristics and gifts that randomly enhance daily life. *Keep reminding yourself to be grateful, each day, for ALL things good or otherwise*, I tell myself. God WILL make good out of everything. I believe that when I or someone else says it. Do you?

Be thankful. Be grateful. Life really does mean so much.

9

My Biggest Enemy

Kelly

Our family of four sat gathered together the kitchen island, praying before digging into our meal of hamburgers, or cheeseburgers for most of us. As I looked down at my plate, I saw my plain hamburger with no open-faced bun, no extras like ketchup, mustard or seasonings, because the bun, ketchup and seasonings contained gluten. My expression showed my feelings about this meal; great displeasure. *What's a hamburger without a fluffy bun, crisp lettuce, a juicy slice of tomato and fried onion, finger-licking-good ketchup, with a dab of mustard to compliment it, and perhaps a taste of mayonnaise?*

I grabbed my fork as Mom watched me from the corner of her eye, as I was still hesitating to dig in. Dad and Troy were already eating with a vengeance. I avoided eye contact with both of them. They were oblivious to my struggle of watching them eat what I wanted to also be eating, but couldn't because of so much being eliminated from my diet just recently.

"Kelly, why don't you have some mustard with it so your burger's not so dry?" I'd never had just plain mustard, it was always mixed with ketchup because they complimented one another. But it was mustard or nothing. *Here goes nothing,* I thought. Much to my surprise let's just say that I fell in love with mustard then and there, and to this day I still love mustard and even horseradish too! This experience was just the tip of the iceberg on my learning curve to altering foods that include ingredients that I couldn't eat and then replacing those with something I could eat! It was a process. And with time, you'll see this, too, changed along with my mindset--being openminded.

24

Changing my diet was NOT easy. Dairy, gluten, and sugar were the hardest categories of foods to give up. But, did I do it without cheating not even one time? Yes! Again, it wasn't easy, especially in the moments I craved eating something that I couldn't have. The first couple weeks were the toughest because the cravings were so strong. My mind was easily my biggest enemy at this time. *Just one bite isn't going to hurt you. One bite won't make a difference.* Being the type of person that likes to do things the right way, cheating just to have something that I craved or wanted wasn't a choice to give into. I had more integrity than that. I'd committed to myself that I was NOT going to give in because my health depended on it, and one bite would make a difference. *Look how far you've come! You can't give in now* were words that would immediately run through my mind when I wanted to give into the cravings. I had my mind battles, my mind being my biggest enemy, but I was ultimately successful in not cheating.

Looking back, I smile at how beautiful a choice I had made from the very start of my journey, a choice that helped me to keep on the straight and narrow path as the days, weeks, months, and years would continue on this health journey.

Two weeks from my initial appointment with the acupuncturist, Mom and I were back sitting in her office. She asked me questions such as: "How have you been feeling in the last two weeks? How is the elimination diet going? Do you feel any different? Better? Which symptoms are better? How is the pain in your left side?"

I responded as she asked her many questions, "Within three days of starting the elimination diet that you recommended, I felt so much better! I had less pain in my left side and abdomen. My headaches decreased. I didn't feel like I needed to cover my head from the light when headaches got severe. I'm still bloated and gassy, although it is less. I have more energy as a whole."

Every couple of months I'd make an appointment with the acupuncturist to see how my pancreas and stomach were functioning. At times they tested okay. Other times, weak. My pancreas, however, never seemed to be functioning as optimally as it should have been. I had other organs that weren't functioning as optimally as they should have, too. My liver, gallbladder, spleen, adrenals, and kidneys were all affected negatively at different times. The spleen, liver, and adrenals were each having a hard time functioning a majority of the time, but not as bad as my pancreas. She'd said they were "stressed."

Over the next two-and-a-half years, I continued to meet with the acupuncturist and took clean food supplements in pill or gel form as well. I didn't have SEVERE left-side abdominal pain during this stretch of time, but there was pain. I was gassy, and ultimately became more bloated over that time. I figured the bloating had to do with food allergies and intolerances, so I'd disregarded the symptoms. I lost over 10-pounds just by cleaning up my diet.

Looking back, I didn't know what it felt like to feel well or healthy. I had lived with headaches, gas, upset stomachs, and bloating since childhood, so those were "normal" to me. I hadn't really saw those as "symptoms".

As the symptoms became more severe during those two and a half years working with the acupuncturist, I lived life without my health holding me back! Rarely did I get a cold or the flu during that season of time! I completed two triathlons during the last summer while seeing the acupuncturists as well. However, my diet was getting more restricted.

I had further foods eliminated from my diet in the course of that time, which included: ALL grains, all night shade vegetables (tomatoes, potatoes, eggplant, peppers, etc.), all hot spices (cayenne pepper, pepper, etc.), all nuts and seeds, sprouted seeds, eggs, and all pork products. I was taking nutritional supplements on a daily basis 2-3 times/day, and they seemed to help. I didn't understand WHY my symptoms were increasing when I was doing everything the acupuncturist had recommended.

I asked her WHY my symptoms were increasing on one visit to her office. Her reply was, "Over time, the food allergies and intolerances should improve. For some individuals it just takes longer." That being said, I kept eliminating foods out of my diet that weren't agreeing with me.

If a food didn't agree with me, I'd have escalated symptoms of gas, bloating, nausea, hot and cold sweats, low back pain, abdominal cramps, abdominal pain on the left side--from under my ribs, down just below my belly button.

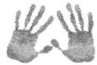

Through the course of these few years, I still lived a "normal" life, doing "normal" things, like "normal" people. I ran, worked, played, spent time with family and friends, and partook of activities I enjoyed and really loved doing. I'd always been active, spending lots of time on the lake water-skiing, swimming, kayaking, and fishing. I liked to hunt, downhill ski, work in the garden (ha-ha, now as an adult--NOT as a child!), help with landscaping projects, and much more. Life went on, and so did I.

10

Words I Will NEVER
Live Down!

Kelly

During the course of the two-and-a-half years I was seeing the acupuncturist monthly, I was washing windows with my dad in the cities. Washing windows is a very physical job. This job helped me gain more muscle and strength than I already had.

Since my diet was restricted, it made going out to eat tricky for supper after work. Finding restaurants with a gluten free menu was key. But even so, I still had to be cautious over ingredients and cross contamination.

I had the winter months off of work so there was more time to do activities such as downhill skiing. My brother, Troy, and I love to ski. We started skiing with the local public-school ski program when Troy was six and I was four years old. Safe to say, we've been at it for a few years now. Troy and I had never been out to the mountains skiing and this February 2012 we were going to get our first real taste of skiing in the mountains! We booked a hotel for a week, bought our ski-lift tickets, made our travel plans, had some food preparations to do, and before we knew it, we had packed up the vehicle and were starting out on our great adventure!

"Colorado here we come!" I shouted, while fist-pumping the air happily in the passenger seat. The drive was long, 14 hours, which was hard as sitting made my low back and abdomen hurt even more. Troy and I took turns driving. I squirmed constantly in my seat. When we made it to our destination, we were both happy to be out of the confining vehicle and ready for an incredible week of skiing, laughs, adventures, making memories, and many firsts.

Skiing in fresh snow up to our knees was INCREDIBLE! Our home state of Minnesota has snow, but nothing in comparison to the mountainous regions of the United States. Our twin-tip skis floated above the snow. Occasionally we dodged trees, ripping a few holes in our coats in the process, jumped a few small cliffs (*um, sorry Mom*), skied along creeks, and half-attempted skiing moguls--which wasn't too lovely for other people's eyes, or our bodies. It's safe to say we lived on the "wild side" those days.

As our week of skiing concluded, my low back was still really sore, but not the same as it constantly was with the abdominal pain tied to it. It was a different kind of soreness. I'd stretched each night after skiing but it just wasn't getting any better; instead, it was getting worse. Towards the end of our last few days, the pain started radiating into the right hip and buttocks region. *Whatever. It'll go away,* I kept telling myself. Well, it didn't go away.

By the time we arrived back home from our skiing adventure, the low-back pain had moved down into both of my hips, but mostly the right side, and now the pain was going down the length of my right leg. Classic symptoms of sciatica. I was having a hard time walking without limping, and again I wasn't one to complain about pain, so I didn't say much about it.

Upon arriving home, our parents greeted us, happy to see we arrived home in ONE piece. Before we shared many stories and laughs with our parents, they saw that I was limping, so one of them asked what was going on. I told them, and the other asked, "Have you taken Ibuprofen to reduce the inflammation?"

I didn't like taking over-the-counter drugs or medications, so my answer was, "No. I've been using peppermint essential oil on my back and doing stretches daily, every night before bed."

"Kelly, a massage would be very helpful for you," Mom suggested knowingly.

"Ah...no. No one is going to be touching my body!" I replied crisply. I didn't even know what a massage really was about. *I'll never live that statement down!*

As if Mom had read my mind, she said, "Do you even know what a massage is?" *How does she know what I'm thinking?* I shook my head "no". She then told me what a massage was and how it would help, explaining what the massage therapist would do to help alleviate the pain.

"I'll see how I feel after the weekend is over," I said. It was Friday. Mom knew better than to take my word for it. She called and made an appointment for me to get a massage the following Monday. I agreed to go. Little did I know that the CHOICE to agree to get a massage would CHANGE MY LIFE, FOREVER!

It was March 2012 as I sat doing my paperwork in the waiting area at the massage therapist's office. The therapist came out from the back room and greeted me warmly. She led me back to her therapy room and asked me questions about my low-back pain.

After our talk, she left the room while I disrobed and crawled between the sheets, feeling a bit uncomfortable. She came back and started working the tight muscles. Sometimes it hurt, but it was a good hurt. We talked throughout the duration of the appointment--me asking questions and her answering and asking some, too.

Afterwards, when I walked out of her office, I'd say my back pain was 80% better. I was impressed that a massage could bring so much relief! Mom paid her and made one more appointment to finish the already-healing work of getting the tightness out of my low back. I thanked the therapist for her help. It sure was nice to feel so much better!

The following Friday I was back at the therapist's office. The appointment went well. Mom and I drove towards home. After about ten minutes of small-talk I asked Mom, "Can I ask you a question?"

"Of course," she answered.

"With all you've learned in the area of natural health, if you had to go back into history and choose a life work to do, what would you do?" I inquired.

She looked out the window as I continued to drive. Within a minute, out of the corner of my eye I saw her break into a big grin. "You want to be a massage therapist, don't you?" she smiled as she asked me, teasingly, but sincerely too.

Laughing, I grinned, confessing, "Yes! I know that is what I want to do, Mom!" She was as giddy in excitement as I was. *Massage therapy is a perfect fit for me,* I thought breaking out in a grin.

I've been blessed with a deep knowing in my heart about certain things. For example: I never knew what I wanted to do for a life work while growing up as a child into a teenager, to now young adult. However, I did know that one day I WOULD know exactly what IT was I was supposed to do. Sometime after I started going to the acupuncturist, I knew that I wanted to do something "natural" in my life's work. There wasn't a doubt about that in my mind, about this KNOWING, but I still didn't know exactly what it would be, or when it would come to fruition. This deep-knowing is a blessing from God. This "knowing" thing has happened many times throughout my life.

Mom and I giddily conversed on the drive and back at home. Then she asked, "Kelly, you know what's next, right?" I looked Mom deep in the eyes and nodded my head…

11

A Golden Year

Kelly

The next step was to find a school for massage therapy.

The first school that popped up in our search was "CenterPoint Massage & Shiatsu Therapy School & Clinic". The website said the school was located in Aberdeen, SD, being only about 1.5 hours away from our home.

The next day, Mom called the school inquiring about information while I was working in Golden Valley, MN with Dad. Right after she'd called the school, Mom called me saying, "You'll never guess who I just got off the phone with!"

Clueless I replied, "Okay, tell me."

"The massage school, CenterPoint! I talked with the admissions counselor, whom was very helpful. Long story short, the school isn't located in Aberdeen, SD. It's right in St. Louis Park, MN! It's only a mile from the hotel you and Dad are staying at! One other important part of our conversation was that their spring term for enrollment ends in two weeks. If you want to start ASAP, you'll have to make a decision rather quickly."

We talked for a while and she filled me in on their conversation. We ended our talk with Mom saying, "I'm going to give you the woman's phone number so that you can talk to her to set up a time to meet, see the school, and talk."

"Okay! THANK YOU, Mom!"

Lots of emotions coursed through me. I talked to my dad, filling him in about Mom's and my conversation. Then, I dialed the phone number she'd given me. The phone rang and the woman answered...

Later that afternoon, my dad and I got a tour of the school. It was a small school with class sizes ranging from 8-20 people. The range of ages of students was 18-65 years old. This is perfect, I thought!

The next afternoon I was back at the school, sitting in on a few classes to get a feel for what massage therapy training was like. While sitting in the classes, my mind went everywhere in thoughts. The one thought that I had the most of my concern was that *I know virtually NOTHING about the human body and anatomy. It's like these students and instructors are talking a foreign language. I love to learn, but this is all so new to me...*

After I was done sitting in on three hours' worth of classes, the admissions counselor I'd met with came to get me from class, then taking me into her office again. We talked and I told her my concerns, fears, likes, dislikes, etc. She calmed my biggest concern and fear, saying, "We teach everyone as if they know nothing about the human body. So, don't worry. Don't let that be an overwhelming concern for you."

Dad sat next to me listening to her answer my questions and provide us with information as well. Then, she asked what I thought about the program and if I'd like to attend school there. I said, "Let me talk with my parents and I'll get back to you with my decision," before leaving.

When we left her office that day, I had all the paperwork to fill out to enroll in the school, if I choose to.

The final decision was made with my parents giving me their blessing--which was important to me, saying, "Go for it!"

I let the counselor know the following Monday, and she said, "Great! There should still be room for you to start in the spring-term group if you are accepted, and then we will get you enrolled quickly. I will have to get back to you within the week to let you know for sure, if you can start with the spring group."

I was excited, nervous, a little fearful, and anxious all at the same time, and the waiting game had only begun.

Short of a week later, it was Tuesday, March 20th, my "Golden birthday", I got a phone call from the admissions counselor saying, "Happy Birthday and CONGRATS! You're going to be starting school in a month!" A big smile broke out on my face. We talked briefly and I hung up the phone, ecstatic about this new life adventure that was REALLY happening!

Later that morning I went to the massage therapist again, for an appointment which was gifted from my parents. On my return back home I was greeted by, "HAPPY GOLDEN BIRTHDAY!" being shouted from short-of-a-dozen ladies that are near and dear to my heart! Mom had thrown a surprise birthday party! Some of the women had made a three-and-a-half-hour road trip to come help celebrate my special day.

Little did I know, I was also going to be blessed with yet another wonderful surprise by one of the ladies. She and her husband used to live a couple houses down from us where our family spent the first 16 years of my life. Mom, Troy, and I played card games with these neighbors. The couple was like family to us.

We shared a beautifully colored tasty meal together, talked and caught up with one another, and then when opening gifts, the one lady who'd been our neighbor years ago said, "Kelly, we have talked about the idea that was brought to us by your mom and you, of you staying with us while you are going to school. We've made our decision… we would love for you to come and stay with us!"

Wow, what a day! First the phone call of acceptance. Next a surprise party! And now this, I thought to myself. Staying with the couple was going to be a good fit.

"Kelly," Mom said, my attention now directed toward her, "I have a song that I want sing for you. It's called 'Find Your Wings'. You are doing exactly this and it's beautiful to see that you are about to FLY." And so, Mom sang, sharing her gift of singing and blessing all of us.

With school only a month away, I faced the reality of a LOT of new changes in my life. Good changes. Exciting changes--and some a little scary. Lots of uncertainties, but another new chapter in life was about to begin!

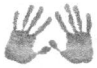

The year of school was more than what I would have hoped for. For the first time in my life (besides when I was homeschooled) I liked school. I enjoyed the challenge, loved the hands-on learning, made new friends, and enjoyed lots of "firsts".

And my health? Well, I continued to go to the acupuncturist semi-regularly, but the left-side pain continued and the symptoms got worse. Over the next year I was getting paler in color and more inflamed on the inside of me. I made it through that school year, "getting by", before the pain took on a harsher degree of dis-ease.

12

ON FIRE

Kelly

In April of 2013 I graduated from massage school.

In June 2013, I opened up my business, "Helping Hands Therapeutic Massage & Body Work". I was a young entrepreneur who was literally jumping right into a new career. It was exciting, nerve racking, full of uncertainties, and all the while enjoyable!

I was juggling a lot of self-imposed challenges in addition to my new business. I was exercising too much; running anywhere between 4-13 miles a day, and biking a few days a week in addition, all because I thought doing a triathlon was important. I was training for not just one, but two triathlons that summer… proving to myself that I could do those. I can look back now and see I was addicted to the "adrenaline high", wanting my next "fix" in the workouts, and then final outcome of both triathlons. My body was not taking the added stress too well.

I had stress building--coming from different areas in my life, mostly from my continued downward spiral of health. Life was a battle physically, mentally, and emotionally. I was angry, bitter and resentful towards certain people, and situations from my past. And, I was still trying to figure out what I could eat that would sit right with my gut. By August, the severity of pain in my left side and symptoms had increased even more-so than it had at the end of massage school.

The pain I had extended from under my ribs to just below my belly button. The left side of my abdomen hurt deep under my ribs where I couldn't reach. In addition, I had a dull, achy low-back pain, mostly on my left side, that extended from the low back then up into the lower third of my rib cage. I had headaches 24/7. It didn't matter if I slept, ate, drank water, used a heat pack, or essential oils, the headaches just wouldn't go away. My stomach was bloated and I was gassy. I had hot and cold sweats during the day, and sometimes at night that woke me up. I was losing more weight and muscle tone. My energy was decreasing. Nausea became a daily battle, hitting me at any given moment in a day. I'd started developing a yellow spot in the whites of both my eyes. My appetite lacked. I had diarrhea many times a day, in addition to "regular" bowel movements. My skin tone had become paler, and I had an appearance of being malnourished. At times all I desired to do was sleep, but I kept up with doing my "normal" daily work, chores, and activities. My hands and feet had been cold in the past, but now my whole body was cold despite we were in the height of summer's warmth. I was fatigued and generally felt "ill".

Mom and I talked about how I wasn't seeing much of any improvements in my health while working with the acupuncturist those last couple months. Mutually then, we decided to put a phone call into the holistic practitioner/chiropractor/acupuncturist that Mom had gone to ten years prior, Dr. Ann.

Mom called Dr. Ann's office and the receptionist told her that, "Dr. Ann is scheduled out a month and a half. Kelly is going to have to wait, unless we get a cancellation." We took the first available appointment. The month-and-a-half wait was painfully long, every day being a battle.

I continued to work, building a clientele in my new business. I was enjoying my new career. I wasn't going to let my health stop me from doing my job. Many days were a real struggle, but I stayed focused taking each day as it came.

During the course of my schooling for massage, I'd met some pretty neat people! One dear friend I'd made during that time was Hallie. Hallie and I kept in touch regularly after graduation. We lived three-and-a-half hours apart from one another. She knew the history of my disease: left-side pain, food allergies, and other symptoms. I went to her regularly for massage therapy after graduation. Often times, Hallie would massage my abdomen, as it helped to decrease the abdominal and back pain, therefore relaxing all the tight muscles surrounding the areas. My abdomen and back muscles were always really tight due to the muscles trying to protect the area that pained me the most.

One fall day in 2013 while Hallie was working on my abdomen, she gently stated, "It feels like your left side is 'ON FIRE', Kelly."

I nodded my head, "yes," and added, "It feels like it's on fire most of the time."

"It feels like a slow burning fire. A very hot fire. A red-hot fire," she murmured. "It's like it's burning deep inside and penetrating outwards." She'd just confirmed to me my very real everyday pain. I later told mom what Hallie had said to me during the appointment, and we both agreed that Hallie is an "agent of healing" and that "she is gifted". I'm so glad Hallie was a part of my healing journey, that I had someone I could be real with and who helped me immensely with relieving muscle tension during every therapy session.

Hallie is a friend that walked alongside of me in the days, months, and years of ill health. She is part of my tribe, and I am eternally grateful for the caring people in my life!

"A real friend is one who walks into your life
when others walk out." -Walter Winchell

13

Fire Confirmed

Kelly

Fall of 2013. Mom and I sat in the waiting room as Dr. Ann walked in. Dr. Ann had olive-colored skin with a beautiful sheen. She over-all had a look of vibrant health. She introduced herself and we went into one of her therapy rooms.

As the appointment started, Dr. Ann asked many questions that I would answer one by one, such as, "Why are you here today? Where is your pain? Describe your pain. What are your symptoms? What does your daily diet consist of? How are your bowel movements? Are your periods regular? Do you have headaches? Do headaches get worse of better when you eat? Are you currently taking any supplements? How much water do you drink in a day? Do you have a history of chronic illness?"

When she asked the questions, it was literally as if she already knew the answers I'd be giving. She appeared to be pretty intuitive. Dr. Ann was intelligent, thorough, and I could tell she truly loved her work helping her patients. Then she asked one more question, "Kelly, have you been working with anyone prior to me for this left side pain?"

"Yes. I have been to a reflexologist, I get massages once a month, and I have been working with an acupuncturist." I replied. Turns out, Dr. Ann and the acupuncturist knew one another! *Small world*, I thought.

Mom was sitting in a chair a few feet away from us. Dr. Ann now gave Mom her full attention, eyeing her. "You look familiar," Dr. Ann stated.

They reconnected after a few shared memory boosts from Mom. I enjoyed hearing their laughter from Mom's memories of when she had been seeing Dr. Ann for her health issues so many years back. Dr. Ann registered who mom was from those memories.

Next, Dr. Ann did some muscle testing with me, using Chinese medicine modalities. She did acupuncture, tapping, and a few other natural-healing methods to see what she would find going on within me. She didn't speak as she worked, other than telling me to put pressure against her arm or move my arm or leg. After a long time of silence, she spoke saying, "Your left side feels like it is 'ON FIRE'!"

I was speechless. I hadn't told Dr. Ann what Hallie, my friend and massage therapist, had recently told me. *Did she REALLY just say "ON FIRE"?* I was silent while my mind reeled. Mom spoke to Dr. Ann while I was lost in my thoughts. *Talk about confirmation!*

It was obvious something serious was going on with my left side. We needed to get to the bottom of it! Then we three talked lengthy about what was going on, what Dr. Ann had found during her examination. My adrenal glands, liver, spleen, and gallbladder weren't working how they should be and were stressed, and my pancreas especially. My digestive tract was very stressed.

Mom next shared some insights as Dr. Ann listened. "Kelly did two triathlons this past summer and has still been exercising pretty hard-core. In my opinion, I think this depleted the little bit of energy that she had left in her body. I believe that's what's aided in her health spiraling downhill so fast in the last months. Is that possible?"

"Yes, it is possible!" Dr. Ann exclaimed. "Kelly's body, her organs, were already compromised prior to her doing the training and the triathlons. The training in itself used energy, but the triathlons used up the rest of her body's reserved energy. This depletion of energy would have ultimately happened in a year or less had she not done the training and events."

Turning to me, Dr. Ann continued, "Kelly, your body is malnourished, tired, and fatigued. You show many signs of having a leaky gut. Our focus now is to get your body functioning properly and back to health again!" Dr. Ann smiled, genuinely. Then, she sat in front of me with a pad of paper and pen. She began writing while making her suggestions of implementing changes. "We need to talk about some lifestyle changes that would help you to become more 'well' in your health."

"Okay," I replied unsure of what she was going to suggest to me.

"In addition to specific supplements and natural remedies that I will be going over with you here and sending home with you, there are certain foods that are going to be important for you to consume daily." *I thought I was doing good already with not eating dairy, gluten, or processed sugar*, I thought to myself.

Dr. Ann made it very clear to me that eating hot and warm foods is what I needed to be putting into my body. This meant eating a LOT of organic homemade soups, soup broths, bone broth daily, warm smoothies, steamed vegetables to the point of mushy in texture, and TONS of steamed dark, leafy greens, eating 4-6 cups per day. I thought, *no more delicious salads,* as they are raw. *How am I going to consume 4-6 cups of dark, leafy greens on a daily basis?* Well, I was going to find out fast!

"An important note… you cannot be using a microwave to warm up ANY of your foods." She added. *WHAT!?!* My mind was beginning to reel. I was becoming overwhelmed with so many big changes. Dr. Ann explained that the electromagnet-radiation waves put off from the magnetron from inside the microwave oven damages the food when warming it up, therefore changing the food while killing the nutrients IN the food. "You're going to have to cook and warm your food in a standard kitchen oven or on the stove top."

Dr. Ann then started telling Mom and me about bone broth and the HUGE health benefits from drinking it daily; which, for one big reason, was how it heals the lining of the gut for someone like me who has intestinal permeability, AKA leaky gut. "I'd love for you to start making your own bone broth, but for right now, if you can't or aren't willing to, you can buy organic-bone broth at the grocery store." Mom took notes while Dr. Ann talked.

Dr. Ann went on to the next subject of steamed vegetables and warm smoothies. "Your vegetables need to be cooked to the point of mushy in texture. The reason is because vegetables have different nutrients in them at

41

different points of their cooked state. Right now, fully cooked by steaming them is what your body needs since your digestive system is not processing food properly. The least amount of stress on your digestive system right now, the better. And for smoothies, they need to be eaten warm."

GROSS! I thought. "By warm, I mean room temperature, or lukewarm." She spoke. My mouth didn't like the sounds of that, but I would do what I was told. "As far as the 4-6 cups of dark, leafy greens, those will also need to be steamed to the point of mushy." We then asked what kind of greens I should be consuming and she said, "Kale, dandelion greens, Swiss chard, mustard greens, collards, parsley, cilantro, beet greens." I had no idea what most of these even were! "Kelly, EVERY food that goes into your body should be organic." Dr. Ann said, looking up from the note she'd just wrote on. "Do you have a food coop where you live?"

Truthfully, I really didn't even know what "organic" was, nor what a "food coop" was. Mom did, since she'd eaten organic vegetables and meats when she'd been going to Dr. Ann years before. I was once again overwhelmed with my new diet regimen. *Will I ever put this fire out?* I thought.

The fire growing deep inside of me was now being directly addressed by Dr. Ann during the fall of 2013. With Dr. Ann's and mom's help, I was on my way to improvements in eating an all-organic diet, and supplementing with nutrients I lacked.

During those first months with Dr. Ann, my energy and overall health seemingly was improving as my ashen skin tone disappeared and I gained some needed weight back... but that was only for a season of time. *Time was something I didn't feel I had much of that fall going into the winter.*

Overall, my health felt out of control. But, with a lot of help from the right people, I would gain my health back, eventually. For now, though, I was literally living one day at a time.

14

Doors Open
Implementing Change

Amy

During the fall of 2013, there were more challenging but good changes implemented into Kelly's life after seeing Dr. Ann on the very first visit to her office. For me, the changes were considered beautiful additions for Kelly to embrace. But I was not Kelly, and I did not have physical pain to deal with as she had. Nor did I have the issues Kelly was going to have to allow to surface in her heart, to deal with past hurts to experience peace in her life. She was on a path towards healing in all aspects. This was going to be something beautiful to witness.

Seeing Dr. Ann had a Deja vu effect. I had learned so much from her ten years prior to 2013, while experiencing poor health myself and in need of practical, healthful guidance in 2003. Dr. Ann had helped turn my health around with healing teas, herbs and roots, chiropractic, acupuncture, nutritional supplements of vitamins and minerals which I was deficient of, and lots of guidance in nutrition and organics vs. GMO foods. These helps, all working together, strengthened my body to ultimately forgo a whole-body detoxification process which cleansed my digestive system of toxic garbage and improving my health tenfold.

I remember one specific late morning, at Dr Ann's office in the summer of 2003. She had been less intense in the sense of her client time schedule. I'd started my normal inquisition, firing questions stored in my mind since my last appointment. She sat on her examination stool next to me, taking more time and care than the usual appointments I'd had with her. "How did you get into this line of work?" I'd asked.

"Well," she said, "when I was 16, I was sick like so many women I see coming through the doors of my clinic, like you. My parents had taken me to medical doctors who were unable to help me change my health with medications. Then, one day they brought me to a holistic practitioner that really helped to change my health, in turn changing my direction in life. Once I'd started on the path to being healthy, I was inspired to be that same kind of help for other women, and men, that want to take a natural approach in improving their health."

"That's a great story! Inspiring!" I responded. She obviously was not on a tight schedule, but I asked her if I was keeping her from other clients. I had more questions.

"No, you are not," she'd responded smiling, her bright, vibrant eyes looking straight into my not so bright OR vibrant eyes. "I have an open afternoon today, so you're welcome to stay and ask whatever you'd like." And so, I did.

Dr. Ann answered ALL my questions. I was amazed by her wealth of knowledge in nutrition and botany, telling me all kinds of facts on how whole foods and plants are used medicinally. We talked for hours. I was thankful for the time she took from her what could had been free time to do her office work or to go home early. She was one amazing lady.

So here I am ten years later, sitting in Dr. Ann's office with my adult daughter as her patient. I secretly hoped Kelly would be inspired by this spirited woman before her who had a matter-of-fact way of speaking to people that CAN be intimidating if you 1) Don't know who you are. 2) Don't want someone else's input, but they give you it anyways. And, 3) You really don't want to change when you know you should to help yourself, and someone is telling you that this is what you have to do in order to improve your situation. For Kelly, this was going to be a challenge to even like this woman, and a stretch of her will to actually implement the changes. I'd hoped for the best, and didn't tell Kelly about the doctor's matter-of-fact ways before her initial appointment.

I realize, to the reader, that it may seem likely Kelly would follow in my, or her parent's and other people she'd respected, footsteps at any given opportunities for growth since she and I had a good relationship for the most part. But that was not the case. Kelly was on a "natural-health" path by her own reasoning through researching and witnessing. Yes, I influenced her in the fact that I'd had great results with Dr. Ann years prior to her own appointments with the reflexologist, the acupuncturist, and now with Dr. Ann, and those positive results which I had impacted my whole family's lives.

Change can be a very difficult task of implementing in the mind of any human being. For instance, growing your own food or buying it from the local grocer, food coop, or ordering it from elsewhere... there are so many choices, not to mention ALL the food in the aisles at the stores to pick from! But also, the challenge to make a change CAN be an exhilarating and hope filled act!

I recall the first time I ever entered a food coop to buy organic produce. Oh boy, I was on brainwave overload... feeling as though I had way too many choices to make with not enough information to know what to buy. Being limited in food choices because of a personalized diet can be a fun challenge. But I admit, it was not fun for me when I first entered the "whole food" arena. It was hard to change, but my health depended on it and so I took the needed steps. I also started ordering from a family-operated coop that was out-of-state that sells organic fresh produce, a large selection of non-GMO foods, oils, supplements, personal care items, and so much more. To this day, we, and others, order monthly from a company that ships our orders on semi-trucks delivering to our area, along with a host of other groups. They travel across the United States to deliver quality food! We also order from multiple companies online, delivering directly to our home, and we buy semi-locally at food coops around the state and near our home.

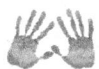

Back to Kelly's appointment, listening to Dr. Ann advising Kelly of needed changes in her diet, this was obviously not new verbiage to my ears. A number of big diet changes had already taken place with Kelly, so to me it seemed that the appointment could had been worse in additional changes, like excluding wheat gluten (and for Kelly all grains), processed foods, dairy, and sugar from her diet. She'd already tackled those! Really, Kelly was in a good place with these changes already under her belt, so I thought the appointment went well. Although, there was the part of her being told that she needed to practice forgiveness and do some work spiritually, mentally, and emotionally toward healing. That process was not new to us, but Kelly was now hearing it from elsewhere and it making an impact on her to address the areas of needed change.

Our major concern at this time for Kelly was the increasing left-side pain amongst the many symptoms she was having for three years already. And, her diet consisting of mostly soup, vegetables, and chicken was concerning as well. She was adamant about taking a natural approach to her health problems. What were we to do? Her dad told her many times that she should go to a medical doctor. Other close family and friends were also telling me their concerns for her. I'd questioned her too, if she thought maybe she should go back to the local medical clinic. She wanted no part of it. Soon, though, after seeing Dr. Ann that fall of 2013, Kelly would be making a trip to the medical clinic, seeing a MD for her severe left-side pain.

15

Choices

Kelly

Journal Entry (JE) September 9th, 2013

I think God is trying to tell me something--to be still and trust in Him. It seems my time is getting shorter and shorter and all the harder to deal with this gut/abdominal stuff going on. Somedays I wonder if cancer isn't eating me from my intestines/stomach.

Changing my diet from conventional GMO (genetically modified organisms) food to organic food wasn't hard. There's a lot of controversy about GMO vs. organic food. I will say just a few things.

First off, eating organic is not a fad diet, it's a lifestyle diet. When people hear "diet" they often think weight loss, calories, low fat, restrictions, etc. Following an organic diet is not associated to those typical "diet" words or the ideas of what they mean.

Secondly, you are the BEST advocate for your health and what you put in to your body. We have the internet at our finger tips to research and learn. Research and find out for yourself what is the truth about GMO vs. organic. You don't have to take my word for it.

When I changed my diet to organic, I chose to make a lifestyle change that I could gladly stand behind. I care about what I put into my body. I have a right to know what is in the food I'm eating, and so do you. I'm not willing to go back to eating GMO foods that wreck-havoc causing inflammation and eventually disease in every area of my body, mind, and being. I'm choosing to decrease disease in my body now, and in my future. I do not want to go through what I've gone through again, out of choice. And, I care about my future health and my loved ones enough to put a stop to illness and disease from cheap food, GMO foods, for future generations to the best of my ability. The thing is, we EACH get to choose how we spend our money in regard to the food we eat.

I hear this statement a lot, "Organic is too expensive." Like I said, we all get to choose what we eat. I'm willing to buy organic because my health and life depend on it, especially if I want to think clearly, be free of depression, anxiety, brain fog, inflammation, digestive problems, be less moody, not have weird symptoms or side effects after eating GMO foods, and feel more balanced as a whole in all aspects of my health. After experiencing these beneficial effects just listed and many other amazing results from eating organic food, I won't go back to eating food that harms my health. Also, organic foods are more flavorful than GMO foods. Eating organic is not entirely perfect, but it's truly the best we can do in today's world that makes foods filled with chemicals and toxicity. How do we know the produce we're buying is TRULY organic? Just look at the label! For produce, the first of five digits to identify the item is the number "9" IF the product is truly organic. Look for the number "9" on the fresh food item's sticker when shopping for produce. Packaged food will have "Certified Organic" labeling on it, whether it is meat, grains, bagged produce, dairy, etc. Look for the "Certified Organic" labels!

In October of 2013, while I'd been going to Dr. Ann, I'd also gone back to the local medical doctor when my left-side pain became unbearable. The left-side pain was so bad at times that when I went to hug people, I made it a point to not let anyone be able to touch, or come in contact with, my abdomen. The searing hot left-side pain ripped deep inside me. My parents were very concerned that there was something REALLY serious going on deep inside my body. They'd voiced their concerns to me, again, about going to the clinic for further testing. I eventually agreed to go back to a medical doctor.

The MD walked into the examination room. It quickly became obvious that the MD had a genuine concern, care, and respect for me, and for all patients. Mom and I, together, told the MD my symptoms and history of left-side pain, along with working with the reflexologist, acupuncturist, and recently Dr. Ann. The MD listened intently and was okay with my trying other routes to get help for my left-side pain.

As I described the left-side pain, the MD drew in a deep breath followed by a grimace that was noticed by both mom and me. The MD took on a more serious tone while asking a number of specific questions about my pain, including: "When did the pain start? Rate your pain on a scale of 1-10, with ten being the worst. Has your pain improved at all? Do you have blood in your stool? Do you have an appetite? How are your bowel movements? Is your left side tender to the touch? Do you get abdominal inflammation and bloating? Does eating or drinking make it worse or better? How is your energy? Does your pain affect your daily routine? Do you have the pain when you sleep at night?"

I answered all the questions and was told to sit on the examination table. My blood pressure and vitals were already taken. The MD wanted to check my other organs and palpate my abdomen. "Does this hurt?" I was asked when the abdominal palpation began.

"Yes, it hurts," I replied.

The MD said, "You shouldn't be having this pain." To this day I still remember the gravely serious look the MD gave first me, then shot at my mom momentarily. Truth was, my abdomen always hurt. Being touched by any amount of pressure, on my abdomen, would make it hurt worse. My breathing had also become pretty shallow because of the pain that extended into my rib cage. Deep breathing was something that I needed to be doing, but that rarely happened because of the pain it inflicted as of late.

The examination ended with the MD saying, "I want to do a few lab tests and schedule an ultrasound as soon as possible. Also, I'd like you to see a gastroenterologist. You need to have an endoscopy done as soon as possible. Are you in the metropolitan area often, since that's where you moved here from?"

We responded with heads nodding a firm "yes".

"Then you can find a doctor of your choosing and I'll give you a referral to see the doctor of your choice. This way, you can get an appointment elsewhere sooner than you would here, since our gastroenterologist comes to our clinic only once a month."

I heard the grave concern in the MD's voice, but again in my heart I was fighting. *I'm not going to be a lab rat. This just doesn't feel right.* I pushed the thoughts aside and said a half-hearted "Okay," in response.

Mom, having been given the grave, concerned, look from a MD while I'd been on the examination table, did not let the Dr.'s clear concern go unnoticed. It didn't sit well with her, my choices, and the MD's concern confirmed her struggle with my choices as of late. I can easily see where she was put in a tough position of listening to me, whom was strictly wanting to follow an all-natural path of healing, and my dad who was telling her I needed to go to the MD, along with other people's concerns she was hearing from. Mom was in the middle of hearing it ALL, and knowing what she knew for herself to be true in her health, she, more than anyone, knew what a tough place it was to be in when people are telling you, well, what they are telling you that goes against the grain of what you chose to believe, think, or do. She understood my choices, and she shouldered other people's doubts in my choices. It was a fine line for her to balance on.

I agreed to and did the in-clinic test that was ordered. Two days later I got the results via a phone call from the MD's assistant saying, "Kelly, the good news is that all your tests came back normal! The bad news is that doesn't help us figure out what the problem is." My heart sank and tears immediately filled my eyes. I'd been in turmoil to go back to an MD, and now this? Another failed attempt to find answers.

I swallowed and asked the MD's assistant, "What did the doctor say about the blood work results? Were there any recommendations for anything?" I needed to know. I had to know, because what else did I have?

"We'd like you to do the ultrasound that's scheduled. We want to see if there are any gallstones or kidney stones that may be the cause of your abdominal pain. And also, we'd like you to see a GI specialist". I shook my head back and forth upon hearing this. Exactly what I didn't want. *I'm NOT a lab rat!* I thought.

50

Another two days later, I, the angry young woman that Dr. Ann clearly saw weeks earlier in her office, in pain, had the ultrasound done at the clinic. Truthfully, I didn't want to do the ultrasound but I finally agreed to it to relieve my parent's concerns, with all due respect. When they did the ultrasound, my right side was X-rayed but not my left. I couldn't understand why my left side wasn't being addressed. At one point I asked if my left side was going to be x-rayed. The answer was, "I'm supposed to x-ray the right side."

I held in my emotions, biting my lip to keep from crying. My mind reeled. My head was pounding more than normal. My thoughts were confusing. I was angry and I left there being very bitter.

When I did get the ultrasound results, again everything was normal. And why wouldn't they be? They x-rayed the wrong side. Talk about a mind battle to hear the "normal" results again. It took a lot for me to swallow and not react when everything in me screamed to react. I felt as if God was giving me a giant hug to keep me from erupting like a fiery volcano.

The MD had also recommended that I go to a GI specialist at the initial appointment. Mom and I talked about that, entirely, in the days after the initial examination.

Huh. The MD really does think there's something serious going on. The MD also knew that time was vital, telling us that I should go to the cities where I could get in sooner. My thoughts jumped back to what the MD's assistant just told me, to see a GI specialist. *I do NOT want to be a lab rat! Here we go, AGAIN!* I thought. *God, what's going on?* I prayed.

16

Repeat Diagnosis

Kelly

I talked with my parents about the GI specialist recommendation. I was adamant that I did not want to do this.

Again, I half-heartedly agreed to see the specialist with ONE condition, that I would be making the end decision of what I wanted to do based upon the results of the initial appointment. They agreed.

Two weeks later, Mom and I were walking into a specialty GI clinic in the metropolitan area. As we walked in the medical clinic, once again the "I don't like this feeling" was hitting me full force. I told myself, *one foot in front of the* other. I thought, *my feet feel like bricks. Why am I here?* I was struggling. I was fighting everything in me to bolt from the building, but I had made an agreement. I intended on keeping my word. To me, my word was my word, and I would NOT break that.

After receiving and filling out my paperwork, it would be another 15-minutes before I was brought to an examination room. In those 15-minutes I'd squirmed in my seat and I battled built-up tears wanting to spill out. I tried with everything in me to keep them at bay. Mom looked at me, started speaking, and the tears tumbled out, one after the next. I was an angry, hot mess. However, I soon composed myself enough so that when my name was called, I wasn't such a dripping mess.

I was asked more questions in the examination room. I felt myself deflating with each question. It wasn't the person's fault asking the questions, it was just me feeling suffocated. I was having a hard time with all of this. I just wanted to be done so I could be alone, by myself, to think and lay down, although riding in a vehicle for four hours made my left side all the worse with having to sit, semi-sit, or lay in the front seat.

After questioning, the GI specialist walked in. I looked up. Introductions were made and then the questioning began again. It seemed endless, but eventually she took my blood pressure, vitals, and palpated my abdomen. As the specialist palpated, I was asked, "Kelly, is there any pain as I press?"

"Yes." I grimaced. It actually hurt a lot. When finished, I was told to go back to the chair I'd been sitting in. I gladly retreated to the safety of it so as not to be touched again!

The specialist started talking, stating, "You probably just have a bad case of IBS (irritable bowel syndrome)." I literally couldn't believe what I was being told. "We can do an endoscopy, though. There are other options, a colonoscopy, a sigmoidoscopy, a MRI, and other ways of testing that we can utilize if need be. We can start with an endoscopy to see if you have a rip, an ulcer, or something else in your stomach or upper GI tract." The specialist then told me, "If you decide to do the endoscopy, I'm scheduled about a month out. If you're looking for a certain day, you might have to schedule out longer than a month."

Mom looked at me. I just sat looking at her. I was still stunned about being labeled IBS. Flashbacks of the MD in September of 2010, when I first went in for my left side-pain and being labeled IBS, were hitting me. *I'm now, again, being labeled IBS? It's as if they don't think there's a more relevant problem.* I was numb to the conversation mom and the specialist were now having.

The specialist left the room and I was immediately led to the scheduling area by the assistant. My head was spinning. Everything was a blur. *The specialist didn't listen to what I told her. She just labeled me, instead, with IBS.*

Mom and I sat down in chairs at one of the scheduling desks. "When are you looking to have an appointment?" the scheduler inquired. I didn't answer, so Mom picked a date. I wasn't comfortable with scheduling a date. We hadn't even discussed it yet, so I just listened. At this point I was ready to cry. With every ounce of energy left in me, I used it to withhold building tears at least until we were out of the building. Those were a long ten minutes between thoughts of disbelief, feelings of anger, and fighting-off tears.

Once we walked outside, got inside and closed the car doors, I let out the heavy building thoughts. "An endoscopy!?! REALLY? Mom, I don't like that idea of getting an endoscopy. It doesn't feel right for me."

"Well, it would be good to see what's going on in your abdomen, Kelly. You haven't had any tests done like this before, so it would be helpful." Mom retorted. I was steaming, a pot that was nearly boiling over. "They would be able to see if there's a rip in your colon, perhaps detect cancer, or an ulcer," She stated.

Her statement wasn't convincing me that this test was a good idea. "Yes, that's true. You know, they could end up perforating my throat sticking that device down there. I'd REALLY be in pain then." I smarted.

We didn't debate anymore. Rather, we discussed and then decided to pray about the possible upcoming endoscopy appointment.

Once home later that day, we talked with Dad, who knew only about the conventional medical route as do most people. He voiced his thoughts about the endoscopy, that I should have it done. After the conversation, we didn't talk about the appointment for a couple more days.

JE November 14th, 2013
Doctors, again, have no idea what is going on in my body. They want to do more tests, first the endoscopy and also a sigmoidoscopy. I'm not looking forward to this at all. I'm a hurting unit, Lord, and I don't know what's going on deep inside my body, but You do. I pray if You want me to do these tests, that You would make it known to me. Somedays the devil is certainly trying to take me down. Please help me, Father. I trust you.

As I've said before, my left-side pain and other symptoms were worse than ever before those many months during the fall of 2013. As for medical doctors, I just didn't trust their "procedures". In the end, my parents and I agreed that I wouldn't be doing the endoscopy. It was MY choice. With ALL due respect

54

to my parents, their genuine love and concern was real and powerful, just like any parent that watches one of their children struggling.

I knew deep in my heart that the endoscopy wasn't what I was supposed to have done. Mom cancelled my appointment. I continued to have bad days, and continued seeing Dr. Ann. I focused on taking each day as it came and making the best of it.

17

Implementing Changes

Kelly

JE November 18th, 2013

I'm frustrated, tired, and weak. I'm nauseated a lot of the time. I was told from Dr. Ann that the state of my liver is VERY bad. Basically, it is on the verge of collapsing. Wow, I'm too young for this. Lord, give me the strength to go on because I certainly can't do this on my own. I don't know the exact reasoning as to why I'm going through this Lord, but obviously you have something bigger and better in store for me.

While working with Dr. Ann, the holistic Dr., there were a LOT of changes that needed to be made in my life. Some of the changes were easy, and others a little more time-consuming, and maybe even difficult, or should I say "patience-testers". Nevertheless, her guidance and direction were appreciated.

I was eating my 4-6 cups of steamed greens each day. I was eating fully-cooked hot foods, cooked to the point of mushy, as she'd told me to. I liked not having to chew my food, but I won't lie, mushy food eventually got old. This was mind-over-matter, and I did overlook that aspect at most mealtimes. I ate home-made soup once a day. Truth be told, I'd actually remembered saying to my mom one day at lunch in my last year of high school, "I could eat soup every single day." Little had I known that only a few years later I would be doing just that!

In addition to eating warm foods, Dr. Ann had recommended eating spicy foods and spices such as: jalapeño peppers, red peppers, horseradish, paprika, cumin, and cayenne pepper. The hot foods and spices were intended to address my sluggish metabolism. Cayenne pepper has a property called "capsaicin" in it. Capsaicin increases heat in the body to burn more calories per day. I needed heat inside my body. Each of the spices suggested could, and would, help me in different ways.

I had completely quit exercising just prior to my very first appointment with Dr. Ann because I didn't have the energy for it, and besides it hurt my left side. Now she was telling me that I needed to move and sweat. Why? Because she said I had muscle dystrophy, muscle weakness and degeneration—a breakdown of the muscle fibers. Since I didn't have much energy to exercise, she said it only needed to be 15-minutes a day to begin with, then to gradually increase the length. Because I was so ill (and prior to this time, prone to over exercising) I needed to find balance with exercise. Each day I would make myself do a short workout that got me to sweat. I'd remind myself of Dr. Ann's words, "Sweating is important to help get rid of the build-up of toxins in your body, Kelly. This will also help warm up your core body temperature."

Another area that Dr. Ann addressed was my liver, which was on the verge of collapsing. To address this, I was not only taking herbal supplements but was told to drink dandelion tea every day. Truthfully, I can look back and chuckle at some of my reactions to hearing things I was being told to do. *Dandelion tea? Who drinks that?* I thought. Well, I learned to, and you know what, I actually LOVED it. In addition to drinking medicinal teas, I was instructed to drink warm water throughout the day to warm me up, and to help in the gentle detoxing process for the liver while taking supplemental herbs and the medicinal dandelion tea. Increasing my daily water consumption was important.

Green tea was another tea that I was told to drink daily. Green tea is loaded with antioxidants, is a great cancer cell killer, improves mental performance, and improves brain function (dramatically with some people). Truly, green tea is one of the best "go-to" teas I continue to drink!

Raspberry tea was also a daily tea to help balance hormones, decreases inflammation, support faster metabolism, regulate hormones, boost/support the immune system, addresses female reproductive health such as cramping before menstrual cycles and toning uterus muscles, and aided in preventing nausea and other gastrointestinal issues that I had. Raspberry tea is loaded with nutrients, vitamins, and antioxidants.

In addition to drinking various medicinal teas, I had started drinking bone broth purchased at a food coop, intended to help heal the walls of my intestines from the damage done from leaky gut. I tried the bone broth for a while, but found that due to certain ingredients, onion and tomato in the pre-made broth, it was making me feel ill after drinking it. So, I stopped. Eventually, in a few months' time, Mom embarked on the journey to making our own homemade bone broth.

I quickly grew to enjoy my daily cups of tea. I also enjoyed the quotes and encouraging messages that some of the tea bags had written on the ends of the strings attached to the bags. Tea gives me a feeling of "joy in the simple things" every day.

Having to drink daily cups of tea, and increasing my liquid consumption due to the supplements I was taking, meant there was no excuse for drinking or eating less. I admit, drinking and eating were a real struggle because they left me feeling even more ill while my organs digested them. I was nauseated every day. Because my pancreas was not doing its job in making enzymes, I was taking supplemental enzymes to help breakdown and digest food, and I was taking Swedish bitters during meals to help activate digestive juices--bile, stomach acid, so I could digest and ABSORB the nutrients FROM the food. I knew I had to eat and drink to live, so I did.

Mom was a big help in reminding me to eat and drink throughout the course of each day. She "had my back", always. Mom was a HUGE asset in making sure I was doing everything that I needed to in a day, encouraging me, and making sure I was eating enough. It wasn't that I wasn't hungry that I didn't want to eat, it was the pain that came from digesting the foods that made me not want to eat. I literally had to constantly remind myself that I NEEDED to eat to get the right nutrients into me, that this is what I HAD to do to reverse my health. Some days were a real battle, and Mom helped to gently remind me and encourage me when I struggled. It wasn't easy for me. And it CERTAINLY wasn't easy for her to watch, being unable to take the pain away as I struggled. However, there WERE times that I had a good appetite!

The night sweats were addressed with a product called CALM. CALM is a "Stress Management Supplement" and is magnesium based. It includes vitamins B-6 and B-12, folic acid, and chamomile and valerian root. Since I was magnesium deficient, and learned from Dr. Ann that a majority of Americans are deficient in magnesium—90%, which causes anxiety and depression. When I am or we are stressed, we use more magnesium to calm ourselves. If we lack magnesium, being deficient, we are actually causing more stress and inviting disease into our lives. CALM helped to lessen the night sweats, for a time, but they never went away completely while I was ill. This product also helped to calm me, bringing a bit more balance to my daily life.

One of the most influential helps from Dr. Ann that I was told to do was to keep a food journal of what I ate every single day. Furthermore, she said I should write down how I felt after eating, and any symptoms I experienced. This was actually something that helped her in our monthly appointments, to direct her as to what needed to be changed in my diet and what was working for me. Food journaling helped me immensely to figure out what foods were and were not working for me or agreeing with me, too. I continued food journaling for the next four years, until I was truly well and healthy again, or for the first time ever.

Dr. Ann elaborated on the food journaling, telling me that I needed to learn to "listen to my body, to what it was telling me. Your body, you, are your own best doctor... if you are listening to what it is telling you." She was the one that really helped me to become more "in-tune" with myself, and listen to what my symptoms were saying. This has also helped to calm myself, not panicking when I experience any kind of change that could cause stress.

I'd, too, been told by the good doctor to work on deep breathing, daily. I tried to do this, but honestly it didn't work due to the even more severe pain on my left side under my ribs and around to my back, a 3-D effect, that resulted from trying to breath deep. This just wasn't possible to do as often or as much as she, or I, would have liked.

I was doing everything to the best of my ability that I was instructed to do from Dr. Ann. Mom was my biggest cheerleader, walking alongside of me every step of the way. After my third monthly appointment with Dr. Ann, I wasn't getting the results that I felt I should have at this point in time, and I was frustrated. I had things that I needed to say. Mom was going to get the brunt of my frustration.

18

One More Month

Kelly

Reversing my health and healing "naturally" was going to be a longer process than I was aware of. It's not like taking a pill for pain relief and 15 minutes later the effects of the drug are noticeable. I didn't fully adapt to that mindset of taking "longer" until after a particularly challenging month.

It was the fall of 2013 that in a moment of frustration I allowed it to grow into verbal anger, directly after an appointment with Dr. Ann. It had been my third month working with the good doctor. I told Mom in the car when I plopped down in the car seat, afterward, and shutting the door harder than need be, "I'm done!"

Silence sat amongst us. When I finally turned to look at her, Mom was looking at me with tear-filled eyes. My angry, hot tears soon poured down my cheeks. I angrily wiped at the tears repeating, "I'm done, Mom. I've done everything Dr. Ann has recommended. I've taken her supplements, followed all her strict diet suggestions, everything. My left-side abdominal pain is the worst it's been. Now, my left side in the back hurts constantly too. I'm sick and tired of being sick and tired!"

Mom watched me quietly as we sat in the car. I tried to control my tears. Then she reminded me, "You've had many good days, Kelly. And on your good days, you tell me that you do feel well. You don't feel bad all the time," she said, pausing. Then she asked me, "What will you do, then, if you quit with Dr. Ann? Do you want to go back to the medical doctors?"

"NO!" I angrily replied. "I don't want to go to the (Western) medical route. They will just want to give me medications, which will make my stomach problems worse. Then they'll do a bunch of tests and they'll all come back normal AGAIN. I'm NOT going to go the medical route." Built-up frustration turned to anger was pouring out of me.

"What do you want to do then, Kelly? What other options do you have? Do you REALLY want to quit everything you're doing?" Mom asked, quietly.

"I don't know!" I hostilely replied. I knew deep in my heart that *I wasn't going to quit.* I was just mad--frustrated.

After a few minutes of utter silence, Mom turned to me, patiently asking me, "Please Kelly, give Dr. Ann just one more month. Please?"

My eyes, swollen and bloodshot from crying hard, momentarily glanced at her looking back at me. With a heavy heart I agreed, "Okay. Just 'one more month'."

"Okay," Mom whispered, watching me sadly. She held out her arms over the center console between us and I fell into them sobbing again. I was a hot mess and mentally exhausted from the wars of decision-making battling in my head. I was also dealing with depression that would grow worse during the next years to come. The battles in my mind were real.

During the agreed to "one more month" I took a wonderful turn for the better with my left-side pain and night sweats, I started digesting food a little better, and I had more energy. Then Mom was crying... crying happy tears while saying, *"'One more month', huh?"*

Looking back, it wasn't until over a year later that we BOTH could laugh, together, over the mention of the phrase "one more month". It took that long for me to see some beauty come from the ashes of that afternoon in her car, letting my frustrations get the best of me. But you know what? The timing was perfect, because I would not only need to understand the concept of giving the all-natural healing route TIME to work its benefits then, but live the concept out in the next three years to come during the worst of worst times.

To those of you that don't know Mom or me personally, or even if you do, many people think that Mom and I have always been close in our relationship. Not so. We haven't always been close. Truth is, growing up I butted heads with her a lot of the time, almost on a daily basis. I was strong-willed and determined. And so was she, so that was difficult for both of us to deal with the other. Mom and I were actually a lot alike. THAT was the problem.

Dad would often come home from his workday to find Mom and me not speaking and mad at the other. He was, more often than not, the mediator for our disagreements. As I got older, the arguments got more heated because, well, I had more of an attitude. By that time, I also knew how to push her buttons, that honestly, I shouldn't had been pushing. Mom had been much more patient with me as a young teenager, which only made me angrier and more defiant in our disagreements. She had changed for the better, but I hadn't.

When I was about 15 years old, we both got to the point where we were tired of our still happening disagreements and arguing. We hit our "rock bottom", so-to-speak. It was time for BOTH of us to change. We talked and agreed that we BOTH needed to work at being more patient, being forgiving, slower to speak, thinking before we speak, to not do the notorious "tit-for-tat", to be more open and honest with each other, and work on our communication skills. Truthfully, it was one of the best things that ever happened for our relationship. And, it needed to happen if we EACH wanted to better our relationship.

In those years of realigning our attitudes, we both had our moments of being tempted to our old tactics, but we overcame, and still do today, together. In my late teen years, 18-19 years old, becoming ill actually helped to continue strengthening our relationship. What I'm trying to say is, we didn't just by chance have a good mother-daughter relationship. We had to both willingly work at it, humbling ourselves to serving the other with kindness, goodness, patience, gentleness, self-control, etc., and through these fruits our relationship grew to be so much more.

Today, our relationship is deeper than it has ever been. We have a mother-daughter relationship that to me is deeply profound. We are the best of friends and have many things in common. We often get told from people, "you two have such a beautiful relationship." Yes, we do. But the thing is, it didn't just happen overnight, or in a month (laugh out loud!). It took and still takes work, and patience, on both our parts. We still have disagreements, but we are able to talk through them reasonably and respectfully. We both talk openly, sharing our thoughts, our hearts, and our perspectives, all so that we can better understand where the other is coming from. We are to the point in our relationship where we both can freely ask for forgiveness when in error, admitting when we are wrong.

Mom was right in asking me to hold on for "one more month" to see some positive results in my health. Thanks, Mom! I could not have gone through these past years without your help, guidance, encouragement, and love. I'm so thankful for our open relationship. You've taught me a lot about being transparent and vulnerable. I thank Papa God for you. I'm so thankful you are my mama, friend, and sister. I LOVE YOU!"

19

A New Heart

Kelly

I continued seeing Dr. Ann monthly for the next one-and-a-half years. I learned SO much from her. Most all of the supplements, foods, and other suggestions that she had me implement into my lifestyle were helpful. However, these didn't get to the deeply embedded root of the problem with the left side pain, so my symptoms were still present. *I was certain my health was in a chronic stage.*

Dr. Ann had talked to me about "...healing in ALL aspects. This means, physically, mentally, emotionally, and spiritually. Kelly, you can have a perfect all-organic diet, but if you haven't healed from your past traumas, hurts, etc., you won't ever be truly healthy. You can't expect to be well without dealing with your past and the hurts that life brings." She paused continuing to look me deeply and directly in the eyes. "Have you dealt with your past, Kelly? I'm not asking you to answer me. I want you to think about this. Kelly, you can't truly heal if you aren't willing to look at each of these different aspects, individually, to become whole and healthy again."

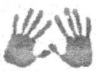

You've heard me reference God and my faith so far in my journey. In order to fully understand what I believe and my relationship with my Papa, God, I need to be REAL with you about how my life has changed. But first, I'd like to say: 1) I'm not trying to make you believe what I believe, nor do I intend to push my beliefs onto you. 2) I'm not religious and have no intentions to be. I simply share my faith, a relationship with my Papa God, with you so you can better understand me and where I'm coming from in my journal entries (JE) and daily life stories being told. In order to understand my relationship with God, I'm going to give just a brief summary of my growing up years.

As a child, I, like many kids, was brought to an institutional church, meaning a building where people come together to worship on certain days of the week. I very much disliked going to church. I didn't care for many of the people, and especially the hypocrisy I witnessed. As I grew into a teenager, our family became very involved with a local church in our hometown. At this time in my life, I despised church even more... having to spend more time there. I was resistant, angry, and bitter. Truthfully, the basis of all these emotions was because I couldn't stand watching classmates put on a church-face--acting a certain way on Sundays and Wednesday nights, and then during the week at school they'd be their totally different real selves. Hence, my choice of words, witnessing hypocrisy. Coincidentally, these were some of the same kids that bullied me and demeaned me at school, adding in my feeling inferior to them. Yet, I was being taught to LOVE them. Wrapping my head around that idea was tough. My parents helped and guided my brother and me in situations that would come up in life at school, and this for me was one of those areas I needed much guidance with. Those fellow classmates' hypocrisy was enough to continually push me further and further away from wanting anything to do with religion.

Eventually, during my 8th-grade school year, our family stopped going to church all together. I was super glad about that! However, Bible studies continued. Church and fellowship meetings were replaced with home-group meetings, so I wasn't quite off the hook. Long story short, I continued to be bitter and angry. It came to the point that my parents realized that I was not coming any closer to God with consistently being around, or in the midst of, "religious activities". They decided to allow me to make the decision to be a part of meetings and Bible studies if I wanted to. Most of the time I passed. But sometimes I'd go because I'd feel obligated.

Fast forward to December 29th, 2011. I was 19-and-a-half years old. This is the day that my life changed for the better, literally becoming a new person, spiritually. Let me explain by going back to that cold, frigid winter night in our home that was no different than any other night.

Mom, Troy, and I were downstairs at our home together. I don't remember what we were doing, but Troy was "lovingly" teasing me, again. Growing up I felt like I was always teased by people, and it was very common coming from Dad and Troy. I didn't like getting teased, and that night I'd had enough of it. I voiced my thoughts. "STOP picking on me, Troy! I'm sick and tired of you guys picking on me. You do it all the time. I've had it with all your teasing. STOP!" I angrily shot at him.

Troy looked at me, bewildered that I was angry. Mom turned her head and looked at me saying, "You guys? I wasn't picking on you, Kelly. And Troy, he was just loving on you in his own way. He wasn't teasing you or making fun of you."

"Yeah, Kelly. I wasn't picking on you or making fun of you. I'm sorry if you interpreted it that way," Troy chimed in.

I angrily got up, grabbed the blanket that I had wrapped around me and threw it on the couch and turned back, walking only a few steps into my bedroom.

"You don't need to throw things because you're angry, Kelly." Mom stated.

"You don't get it," I curtly said to her. "I'm sick and tired of being the one who gets teased, picked on, and made fun of. I ALWAYS get the brunt of it. I'm not putting up with it anymore." By this time, I was in my room talking through an almost closed door.

Troy then said, "Kelly, I wasn't intending to pick on you."

"Well, you were picking on me." I said, unrelentingly.

"I'm really sorry, Kelly." Troy had stated. Then I heard him say to Mom, "I wasn't picking on her, Mom."

"I know, Troy. It's not you that's the problem. It's her heart. She needs a change of heart. She needs a new heart." Mom replied. The two were talking softly so they thought I couldn't hear what they'd said... but I did hear them, clearly.

"Bull!" I muttered under my breath. Tears started forming in my eyes. The lights went off in the living room and they both went to bed. And me? I did not go to bed.

If there are two sentences that can and have the ability to forever change a person's life, they are, "I love you" and "I forgive you".

It was after 10pm. I was alone in my bedroom. I knelt by my bed and soon broke down. My gut-wrenching sobs were muffled by a pillow. The sobbing was deep, and the sorrow I felt was going deeply into my inner being. My heart was broken. It was time to talk. I cried out to God, utterly broken, for the first time in my life. My heart and whole being hurt. I needed peace in my life. For the first time, that night in my bedroom, I was aware that I needed to ask for forgiveness. I didn't hear God, and I didn't see God. However, I could feel God's presence. It was like I was being held in a warm hug. Between sobs I spoke to God, apologizing for many things I knew were wrong. I told God, "I'm angry, bitter, unhappy, have a hardened heart, am holding unforgiveness toward others, and the list goes on, Lord. I need your help, God. I'm sorry."

Immediately upon speaking out, I felt a peace deep inside my heart that spread throughout my whole being. Never in my life had I felt a peace like this before. It was unreal. To this day, I still have that peace and I thank my Papa God for it.

The next morning, I got up feeling peaceful. I wanted to tell my parents and brother the good news because they too, had had similar experiences in their lives. But I also wanted to see if any of them would notice how peaceful I was!

A woman once gave me a gift, a ceramic green painted, fall colored leaf, which had written on it "I love you so much. Love, God." She has no idea how often I would go to read this during both the day and middle of the nights when I couldn't sleep when I was sick. I'd stand tracing its letters, being reminded that I am never alone, and am loved more than any person can imagine is possible. In the days, months, and years to come it was something that I gravitated toward for comfort, a reminder, and to be with my Papa God in mind and heart. *To the woman that gave this gift to me: Thank you. I truly treasure it, and you. Thank you for your kindness, prayers, friendship and love.*

Over the course of a few weeks after that night in my bedroom talking to God and receiving forgiveness, I became a different person. I was happier, less moody, talked more, laughed and smiled more often, and became more pleasant company. I was peaceful and didn't react right away when I got upset. I even apologized for being wrong at times--which prior to that, was unheard of.

I still remember the day that I told Mom about this new, wonderful, change in my life. We were going to have a family prayer meeting that was "optional" for anyone to be present. Now as I said before, prior to this new change I would more than likely not show up for any meeting, but on that night, right as the meeting started, I walked through the door much to everyone's surprise. Towards the end of our time together, I took a turn to pray.

Later that night Mom asked me privately, "What's going on with you? What was that, your prayer? That wasn't the Kelly I know."

"I'm not lonely anymore, Mama. I've got Jesus. He's with me all the time." I said, smiling. She looked at me in wonder. I said no more, until moments later when she and I were standing in the kitchen cleaning produce. I turned and said, "Do you think there has been something different about me lately?"

Mom smiled while looking at me saying, "Why, yes! Troy and I were just talking about that recently. I'd told him, 'It's almost as if Kelly's a new person!' Dad and I talked about this too."

"Well, I AM!" I stated.

"Oh, KELLY!" She dropped the potato she was washing, water flying as she grabbed me into a big hug and kissed me. Happy tears poured down her face and we stood hugging one another.

William Paul Young, author of the popular book, "The Shack"[1] and other spectacular reads says, **"In order for forgiveness to take place, something has to die. If you make the choice to forgive you have to face into the pain. You simply have to hurt. Forgiveness is so difficult because it involves death and grief. In order to forgive we must embrace love."**

Young states it well. Forgiveness is so hard because it means we do have to face into the pain. On that cold December night, I became a new person with a new heart, receiving true unconditional love and forgiveness for the first time in my life. Do I deserve it? Absolutely not, but my Papa God loves me more profoundly than anyone ever will, and more than any of us can know. Child-like faith. It's truly that simple. My child-like faith is sweet, innocent, direct, simple, and pure. Every day of my life is a hands-down, beautiful dance with my Papa God, my best friend, and I wouldn't exchange it for anything. All these years since that night, my relationship with my Papa God has grown to much more than I could have ever imagined. And you know what? It's rarely dull…and it's never religious!

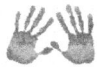

Dr. Ann's gentle reprimand for healing in ALL aspects to be WHOLE hit close to home that day at her office. I'd gotten right with my Papa God a few years prior to seeing her that fall of 2013, but in the days, months, and years to come, forgiveness and healing were going to continue. Both are like peeling the layers of an onion. Some of those deeper layers of pain that I hadn't even known existed were going to come closer to the surface.

---

[1] "The Shack", by Wm. Paul Young, 2007, www.theshackbook.com

20

Will I Survive?

Kelly

JE December 13th, 2014

Mom and I both truly believe I have cancer. However, I have been given no "diagnosis". All the natural ways of healing that I have been doing are addressing my state of health as if I have cancer. Hmm. I have looked like death's walk for the last month-and-a-half in reference to my state of health. Thank you, Lord, for being with me every step of the way. I continue to give You all the glory and praise as I struggle through each day.

A summary of the remainder of time when working with Dr. Ann. Since Dr. Ann wasn't a medical doctor, but a Chiropractor who specialized in many healing modalities, she didn't practice in "diagnosing diseases" like cancer, I never asked her if that's what she was treating me for. I didn't have to. From doing my own research, I verified that I had every symptom of pancreatic cancer except for blood in my stool. Deep in my heart, I knew pancreatic cancer was the core issue.

While working with Dr. Ann, Mom and I had started to do our own research to better help my ill state of health. Dr. Ann had encouraged this too! "Don't take my word for something," she'd stated, "find out for yourself what is true. You, yourself, are your own best doctor," she continued. "I'm here to help you in your journey in whatever ways I can." This was when Mom and I really started to learn about health and healing in deeper ways. Our research was diverse, not limited to: leaky gut, food as medicine, essential oils, cancer, gut microbiome, the gut-brain connection, GOOD fats vs. BAD fats, auto-immune diseases, healing teas, and more. Safe to say, we were "research junkies" to help ourselves understand what was going on specifically in regards to my health. We learned a lot.

JE January 1, 2014
I had a revelation of what all of my journaling these past few years, and years to come, is to be used for. Lord, you want me to write a book about what I have been going through. Okay, I will. I have NO idea what or even how this is going to get done, but there is one thing I KNOW: With You, Papa God, ALL things are possible!

The winter of 2013-2014 was rough for me physically and mentally, as I didn't feel well. I was battling depression, and continued to juggle my health issues, work-life, home-life, and trying to not let any of life's struggles take me down. I continued to do everything Dr. Ann had said, and was also working at my business in massage therapy--growing my business clientele. When spring came, I was glad for the warm weather and change of seasons!

My symptoms at this time included, but weren't limited to, the following:
- Headaches (present day and night).
- Hot and cold sweats (day and at night).
- Nausea (whenever I ate or drank anything. I'd wake up to this at night, too, while my digestive system was attempting to do its job).
- My stomach made a lot of loud "digesting" noises 24/7.
- Diarrhea (5-15 times per day)
- I was pale in color, having a gray tone. Mom called it "ashen".
- Sleep was light and short lived. I could only sleep on my left side curled up in the fetal position because of the intensity of the left-side abdominal pain. The times I'd try to slowly roll onto my right side brought such pain to my left side I couldn't handle it. Sleeping was exhaustive.
- The pain in my left side extended from under my ribs, mostly on the left side, extending down to the belly button. My left side was on FIRE. When the severe pain would start, my whole abdomen would begin to hurt, but more-so on the left side. The pain under my ribs radiated into the left side of my back. It was a 3-dimensional type of pain, stemming from deep inside the left middle part of my ribs.

- I was dizzy and light headed. At any given time, a room could spin, even if I was lying down.
- I lost more weight, getting to be too thin and malnourished looking.
- I'd wake up daily, in the early hours of the morning, to a searing, ripping pain in my abdomen that left me breathless and tearful.
- I had yellow, raised spots in both of my eyes, and a hazed, yellowish color where they should had been white.
- I could no longer sit comfortably. The sitting position brought such discomfort that car rides were dreaded. When it was time to go on road trips 3-4 hours to the city, Mom would drive while I semi-laid and curled up in the front seat attempting to get comfortable (which really didn't work). Sitting just hurt.

JE April, 2014
I'm really tuckered out. I have been virtually exhausted all the time. It has been continually getting worse. I've been trying not to let the tiredness get to me, but it's caught up with me. My gut has been really bad. It's been raw, uncomfortable, and hurting. My eyes are so tired. Headaches are rough, consistently getting worse...not sure how that is possible since I have them 24/7. I'm so tired, Lord. Help me.

Each day I woke up feeling like I'd not slept. With what little sleep I'd get at night, it hurt when I'd sleep so I never felt real relief and rejuvenation from a night's rest. Waking up to ripping and searing pain in the wee hours of the morning left me breathing very shallow. The pain ultimately left me curled up in the fetal position on my left side, praying while tears trickled down my face. I was now beginning to learn how to cry "beautifully" since sobs and deep breathing while crying were out of the question due to the pain it could inflict.

Good things were coming out of my pain, despite its difficulty. I was learning much about patience. Each day and night were a battle, but with one foot in front of the other, I'd make it through the days.

In August 2014, my parents celebrated their 25th Wedding Anniversary. Family, friends, and relatives had come to help join in the celebration. Nearly everyone had arrived to our home and the celebration was about to start. I had some color to my skin since it was summer, and a little redness to my cheeks so I didn't look sickly to most people. I truly wasn't feeling well, but to me that didn't matter. I was here to help celebrate and be of good cheer. Most people had no idea the severity of how sick I was.

Before the festivities got rolling, Mom came over to me while we were outside preparing for guests. Our eyes locked. I looked deep into her heart as I looked through her eyes, and she looked deep into mine. I extended my arms and we met, embracing one another in a hug. Hugging meant NO ONE could touch my abdomen as it hurt. "I love you, Mom." I spoke.

"I love you too, Kelly. I'm so happy in my heart that you are here with us. I don't want to think about how this would have been without you with us today." Mom said.

"I am too. I knew you were thinking about that when you walked up to me." I laughed, growing serious. "Thank you, for not giving up on me. For loving me, despite everything we've gone through together. I love you more than words can speak, Mom." I continued to hug her.

"Oh Kelly, you're my miracle baby. Thank you." We gave each other one last squeeze, then dried our eyes. It was our special moment.

My parent's celebration was wonderful. It was filled with love, laughter, smiles, friends, family, warm weather and sunshine, and lots of wind! Many beautiful memories were made, and many of those were captured on camera. Mom asked a mutual friend of ours, an artist and photographer, to make a video of the pictures afterward.

After Mom received the video and was viewing it one day at work, and I in the office area as well standing by, she had paused the video. In doing so, two images over-lapped to make an effect of "a message" within the double image. We both turned to look back at the screen, and what we saw was clearly a message that left us speechless. A question, a reminder, and a loud answer stood out, all concerning me. I was also IN the picture, another focal point that helped me to know this message WAS FOR ME! See the double imaged photo on the next page.

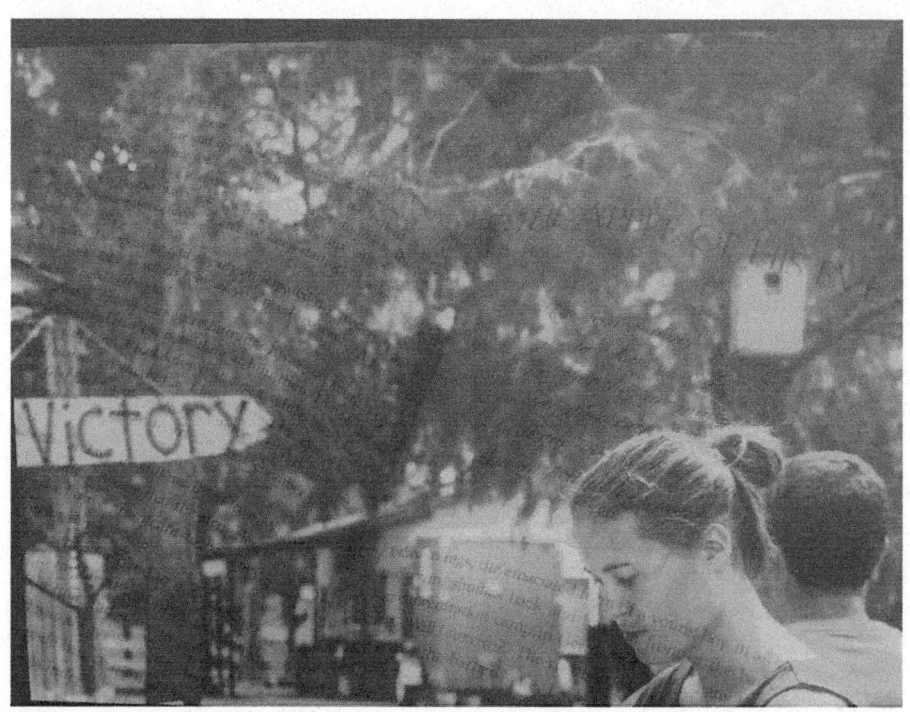

Victory, center high on the left, stood out. **The Apple of His** (Papa God's) **Eye** near the top going to the right--a chapter title in the book, "A Match Made in Heaven"[2]. Mom had the book laying out on a table the day of the party, specifically on this chapter, "Apple of His Eye" which stood out, too, in the double image. In small print, center near the bottom, were the questioning words, **"Will I survive?"** that also stood out to us as well.

The story in the book Mom had the pages opened to was of a young girl and boy who'd met at a Holocaust camp during World War II, each on the other side of a fence separating them. In the story, the children, although separated for many years after the war ended and not knowing how to find each other, were brought back together as adults by a preset-up blind-date in New York city. By chance? Or, by God's hand at work? *What were the odds of that?*

[2] "A Match Made in Heaven, A Collection of Inspirational Love Stories" Volume II, by Susan Wales & Ann Platz, Guideposts edition pg. 111, Multnomah Publishers, ©1999. Told to Susan Wales by Herman Rosenblat, the young boy in story, who tells his life story In "The Will to Survive" published by Adam's Media Corporation, Hollbrook Massachusetts.

Mom loved the story, and was why she had it sitting out at their anniversary party. There's obviously more to their story, but I won't ruin it for you if you choose to read it for yourself!

Mom and I were both awed at what so easily stood-out on the screen's double image before us. We took a screen-shot of the double image shown on the computer screen. The messages spoke to both of us in the same sense as "God's hand at work" in my life and in the details of the children's lives in the story, they BOTH surviving their horrid ordeal and then their paths crossing again as adults. God's hand works, and who will reverse it? Not one.

I felt the messages for myself, personally—me wondering *WILL I SURVIVE* my health crisis. Then, me feeling I'd have **VICTORY**! And I being reminded that I am the *APPLE OF HIS EYE*--which we all are the apple of His eye.

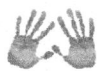

Because of no new developments in healing, my time working with Dr. Ann had come to an end the fall of 2014. Left with no insights on who would be able to help me, Mom and I both wondered, *what's next?*

21

What's Next?

Kelly

Mom and I talked about finding a new doctor to help me with my left-side pain. We decided to look online for a Functional Medicine Doctor (FMD). She found a handful of them, the closest being four hours away. The FMD we picked not only practiced holistic and alternative ways of healing, but also incorporated Western Medicine in his practice. That was part of the reason we thought he would be a good fit--to incorporate both Eastern AND Western medicine, to get to the root of the left side pain.

Mom called and set up the appointment for mid-November 2014, one month after my departure with Dr. Ann. We both spoke to the FMD on the phone. He had many questions he wanted to ask me prior to the physical appointment. He also emailed paperwork for me to fill out for when we'd meet him. The month between leaving Dr. Ann and meeting the FMD was a long one. I continued to battle all of my symptoms and pain.

The day before the appointment finally came, a snow storm was coming in, so Mom and I drove the four hour drive the evening before, staying overnight at a hotel five minutes from the FMD's office, to be there on time for the morning appointment.

The next morning the city folks woke to over a foot of snow. We were only five minutes from the FMD's office but gave ourselves ample time to get there. Just as we arrived to the parking garage at the office building, my phone buzzed, notifying me of a phone call and voicemail. I looked at it, curiously, as I didn't recognize the number. My phone hadn't even rung. *Weird,* I thought. I listened to the voicemail, "Hi Kelly, this is Dr. Jake. Unfortunately, due to the weather and the slow traffic I won't be able to make it in for your appointment this morning. I MIGHT make it in for my afternoon appointments, but I'm not even sure about that yet. Sorry. You can call the office to reschedule your appointment."

I was devastated and angry. With a roaring vengeance I cried out, "You've GOT to be kidding me!" Mom looked at me, bewildered. I told her the voice message. Tears pooled, then ran down my cheeks. I angrily wiped at them. I gave Mom the phone and she listened to the voicemail. Then, she called the doctor back. He didn't answer, so she left a message for him.

A few minutes later the phone rang from the same number, so mom took the call. He said, "I'm unable to get into the office. I only made it two miles from my house. The roads are icy, stopping traffic over the bridge. I don't know if there's an accident or what. I probably won't be coming into work at all today. Call the office and they'll reschedule your daughter."

Mom responded, "It's been almost a month of waiting to get this appointment for Kelly. My daughter is sitting here next to me in excruciating pain, and you're telling me to simply reschedule her? We drove here last night from four hours away to beat the storm. Can you see her this afternoon?" The conversation elaborated, then came to an end, he being unwilling to commit to an afternoon appointment.

Because of his shortcomings in communicating, we researched him in depth right there in the parking garage, finding out that he wasn't what he claimed to be. He did not have the credentials of a FMD, but that of a chiropractor who did some Eastern therapies in his practice. Needless to say, I didn't end up seeing him that day, or ever.

Where would the road lead to next? As we pulled out of the parking garage and into traffic, tears silently and softly trickled down my face. *Why is this happening, God?*

Stopped in traffic, Mom leaned over and gave me a side hug. I fought the sobs that wanted to surface, but that would make my left side hurt more. I squirmed in my seat. Silent tears continued trickling down my cheeks. Mom had her tears, too. I clenched my jaw and tried to breath. Inside the car was silence as

I sat staring out the window, feeling numb and detached. She called to let Dad know of the morning's flop.

Frustration, anger, bewilderment, and more emotions flooded through me that morning. I fought off the *"of course this would happen to you"*, and *"another dead end"* thoughts. I'll admit it wasn't easy to find anything positive in the situation. I was in turmoil while riding side-saddle to Mom who was in the driver's seat.

After much silence while driving the freeway at minimal speed, Mom spoke-up, "Kelly, do you want to see if Dr. Daniel (our family's NUCCA Chiropractor) has an opening for you? Maybe that would help?"

I continued staring out the window. After some thought I replied, "I guess I could do that. Seems I can't stay in alignment very good since I've been so sick. I reckon that might be a wise choice." I called the chiropractor's office. He had a pretty open schedule, with having clients cancel, so I got in immediately.

I'd started going to our NUCCA[3] chiropractor back in 2011. I'd gone to other chiropractors before Dr. Daniel, chiropractors that weren't trained in NUCCA like Dr. Daniel is. NUCCA (National Upper Cervical Chiropractic Association) is a non-invasive, gentle, unique type of chiropractic therapy. The doctor does his adjustments from the cervical atlas (first bone in the neck), using a non-invasive (no cracking of neck or body parts) method to adjust and bring balance back for the patient. After my very first NUCCA appointment, I'd felt the difference immediately. For the first time in years, I got long term relief for my right shoulder pain, which stemmed from a high school alpine skiing competition injury. Along with MANY other benefits, NUCCA therapy got my head back on straight, relieving pinched nerves to open the highways of communication so that my brain could get messages of healing through the nervous system, to my shoulder.

---

[3] What is NUCCA, https://nucca.org/

Many years later, now that morning of the snow storm in Dr Daniel's office, he asked me, "How are you, Kelly? What's brought you in today?"

I told him about our morning, my presumed appointment with the assumed FMD, and my frustration. I said, "I honestly don't know where to go, or what to do next. I'm certainly not going back to that guy." Dr. Daniel looked at me, astonished. Turns out, he knew of the guy and confirmed that he wasn't a FMD at all.

Throughout the course of our conversation, Dr. Daniel said he knew of a FMD located only ten minutes away from his office. He told me a testimonial of someone he knew that had gone to this FMD he was referencing. "I'll get the name of the business when we are done here." And with that said, he did his thing and got me back in alignment.

Being so sick, my body was constantly fighting itself to stay in alignment, adjustments lasting for a short amount of time. With NUCCA chiropractic, the long-term goal of the chiropractor is to see you only once or twice a year. Why? Because once the vertebra's atlas and axis are back in alignment, your body should be able to hold its alignment. Being in alignment, with no restrictions or impingements, healing should happen. There are exceptions to this 1-2 times a year, given a patients' injuries, state of health, etc. My ill state of health, and having my body constantly fighting itself, meant I was seeing Dr. Daniel every few months.

After the appointment, Dr. Daniel gave me the name of the nearby FMD saying, "I'm really sorry you got stood-up, Kelly. I'm glad you came in today. I hope this information is helpful."

I smiled, touched by his apology that wasn't even his to issue. "Thank you for the information and for your help. I feel better than I did when I walked in. And thank you for caring." It was nice to have some relief from my constant headaches. They never totally went away, but I'd take whatever relief I could get.

Later that afternoon, Mom called the new FMD's office on our way back home. He was scheduled out a month. Long story short, after much talk the

FMD agreed to see me the following week. I can't begin to tell you how relieved I was. *Help and answers are right around the corner,* I thought.

JE November 12th, 2014

I'm sick, so very sick. It started last night near bed-time and has been bad since then. It has been well over 24-hours. I have had hot and cold sweats. I feel like my gut is ripping apart. The cramps are horrendous when they grab me. I feel like I'm going to vomit and go to the bathroom at the same time. My entire body aches, and low-back pain is constant. I've had major headaches that don't go away... for a LONG time now. Not getting very much sleep with all this plus all my other symptoms...sigh.

22

Mr. Rabbi

Kelly

Days, weeks and months of being ill were not easy. I'd wake up in the morning wanting nothing more than to just go back to sleep. But that wasn't a choice for me as I had a business with a steady growing clientele to run, and three loving pets--two cats and a rabbit that were relying on me to take care of them. All of these were GOOD motivators to make me get out of bed in the morning!

Mr. Rabbi, pronounced *Rabb-ee*, is a mini-lop rabbit. He had come to us on Labor Day weekend 2014. His first owner, whom we knew, no longer wanted him, so I willingly became his new owner. Our family had raised mini-lop rabbits, along with many other animals, while growing up. I knew how to take care of a rabbit.

When I first got Mr. Rabbi, he wasn't very friendly. He didn't want to be touched, picked up, or pet. He'd hop to the opposite side of the hutch when I'd go to see him. Prior to him coming to our home, he was eating store bought rabbit pellets. He lived in a hutch that was spacious at his other home, and his hutch living didn't change when he moved to our home—we were given his hutch when taking ownership of him. The only change was his diet. I'd done research on what a rabbit's diet could be. I decided that Mr. Rabbi was going to eat an ALL-organic diet. This consisted of dandelions, kale, collards, Swiss chard, beet greens, carrot tops, apple chunks, raisins, dried apricots, dried cranberries, walnuts and pecans.

Mr. Rabbi LOVED his new array of fresh foods! As he'd munch on his food, I'd attempt to pet him. It didn't take long for Mr. Rabbi to enjoy our special time together. Each morning and night when I fed him, he would eat and I would lovingly talk to him while petting him. Within a month's time, Mr. Rabbi started to greet me when I brought his food to him. He WANTED to be pet, even more than he wanted his food! Eventually, he let me pick him up and hold him! His heart would beat very fast against my chest (this is normal for rabbits), as he nuzzled his head into my neck.

My family and I witnessed Mr. Rabbi's demeanor change, all because of his diet. I loved the little white rabbit. He grew to love me, too, just like my cats, especially Goofy--my Calico cat who had come to us years before. More on Goofy later. Each time I went to feed Mr. Rabbi, Goofy would slowly walk behind me. She'd sit a distance away from the hutch watching the rabbit intently. And Mr. Rabbi would do the same from inside his hutch, watching Goofy.

As Mr. Rabbi grew more friendly, I decided that it wasn't fair for him to have to sit inside a hutch all day and night. We have a big yard with lots of flower beds, coverings so he could play and sit under safely. Dad built a little door and ramp for Mr. Rabbi to go in and out of his hutch. When I'd go to feed him in the morning, I'd open up the little door. He'd come hopping right out and hop in circles around my legs. It didn't take long before Mr. Rabbi was putting his front two paws on my legs, wanting to be pet. I'd reach down to pet him and then he'd run in circles in excitement. After putting his food inside his hutch he'd follow me back up to the house, hopping between my legs, often times tripping me up!

Mr. Rabbi had become a completely different rabbit from when I got him. In time, he followed me EVERYWHERE when I'd go outside. And soon after that he started following everyone in our family around when they were outside too.

When Mr. Rabbi first came to us, Goofy, my indoor/outdoor cat, wasn't keen on having a him around. Now that Mr. Rabbi was freely hopping around the yard or elsewhere, he was a REAL pest to her! He'd follow Goofy around the yard trying to play with her. She didn't like having him follow her everywhere, especially when she wanted to go hunting. Goofy had her daily routine and Mr. Rabbi was messing it ALL up!

Over time, I believe Goofy grew to love Mr. Rabbi. It wasn't uncommon to see the two friends laying side by side watching life outside happen together. Everywhere they went, they would go together. They were a team, kind of.

Somedays, the two would be gone on an adventure, wandering around the neighborhood together. Sometimes I'd have to go out looking for them if they hadn't come home before the sun was about to set. Other times, I'd find them visiting some of the neighbors, who didn't actually love animals but soon came to admire (and maybe even love) the pair. The two became the talk of the neighborhood, and even to visitors that drove by to the boat launch right next to our home. Mr. Rabbi loved to make friends with both people and animals!

One time, Mr. Rabbi brought home a new friend he'd met! For REAL! Mom had opened the front door one beautiful, sunny morning well after I'd let him out of the hutch earlier that morning, and there sat Mr. Rabbi with a small cat next to him. Mr. Rabbi hopped up to Mom, then turned back to the cat and hopped back over, sitting right next to the cat again. NO KIDDING! Mr. Rabbi looked at Mom and then the little white and gray cat cried out, "Meow, meow."

"Kelly! Come see what Mr. Rabbi just brought home!" Mom called to me. I walked past her peering through the open door.

"Oh! Mr. Rabbi! You brought home a new friend!" I smiled, laughing. The little cat was in rough condition, with dried blood on it, an ear partly missing, and moisture oozing from its eyes. My heart went out for the little cat. Mr. Rabbi excitedly hopped around his new friend. I watched the cat as it hesitantly walked away from us, slowly walking across the road to the neighbor's yard, with Mr. Rabbi following closely in its footsteps. No idea where the two went, but Mr. Rabbi came home alone later that morning.

Mr. Rabbi was with us for just over two years before he passed away. During the course our time with him he taught me a lot. He was a big part of motivating me to get out of bed in the morning when I was so sick and depressed. He showed me unconditional love, in turn, helping me to start living my life more this way too. With the simple joy he brought to my life, I really began to learn the concept of "joy in the simple things" on a daily basis. And that is a life lesson game changer. Mr. Rabbi confirmed to me, too, how our diets impact each of us, by my changing his diet and his good results from doing so. Our diets do matter in every way of living our lives.

Mr. Rabbi and Goofy, together, gave me ample opportunities to go on adventures with them. Since I was so sick, vacations away from home weren't a possibility for me due to many digestive aspects. But with these two I could have as many adventures as I wanted, all in our backyard. We soon became known as the "Three Amigos". We'd go out for walks; a girl with her cat and rabbit. Needless to say, they helped bring out the best in me when I certainly didn't feel up to it.

Mr. Rabbi, as have all my pets, aided in my health journey, helping promote healing for me in his own unique way of bringing me joy. Mr. Rabbi was a one-of-a-kind rabbit that would have made an excellent human being. His time with us was nothing short of a blessing, a joy, and filled our family and neighborhood with lots of love, wonder, and laughter.

23

Rubbing Shoulders

Amy

In the fall of 2014, our family's chiropractor, knowing of Kelly's health struggles and her gluten sensitivity, passed along to both Kelly and myself an email from a doctor, one of the world's leading gluten specialists. The email contained information on an upcoming online webinar on the topic of gluten, with an offer to sign up to hear daily presenters, for free, including more than two dozen speakers. We were interested.

We signed up for the webinar, and when the time came to hear the speakers' interviews with the doctor hosting the webinar, we listened to multiple interviews via email links sent to us daily that were pre-recorded. Most all of the guests were MDs, including multiple Neurologists, a Cardiologist, multiple Functional Medicine doctors, and Autoimmune and Celiac Disease doctors who research these diseases. One of those doctors even suggested autoimmune diseases and celiac disease CAN be reversed according to his findings, and who also believes that no person can fully digest gluten. Other speakers were clinical nutritionists, an entrepreneur of health and superfoods.

What IS gluten? Gluten is the generic term used for the storage of protein in grains, specifically found in wheat, rye, and barely. The gluten protein is the toxic substance that causes an immune response in individuals with celiac disease, but in a recent 20-plus year span has shown itself a nuisance to gut health--gut microbiome, in a large population of people world-wide. One may be familiar with the term "gluten sensitivity" which has been around for quite some time.

Some of the other speakers were leading activist and spokesperson on the health consequences of GMOs and pesticides in our food system impacting our guts AND brains. All of these professionals educated us on the subjects of: The "Gut & Brain Connection", the gut being our FIRST brain, "Intestinal Permeability", also termed "Leaky Gut", the dangers of GMOs in our food system, and the impact GMOs have made in the health of Americans and worldwide, how doctoring with prescription drugs leads to toxic overloads and is missing the mark in treating symptoms and disease, along with much more healthful information, including food as medicine and nutritional healing.

After we'd heard the entire webinar, we invested in a full copy of it for future referencing, and also for the purpose to share it with others. We learned so much from this doctor and his guests, a tribe of teachers.

> **"Knowledge is power. Information is power. The secreting or hoarding of knowledge or information may be an act of tyranny camouflaged as humility."** -Robin Morgan

Why do I write about this kind of information? Why do I often times share troublesome health misconceptions while visiting with those I do life with, or share on social media? Because I care about people, and the damage that is being done to us as people, and in animals, by government run farming, large corporations, and the pharmaceutical industry, "Big Pharma", who are making all kinds of profits while unknowingly or knowingly making us eaters and prescriber's sick. But please, don't just believe me, do the research for yourself.

Also, I share information because I, myself, was a toxic-infested human being in need of help to change my mental and physical health in my late 30's. Thankfully, I chose to step out of my comfort zone, get myself informed, change my thinking, and in doing so I learned how to change my health, slowly but gradually, with all natural approaches, supplementing with nutrients that I lacked and then detoxing my body of built-up toxic garbage--pathogens that first caused inflammation and then mental and physical illness and ultimately will cause disease.

Autoimmune diseases, heart disease, cancer, depression, and more are killing us, literally, daily. The time has already come to exposing the negative effects of nutrient-dead processed foods, added hormones in meats, chemicals sprayed on crops--directly affecting fruits, vegetables, and grains that are part of so many processed foods, and the deadly impact these practices have on our health. It's become one of my passions to gather and share information to help others change their health for the better, if they want to. Bottom line: It's up to us to research and implement healthful changes, independently and corporately, and having accountability if it is actually wanted. We've got to WANT to change our health situation to even begin to change at all, and part of that is educating ourselves, acting on the knowledge we've gained, and making daily choices to live a healthier life.

The minority of people wanting changes in our food supply is growing in number. Americans are waking up and starting to hear the call to not only clean-up their diets but to challenge the USDA practices and the dysfunctional "Food Pyramid" directive. People are seeing the need to grow their own food or find acceptable resources to buy wholesome food from. I'm expecting to see the minority in this arena of food quality grow into a majority before I die.

All this to bring me to my main point: The importance of really taking time for talking to the people we are "rubbing shoulders" with. This statement has become an action term with my family of four over the years since I was ill and turned my health around. "Rubbing shoulders" means that we are paying attention, listening, and talking to those who come into our life, really taking time to get to KNOW these people and hear what they have to say. They're in our life for a reason, whether that be to connect us to themselves or others through their connections, for them to be a part of our lives now, or for an extended period of time, all for reasons unknown to us, mostly!

Life is about relationships. We CAN learn from every single person we come into contact with! We all have something to bring to the table for others, too, if they are willing to pursue further opportunities of relationship, knowledge, or growth from even someone whom may be deemed "less than", including yours truly! And you know what? It's FUN to get to know the person next to you and connect with them on some level! Seems as though there is always a common connection, utterances of "It's a small world" come to mind!

"I define connection as the energy that exists between people
when they feel seen, heard and valued; when they can give

**and receive without judgement; and when they derive
sustenance and strength from the relationship."**
-Brene Brown

So, I ask you, who are you "rubbing shoulders" with? Are you paying attention to those people coming into your life, sporadically, on the job, at the gym, in the pew next to you, etc.? Those people are not randomly brought to you. You have something to share with them. Of course, we all have a choice in relating or not. We can either not take the extra time, or perhaps live in fear of stepping out of our comfort zone, to start a conversation, OR we can invest a few minutes or more and possibly be blessed by the time we spend in getting to know the one next to us!

Being blessed by another human being and being thankful for meeting so-and-so are common prayers of mine. I'm blessed to have, and thankful for, so much change in my adult life, and for the people who've helped bring about those positive changes. I'm thankful for the hands of God putting people in my life that have motivated, helped, encouraged, taught by sporting a life well-lived, and all those who've impacted me to making better choices for myself and ultimately extended into my family.

One of those people who've blessed us, who comes to mind because of writing this today, is our family's NUCCA, chiropractor, Dr. Daniel. He chose to get to KNOW us during the time our lives intersected at his office, and he still does. And then he shared the email from the gluten specialist who aided in bringing information on a gut healing program to help save Kelly's life and guide her into optimal health, among other helpful insights, pieces of information, and recommendations over the years. From that one email on the subject of "gluten" came a whole lot of information and connections to aid in changing our family's health, specifically Kelly's health. *"Thanks, Dr. Daniel, for rubbing shoulders with your clients. You definitely rock!"*

24

Deeper Underlying Issues

Kelly

In mid-November, 2014, I meet my new functional medicine doctor (FMD) that was referred to me by my chiropractor. As Mom, I, and the FMD sat together in his office, he asked me many questions. The questions were virtually the same as the ones I'd been asked in the past, "How long have you had this left-side pain? Where does it hurt? What are your symptoms? How are your bowel movements? Are your periods regular?" Etc. etc. etc. After a good length of questioning, he had me sit on his examination table. It was time to have my vitals checked and have my abdomen palpated. I was NOT looking forward to that.

As the FMD palpated my abdomen, I resisted the urge to tell him, "STOP! It hurts!" He needed to do his job to figure out what was going on, so I let him. I held in my reactions as best I could to the very real pain from the uncomfortable pressure. "Does this hurt here?" He'd asked.

"Yes. It hurts." I replied. A couple times I grimaced as he ever so gently palpated. Even his gentle touch hurt.

After the palpating, the FMD had us go back to his desk, sitting in chairs again. He stated, "Nothing feels abnormal. I think I'd like to do three tests giving us insight to the problem of your pain." He proceeded to tell us about the three tests: 1) A Comprehensive Stool Analysis Test (CSAT), 2) a Small Intestinal Bacteria Overgrowth (SIBO) test, which is a breath test, and, 3) a Food Allergy test. "These three tests will be helpful to expose a possible bacteria overgrowth, parasites, H-pylori, candida, an under-or over-abundance of good and bad bacteria, salmonella, and a number of other things. You can do all but the food allergy test from your home," the FMD stated.

Mom and I agreed that I should do all the tests he recommended. He went to the front office, grabbed his packages of tests and came back in. He said, "I'll send these tests home with you," while he opened each one up for us to see. Next, he explained exactly how to do the SIBO breath test, and made clear how to do the other test he had for me. "When you complete the SIBO breath test and the CSA test, you send the specimens via pre-paid shipping labels back to the labs I use to run the tests. The third test you will need to have blood drawn at a local clinic, then they can send it to the lab I have labeled on the packaging for that test packet. Once I get all the test results back, we'll go over the results next time you come back, in three weeks."

I knew I had leaky gut. The FMD had confirmed that during the first part of the appointment in saying, "Kelly, your diet is absolutely amazing! You're eating organic, fresh, whole foods! No processed foods. No Dairy. No grains. No sugar. You obviously have many indicators (symptoms) that point to leaky gut, but you ARE doing all the right things to heal the gut."

My daily diet consisted of vegetables, a few fruits, a few servings of grass-fed, pasture raised, no hormones infested meat, homemade soup, and homemade bone broth. The FMD knew that what I was eating wasn't the reason for my left-side pain. "There's a deeper underlying issue for the left side pain," he'd said.

The FMD had also recommended nutritional supplements, which I purchased before we left his office. We were there for over an hour, a standard amount of time for seeing a functional medicine doctor on the first visit. As I walked out of his office I thought, *Alright, I'm finally going to get some REAL answers from these tests! I'm truly going to find out what is going on inside my body.*

I started taking the nutritional supplements and other "aids" I had purchased the very next day. Just like every other time in the last two years when taking supplements, some of those "aids" being "detoxifiers", made me feel worse (bloated, increased tension headaches, searing abdominal pain going straight into my back, and A LOT of gas). This time was no different. If I knew anything, I knew by now that I needed to take the supplements even if I felt worse. Over the next three weeks I had some really, really bad days. For the most part, there were no positive changes in my symptoms. If anything, my "regular' symptoms were worse.

JE November 27th, 2014
I'm so very pale. I'm utterly exhausted all the time. I'm so weak and all I want to do is sleep. I know that I can't do that though, because I need to stay moving. I need to try to keep my body temperature stable, try to get stronger and utilize what muscle I have so that they don't atrophy. This is really getting hard on me. I feel like I'm slowly sinking and can't grasp the surface of what is really going on inside my body. Help me Papa, give me the patience and strength to go on.

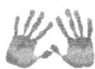

Bone Broth
Mom started making bone broth in 2014 when Dr. Ann had told us, "Homemade bone broth is easy to make. There are different recipes, according to preferred seasonings. If you want to make your own, find a recipe that works best for you AND your body. I will send you home with some recipes. You can find more on-line. Organic grass-fed beef bones or organic free-range chicken carcasses are the base for bone broth. Chicken feet are a must! Use clean filtered water, the best you can find."

Chicken bone broth is what we make most always. Beef BB doesn't appeal to us as much. We use chicken body cavities, necks, and already cooked bones from other meals of roasted chicken we'd had and then froze them. "Chicken feet makes the broth even more nutrient dense from the extra collagen in the feet, which is great for intestinal healing of leaky gut." Dr. Ann had told us. She'd continued, saying, "Bone broth is historically proven to aid in healing of digestive issues, allergies, immune system health, bone and joint health, brain health, and skin conditions." All I can say is, WOW, that's one healthy broth!

As we began daily consuming bone broth at home, Mom didn't care for the taste, but she drank it anyway. Over time, and cooking it with extra ingredients such as more vegetable scrapes/peels and cooking herbs, she grew to like it. I liked the taste of bone broth from the start, but I grew fonder of it as time went on.

We add ghee (clarified butter—contains no dairy) and coconut oil to every individual cup we drink daily, to help promote: healthy brain function, weight loss, reduce brain fog, reduce the risk of developing dementia and Alzheimer's, and to over-all help our bodies function optimally. We also add a ½-1 tsp. of sole--saturated Himalayan Sea salt in purified, clean water, setting in a jar. And, an extra serving of collagen powder (in a non-invasive processed form) to each morning cupful.

As we continued making bone broth, we learned that collagen, found in bones, the joints, and the feet of chickens, contains "gelatinous matter." Collagen is the substance that holds our whole body together! Not only does collagen give skin a beautiful glow, it strengthens and makes skin more elastic. And, it replaces our dead skin cells, reduces wrinkles, and revitalizing skin from the inside out! Collagen promotes better digestion, stronger bone and joint health, healthier hair and nails, reduces the speed of aging (Mom thinks THAT is important), gives greater flexibility and mobility to our bodies, improves sleep and brain function, makes tissue repair happen faster, increases energy, and improves all around body function. Our bodies LOVE collagen!

During the first year of drinking bone broth, I often thought to myself, *my health is changing for the better every time I drink this, even if I don't see my symptoms changing.* I believed that my health was changing, simply by sipping on this daily hot drink. My brother and grandma drink it too! Grandma makes hers from scratch and shares it. I'm so proud of my grandma for doing that, and for my brother who takes the time to drink it.

Bone broth is like our "morning coffee"! We can kick-start our day with this nutrient dense drink, helping ourselves to heal from the inside out!

25

Interesting Results

Kelly

December 2014. Three weeks after my initial appointment, Mom and I were back sitting in the FMDs' office. After greeting us both, he asked, "Has there been any changes since I last saw you, Kelly?"

"No. The supplements only make me feel worse. I'm still taking them though." I stated, honestly.

"Do you know which supplements are making you feel worse?" He inquired.

"All of them." That was the truth. My response perplexed the FMD. However, he moved on. With a copy of my three test results in front of him, he handed Mom and me a copy to share. I was anxious to hear the results!

"I find these test results very interesting. Everything came back 'normal'."

My heart deflated immediately, but I continued listening as he went on. "Did you follow the directions correctly on the SIBO Breath Test, Kelly? I was sure the results would have been positive for SIBO." He spoke.

"Yes, I followed the directions. I did exactly what it said." I stated respectfully.

"I wouldn't have ordered that test if I thought you were going to test negative for it. Are you SURE you did it accurately?" He asked again.

"Yes." I crisply replied.

"I read the instructions, too. I watched her take the test. She did it right." Mom added. I was glad Mom shared this because I was getting irritated that he was implying I did the test wrong.

The FMD moved forward to the CSAT results. "There is nothing overly abnormal that showed up in this test either. Your gut flora isn't quite 'normal'. This means that some of the flora—bacteria, are a little too high or a little too low. However, that being said, none of the bacteria were 'abnormally' high or low." He proceeded to say, "I'm not too concerned about the slight elevation or lower level of the bacteria, since the results weren't in the 'abnormal' range."

Next, the FMD went over the Food Allergy test results, which indicated virtually everything we already knew. I was allergic to some foods, and intolerant to a whole lot of foods. FYI: **Food allergy tests** are accurate regarding specific nutrients. **Food intolerance tests** are inaccurate, because they are only testing the foods we've recently eaten in our diet, foods that our body are already reacting to **today** (not last year, or three months ago. Not tomorrow or next week. Only today)! There's no accuracy in testing for food intolerances, with the exception of doing an "Elimination Diet".

The FMD came to the conclusion that I should continue with the nutritional supplements specifically for my leaky gut, and some of which were detoxing me. He also recommended that I try a FODMAPS diet, which is an elimination diet. We told him that I'd been unofficially doing that for the past two years. I also stated, "I'm not going to add any foods back into my diet that I know cause me problems digesting. It's too painful."

We all agreed to not have me go the route of adding those foods back into my diet that I knew were grievous. In addition, he said, "Keep doing what you are doing, with all organic food. Staying grain, gluten, dairy, and sugar free like you're doing is perfect, Kelly. Keep drinking your homemade bone broth daily, too."

He wanted me to do a phone consult in a month, that way I wouldn't have to drive four hours to the appointment. I appreciated his thoughtfulness and agreed. "If you need to talk to me sooner, if something comes up, please don't hesitate to call the office." He'd spoke. Then, I purchased the new recommended array of nutritional supplements hoping that they would help. Having paid for my appointment, we departed his office.

Reflecting upon first hearing and seeing with my own eyes the test results, my heart had rejoiced that there wasn't something serious going on with my digestive system. But yet, the results didn't give me any insights or answers to my left-side pain and symptoms, and that broke my heart.

When Mom and I walked out of the FMD's office building, Mom stopped walking while looking at me. Tears had pooled, spilling down my cheeks as we'd been walking. Mom reached out her arms and drew me into a hug. I cried, but with-held sobs as there were many cars in the parking lot and I didn't want to make a spectacle of myself if someone were watching. I withdrew from her embrace, catching a few breaths of crisp, cool air while walking to the car before getting in. Once in the car and settled in, there was dead silence for minute. That minute felt like an eternity. No words needed to be said. Mom knew my heart was broken.

"Kelly, it was good you had those tests done. Yes, I know we didn't get ANY insights on what is happening from the results, but these supplements might be exactly what your body needs. They will help heal your leaky gut." Tears continued to flow. I cried in silence. I was really beginning to get the hang of "crying beautifully"! I knew myself well enough that if I spoke, I was going to start sobbing and I couldn't handle the physical pain that inflicted. After a couple minutes of silence and a gigantic headache brewing beyond the norm, I'd gotten ahold of my emotions. "Do you have anything you want to say?" Mom gently probed.

"I'm frustrated. Angry. And, I really don't want to talk about it right now." I responded bluntly.

"I understand." Mom replied. She, of all people, did understand. We let the silence sit between us as she drove to our next destination, for groceries, before driving home.

After shopping and packing the groceries into the car, I was ready to talk. We talked the entire 4-hour drive home.

26

Adventures With Goofy

Kelly

Years ago, while being a very young teenager, on a cold, snowy, December afternoon, a stray kitten arrived at our cabin which is now our residential home. The kitten sat outside crying under an evergreen tree, shivering, curled in a tiny little ball of fur. My parents could hear the little kitten's mournful cries from inside the house. It wasn't long before they ventured outside to investigate, meeting the scrawny but darn cute kitten. Her cries sounded like "eh" instead of "meow". They decided to bring her indoors for some food and water.

Once inside, the kitten ate with a ferocious appetite. I LOVED the cute little girl. She was a long-haired calico cat with beautiful markings. She finished eating her first meal with us and proceeded to explore her new "to-be home". It didn't take long before the little kitten was overtaken with drowsiness on her full tummy. All the while our attention was given to her, my other cat, Bun-Bun, eyed the stranger from a distance.

The little kitten had a personality that, over time, gave her the name that she continues to live up to today, "Goofy". Throughout the years, Goofy and I have formed a tight bond making us an inseparable pair. Let me explain further.

Goofy is an indoor and outdoor cat. If there's work to be done outside, she's right at my side. If it's time for bed, she's curled up in a little ball next to me, purring softly. And when there's adventures to be had, we are off on them together! Needless to say, we are a team. If you ask for one of us, you'll almost

96

always get both of us! Goofy loves to run and play, leading or following. But when she's tired on any outdoor adventure, she rides on my shoulder.

Goofy has taught me a lot about relationships, and I've taught her a lot of different things through the years too. I readily admit, some good teachings and others, well, maybe more of an inconvenience... like when I taught her to open lever-handled doors!

I still remember the first time Goofy let herself into the house we now live. At the time the house was our cabin, and all our pets traveled with us from home to cabin and back. I'd been teaching Goofy to open the door on her own, through the house-entrance door from the attached garage.

Our family of four were sitting together at the table eating supper and talking, when all of a sudden, we heard the door handle being jiggled from the garage side where we knew Goofy was. The jiggling noise was not new at the time, as she experimented with trying to get in, often. Goofy normally moved the door handle as I had been teaching her to, making noise while doing so! But, on this day, to everyone's astonishment, the door opened! By pulling down with her two front paws, at the same time her weight pushing against the door, she succeeded in opening the door! I'll never forget the look on Mom's face as she turned to me saying, "NO! You did NOT teach her to open the door. KELLY!" Dad was laughing hysterically! The look on Mom's face was PRICELESS!

Sheepishly, but with a big ole grin on my face, I chimed right in saying, "I sure did!" I complimented my cat as she came strutting up to us, "Way to go, Goofy!" I leaned down, scooping her up in my arms as Mom sat there shaking her head. And that, my friends, is how Goofy became an official indoor cat! She could let herself in whenever she wanted. And from then on, she did just that!

Throughout our time together, just like I did with Mr. Rabbi, I changed Goofys' diet to an all organic, dairy and grain-free cat food. She eats virtually what I eat, although a bit different in form and packaging, hers being dried.

Up until just this last year, 2018, Goofy was free to go outside alone. Every morning she'd be let out. Mom and I used to joke, "Goofy always knows when it's time for breakfast," as she'd come around the house from the deck after her morning adventure, right as Mom and I would sit down to eat. It didn't matter what time breakfast was, she just seemed to know it was breakfast time! She was ALWAYS right on time. I'd open the patio door and she'd walk up to my chair, then jump up sitting in her designated portion of it. I'd shut the door, turn around and join her, both of us sitting comfortably. To this day Goofy sits patiently, waiting for breakfast to begin while we do morning grace, hoping she'll get some yummy table food. She always gets a little something. She has also learned more about using her manners at the table!

Goofy is truly a pet with great character. She would make one spunky, children's storybook character! "I think it would have to be a series, because we've got so many fun stories to tell!" said Mom. Goofy has got spunk, zest, attitude, and TONS of love. To me, she's not just a cat, she's become like a little sister to me, and a friend. Our bond has grown deeper and deeper through our now 13 years together. When I was sick, she knew something wasn't right with me. She was my daily alarm clock, but some days she let me sleep in a little later… and how she knew the days that I needed that extra sleep I'll never know.

It's been said that "pets know things." I truly believe that. All of my pets have been that way. Goofy is no exception, but we've got a connection that's deeper than I've ever had with any of my other pets.

Now-a-days, our outdoor adventures look different than they did years ago, although we still go on endless amounts of adventures together, and we share meals together. She's still my daily morning alarm clock, too. However, she no longer has to open doors to get into the house. Truthfully, we had to replace the door handle, a lever, to a knob because she perfected the art of opening the garage door and wouldn't shut it, which became problematic. When she goes outside, now, she has to have someone with her at all times. So, like I said, we continue to have our adventures, having one every morning before I leave for work or get started at home with a day's doings. And then again, when I return home in the evening on workdays, she is waiting at the door for me. With my work schedule, I don't always get home at the same time every night, but she's ALWAYS either looking out the window for me, or waiting at the door to greet me and hoping for one last adventure before bed. Upon seeing me she says, "eh, eh, eh", because she still doesn't "meow", and I "eh" back… and our conversation goes on and on as we walk into the kitchen together or head outside for one last adventure. I then get her food ready and she eats. Immediately upon finishing supper, she walks into the bathroom, jumps on the vanity for a drink of fresh water from the faucet that I turn on for her, and from there on out we spend the rest of the night close by each other's side. It drives my family nuts, sometimes, because they are virtually "unnoticed" by Goofy once I arrive home.

I've learned a great deal about the dynamics of relationships with our friendship and sisterhood. Some examples are the "give and take" balance in relationships. The importance of sticking to your "yes" and "no's". Listening and not reacting when irritated or frustrated--she can be really persistent at times. Speaking respectfully when I'm feeling impatience. Learning to be more patient and loving, especially when I just don't feel like it. To spend time together, but also have needed healthy time apart--you're welcome family... you can have some quality time spent with her too. Absence makes the heart grow fonder, and I've found that to be true.

As I stand here writing today, Goofy is laying here right next to my computer. And why wouldn't she be? She's been a part of all my healing journey. I'm so blessed to have a furry little friend that makes my world a better place to be in. She's brought out youthfulness, silliness, laughter, and joy that for a great many of years I didn't have a whole lot of.

Today, I'm so thankful to be able to live, laugh, and love. I can truly contribute a good portion of this to Goofy, who has helped me to be more down-to-earth, to be kind, and to feel free. She's a pure blessing, who's lived life through the thick and thin with me. Goofy is my furry friend that has never left my side through it all. That is an expression of LOVE and FAITHFULNESS.

27

Living Loved

Kelly

The same day I'd first met with my FMD (functional medical doctor), mid-November of 2014, I started taking the new supplements he'd sent me home with. Just like times prior with starting new supplements, my symptoms got worse, making me feel miserable. I had headaches 24/7. I was bloated, and gassy. My left-side pain went from just under my ribs down to just below my belly button. My entire abdomen hurt, with the most pain starting right under my ribs on both sides, but the left side was always worse. I'd use my "Thera Cane" (a self-massaging tool) to dig deep into my abdomen and back, trying to reach the painful spot. I never really found total relief that way, although loosening the muscles helped.

Sleep was elusive during this long season too. It took me at least an hour to fall asleep because of the constant presence of pain. Finding a comfortable position lying down, or otherwise, was impossible. I couldn't sleep on my right side at all. I slept on my left side in the fetal position. I'd finally sleep for a few hours, but since my body was so aware of the consistent pain, I'd wake up a lot during the night, and in the wee hours of the morning to the red-hot searing pain IN my abdomen, which would jab straight thru my abdomen into my back. Trying to fall back asleep while battling the pain was exhausting. And when I'd get out of bed in the morning, I never felt truly rested. Often times, I'd feel worse when I got up in the morning than I did when I'd went to bed the night before. It was draining, both physically and mentally.

Other areas of concern were that I had diarrhea, and had undigested chunks of food coming out in my stool. I was malnourished even though I was eating nourishing food. I was pale. I had no stored energy. I was constantly cold. I had hot and cold sweats both day and night. I battled nausea numerous times each day. And then a new symptom started. Burping. I started experiencing acid reflux, which I'd never had before. Eating and drinking anything made my symptoms worse shortly after ingesting. And the new supplements? They just enhanced my symptoms. I had dark circles under my eyes. Also, my eyes each had a yellow spot in the area between my pupils towards the top of my nose. The whites had long-since been white, but rather were an ominous, cloudy, yellowish-gray color with tiny veins of red threading throughout.

I truly felt like I was existing, not really living my life. The pain from my left side was so severe at times that I was left totally immobile. I was ready to be with my heavenly Father IF it was my time. I, myself, had come to terms with that, mentally.

Sometimes Mom would come into my room during the middle of the night to make sure I was okay, her knowing of my symptoms and day to day emotions. There were times that she had checked to make sure that I was breathing during the night while I tried to sleep. My breathing was so shallow that she would put her hand on my back to feel for breaths being taken. Or, she would wake with a strong urge to pray for me and then come and check on me, praying over me as well.

During the night I would sometimes wake myself up by my own cries from pain. My brother, Troy, who had a bedroom next to my own, would awaken to those cries sometimes. My faithful two cats, Goofy and Bun-Bun, never left my side at night in my room (at least that I know of). They would lift their heads up when they heard whimpering, watching me closely. Those two were the best company.

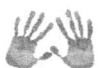

I've shared how Goofy came to our family already, in "Adventures with Goofy". However, my other cat, Bun-Bun, came into our family before Goofy. He first came into our lives as a stray kitten, too, like Goofy did. He was only about six months old, hanging around a restraint/lodge next door at the cabin, and curiously wandered into our yard when we were at our cabin on the weekends.

One particular weekend, in December of 2002, it was unanimously decided that the scrawny, furry, black cat should come inside for a meal. Bun-Bun not only got good food into his tummy, but he also received a bath! He loved the bath! No clawing or fighting us, much to our dismay. Our dog Sam, a Samoyed breed, whom was sitting in front of the fireplace that night while we all slept, welcomed Bun-Bun into the family by allowing him to come and lie with her on her pillow (or so we like to think that's how it happened)! Imagine, 5-6 pounds of long black fur curled up in a ball next to 95-pounds of fluffy white fur! Anyhow, that's how my parents found the pair the next morning.

Mom had said, "They are ALMOST total opposites; large, white dog VS. small, black cat. Looking at them you could see there were no boundaries or color or size!" Both of their long furry coats and LOVING hearts were their common denominators. Sam had a big, BIG heart! Needless to say, Bun-Bun was officially a part of our family that weekend, being loved by ALL.

Sam, our dog, passed away a good while after Bun-Bun, and later Goofy, joined our family. During their time together, Sam and Bun-Bun were the best of friends. Bun-Bun became mostly my pal, too. He and I formed a special bond. I was ten years old when he came to us, so we really grew up together.

When I was sick, Bun-Bun in his later years then, knew something was wrong with his girl. Often times, when he was nowhere to be found, and I would had loved to have found, he'd come out from who-knows-where and find me. His timing was always impeccable. I recall those times when I'd be lying on the floor curled up in the fetal position, in pain, and there he'd come walking up to me, his deep purr making his presence known. He'd gently nudge me with his head. I couldn't begin to count the times he'd let me cry softly into his fluffy fur, or he'd let me stroke his fur to calm myself. He was a pure bundle of soft, fluffy fur, with a big, big heart full of love!

Bun-Bun always slept on my bed close to my feet. This was something we'd started doing sometime shortly after he joined the family. He was my protector, my guardian during the night. Those later days, with me being so sick, he'd continue to curl up in a ball tight against my feet keeping them warm. How did he know my feet needed warming because they were so cold? His intuitiveness didn't stop there.

As I laid in bed sick, he'd walk next to me smelling me. There were times he even put his furry front paws on my chest and would lean into me, as if to really make sure I was breathing. He'd wake me up when he'd do that. All the while he'd softly purr, then he'd see my eyes open and I'd lift my hand to pet him, the decimals of his purrs rising to those occasion! There were rare moments that I would be semi-sleeping on my back, and Bun-Bun would gently walk onto my abdomen and sit. He'd wake me up doing this. And YES, his little weight hurt too, but I allowed it because of what he did, shocking me the first time he did so, leaving me speechless. He'd start gently pushing his fuzzy front paws into my left side, just underneath my ribs where it hurt. One paw digging, then the other. I'd say, "It's like he's trying to knead dough!" He'd do this for 1-3 minutes, and every time, right when I was just about ready for him to stop, he'd stop without me having to tell him. Then he'd look at me and gently walk off of my abdomen. Animals KNOW when their humans are hurting. And how did he know EXACTLY where to "knead" my dough? *Hmmm...*

When I first got sick, Bun-Bun was around eight years old. For the next seven years, he was by my side, never leaving me during the night, always watching me closely during the day, too, when I was home.

Fast forward. During the very end of Bun-Bun's life, around September of 2016, I noticed he wasn't eating much. As the days and weeks went on, his health continued to diminish fast while my health had been reversing for a year. Interestingly, when I had been having good results with a new and even more different doctor, Bun-Bun had quit seeking us out, never purring and seemingly not wanting to be around us very much--I'm sure because he didn't feel well. I sought him out to tell him the good news about my health, being WELL and getting healthier. I found Bun-Bun downstairs, curled up in a ball in front of the fireplace. He saw me, looked me deep in the eyes, then getting up ever so slowly he walked right over to me. I waited for him so as not to spook him. He made his way over to me and I pet him. I then spoke softly and gently, telling him my good news. He started purring while turning to look at me. I swear he knew what I was saying. The look he gave me made me think he really understood what I'd told him. He got the news HE was waiting to hear!

The next day his breathing was very bad. We could tell that it wouldn't be long before we'd have to put him down. The following day, we shared one last special moment and I told him, "I'm really going to miss you Bun-Bun. Thank you for hanging on until you could hear the words both of us were waiting for with my health. I can never thank you enough for your love and support throughout this journey. You helped make EVERY DAY possible. Thank you. We both know it's time to say goodbye. See you later Bun-Bun. You can go now, buddy."

That day was in October of 2016, just days after I got my clean bill of health, that Bun-Bun passed away. I truly believe he held on to the very end because he wanted to know I was really going to be alright. His passing was bittersweet.

28

A Close Eye

Kelly

Another month went by and none of my symptoms were improving. In fact, they'd gotten worse in intensity, so I decided to quit taking most of the supplements I'd started weeks prior. I'd try some, again, after some time passed.

During the course of this time of my illness, I was still working full time. I was self-employed as a massage therapist with now a full clientele. I worked four days per week, filling nearly 40-hours with office work, creating advertising info, and therapy sessions. Massage therapy sessions could be half an hour up to two hours in length. Since I was having diarrhea 5-15 times per day, the two-hour massages were tricky. Thankfully, I ALWAYS made it through the session, thanks be to Papa God.

Mom was the receptionist at my business during this time, also. She was, and STILL is, a HUGE help to me. She'd warmed up meals in the countertop toaster-oven for us, made sure I was eating food and drinking enough water, kept laundry going, helped with various business aspects, checked clients in and out, and all those numerous receptionist duties like answering the phone, answering questions, and scheduling clients.

I didn't feel I had the full needed amount of energy to do my job, but I didn't dwell on that. I focused on taking one client at a time. Most days I didn't know if I would make it through the morning, let alone the end of the work day. I was pretty much exhausted before I started working each day, so focusing on each client was key. Knowing that I was helping someone else get relief from their pain, honestly, kept me going. The work wasn't about the money. I loved my job of helping people become free of bodily pain.

To this day, I continue to love the work I do. Helping people in physical pain that come to my office is really rewarding. I get to administer healing with my clients as they work through their pain, aiding in their pain-relief plans. Seeing the frowns when arriving, turn to smiles when leaving, is so rewarding and awesome to witness. People smile more freely, without hesitation, when they feel good.

At the end of my work days, I'd drive 20 minutes home. I'd be utterly exhausted after work while I was ill. Once home, pets being cared for and me being showered, I'd curl up in bed in the fetal position, laying on my left side often unable to sleep. Mom would always say to me, while hugging me goodnight, "I love you, Kelly. Hang in here. You're doing awesome!"

I continued to struggle in daily life as another month slowly passed before my third appointment with the functional medical doctor.

Finally, the FMD called for our phone consult, digging in right away asking me, "How are you feeling Kelly? Have your symptoms gotten any worse or better? Give me an update."

I told him, "I quit taking a couple of the supplements because they're not working. The supplements make all of my symptoms worse. I've stopped and started taking them a couple times, but each time I felt worse when taking them." I felt like I was reliving the last consult that I'd had with him, telling him the same things.

"Which supplements are doing that?" He probed. I told him which ones, and he went on. "I want you to start taking those supplements again, but in smaller dosages. Try taking a quarter of the full dose for a few days. Also, introduce one supplement at a time to make sure they're each doing their job."

I was very skeptical. However, I agreed. He wanted to schedule another phone consult in a month, after the holidays were over. I agreed, hesitantly, and he scheduled the appointment. Then the phone consultation ended.

Mid December 2014. The holiday seasons were always busy at work. Mom was busy scheduling clients, selling gift certificates, and doing her normal receptionist duties, and warming up a meal or preparing a snack for me too. Even though often times I didn't want to eat, she would smile and hand me a small portion to eat. I would smile back, thanking her. Mom kept a CLOSE eye on me while I worked throughout the busy days. Truth be told, she was there not only to help me in my business, but because I really did need someone keeping an eye on me. She had my back!

Clients would come in and then go after their sessions. With each client, I was that much closer to the end of my work day. I know it might sound crazy, but despite my being sick, I loved my job. I loved hearing my clients talk about their families, children, grandchildren, childhood memories, personal history and news in their lives. My clients didn't know I was sick, or if they did, they weren't saying anything... nor was I. I didn't want them to know I was sick and struggling health-wise while I worked, but I'll get into that later.

My diet was, and is, all organic, using whole foods as medicine. A typical day for me included eating and drinking a variety of foods: bone broth, chicken veggie soup, steamed dark leafy greens--either kale, collards, spinach, chard, or mustard greens, steamed vegetables--carrots, cauliflower, broccoli, snow peas, brussel sprouts or green beans, boiled chicken or turkey, avocado, and maybe some dried fruit--raisins, blueberries, cranberries, and mulberries. All these foods were providing me with vital nutrients I needed, but again I was absorbing very little of those. But what little I was absorbing was helping me function.

All day, every day, I was in pain. I was ready to go home to be with my Papa God, IF it was my time. Thanks to the food, Mom, my pets, and my family's continued love and support, the bone broth, and the few supplements I was taking, and by the pure grace of God, I was alive.

I was still very depressed at this time. I was frustrated that I wasn't feeling better as fast as **I thought** I should be. And, I was struggling to make it through each day, no matter what the day consisted of. At this point I was pretty low in spirit, and was not enjoyable to be around. This digestive illness was hard on me, and hard on my family members. The pain I was enduring almost felt as if it was taking the life out of me. I had yet to come to peace in FULLNESS with accepting that this was happening for a reason. Yes. I knew it was happening for a reason, but I didn't believe it in **fullness.** I was still putting MY expectations of what **I wanted** for results in my own time frame, not my Papa God's. I had a LOT to learn.

God was using this illness to grow and change me for the better, IF I was willing to listen, abide, and learn from it. Your life, your choice. What choices would I make? I had a lot to learn, and it was going to get worse before it was going to get better, if that even seems possible.

29

Please Do Tell

Kelly

JE November 28th, 2014

My gut is not good at all. The left-side pain is terrible, and ALL the symptoms that come with it. My eyes are yellow and have distinct raised yellow spots, one in each of them. My health is steadily declining. Help me, Lord, please! Answers soon? Please Papa, show me in some way, shape, or form. I just had one of those moments where you just cry, straight out, "Why?" A dear friend said this to me recently, "Kelly, I would give you one of my organs, blood, or anything that would be helpful for you."

Mom and I had a conversation earlier, back in the late fall of 2014 between the span of working with Dr. Ann and before working with the FMD, discussing the subject of people in my life knowing about my health situation. "Kelly, our friends and family know that you have food allergies and intolerances. Some of them know more of what you've been experiencing, the pain, and the things that you and I have shared with them."

"Yes," I'd questioned?

"Well, I want to ask you if you want people to REALLY know what is going on with you? The reason I ask is because some people have been asking me how you are. They are concerned about you. I want to respect your privacy. Do YOU want to tell people when they ask you about the all-natural way of healing you've chose? I'm asking because individuals sometimes voluntarily share their opinions about what THEY think you should do, and I know it can be hard to hear at times, because it's hard for me to hear and not say anything. You and I both know you don't have extra energy, and I'm

109

wondering if you want to exert any energy into having to deal with people and their opinions? That "battle-of-the-mind effect" from too many choices to think about, you know…it's real, the battle.

Oh man, she has a GREAT point. I really haven't told but a couple people how sick I really am. None of my clients know. My clients, family, and friends know I have food allergies and intolerances like Mom said. And some family and friends know that I don't feel well. Do I really want to open up by telling people my health situation and be bombarded with opinions, ideas of "you should try this" or "you should do that"? My mind was already catching-on to what Mom was getting at. I was REALLY glad she brought this to my attention.

"Mom, you're right in asking. I hear where you are coming from and appreciate your concern. I think you have a very important point that needs an answer--one that is right not only for me, but for you too. You shouldn't have to field people's questions, their thoughts, or their opinions. Obviously like you said, I really can't and don't want to add onto my plate right now, dealing with people's questions or opinions. I don't have the energy and time, nor do I want to convince people of my choices. It's MY choice to do what I'm doing. I think for both of our sakes we shouldn't tell people all of what I'm battling." I'd stated.

Mom nodded her head in agreement. "Kelly, you really don't have extra energy to exert in explaining your health choices to people. It's probably in your best interest. I think this is a wise decision. Besides that, having depression on top of this, it could really bring you down with worrying if you're making right choices for YOU, when people tell you it's wrong, or even dangerous what you are choosing." I thought for a while, then she added, "Kelly, there are some people that I think SHOULD know about your critical state of health. You know, those inner-circle people that care about you deeply." I nodded for Mom to go on. "Grandma should know more. She loves you and is always praying for you. Your school friend, Hallie (the massage therapist). Our friend (a woman that's like a grandma to me), and your auntie Lori, too."

I looked at her while thinking about the people she'd listed. *She's right. These are the people that care deeply and won't put their judgement on me for the choices I'm making.* "You're right. These people should know."

110

I'm the type of person that tells the truth, to the point of sometimes being blunt. Not telling people what was going on with my health wasn't necessarily easy when questions did arise. I learned to kind of dance around questions, to avoid outright lying or being rude, by being vague. To my extended family, friends, clients, that didn't know I was this ill, I'm sorry if this hurt you, that I wouldn't and didn't tell you the truth about my state of health. I, in NO way, shape, or form am trying to justify my choices when I say, "I was honestly looking out for the best interest of myself. I didn't want to add onto the mountain that I was already climbing daily."

Mom and I knew how we, ourselves, want to jump in and help when a loved one is ill. "Helping" people seems to have good motives behind the intentions, but I, we, truly felt we couldn't deal with any extra well-meaning we knew, especially since I was not taking a Western medical route. It was my choice, and I can honestly say that this choice of going "natural" was the **best** decision for myself. Also, we didn't AVOID talking about my health with people that asked. We just didn't explain in FULLNESS the depth of what was really going on in my health. My clients didn't know because I did not want them to feel any guilt about me working on them when I was not feeling well. I truly wanted to help them in their journey to wellness, if this was the one way which I could help people. And, they also gave me an extra motive to get out of bed each morning!

To some people, I looked the "state of health". You know, the worldly view of "skinny--in shape and looking good". Some people told me this even when I was very sick, because to them I did look fine. Other people, that spent more time with me, that saw me more often, picked up on "something wasn't quite right" with me, and they'd ask. And then there were those people I saw real often that still had NO idea that I was even sick, which goes back to, I looked good and healthy--in their eyes.

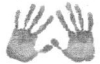

I've learned that everyone has their own idea of wellness, health, being healthy and being well. But, that's a subject for another time. The point is, I wasn't sharing a lot about my health during this time, but there would be a time in the future to share. And that future time, well, is now! I want you to hear my story, all of it, IF you want too. No obligation. To you, the one reading here right now, "I truly hope and pray that my story touches your life in some way. Maybe you can relate. Maybe a loved one is going through something similar. Or maybe you're just curious as to what REALLY happened while I was sick. I don't know your motive or desire for wanting to read my story. But there are a couple things that I hope and pray from the bottom of my heart... that you would learn and take away things from my story, knowing that there are other options of healing, more than even what I've written about here. Also, that through my being completely transparent and honest, that you would know me for the REAL person that I am. In addition, that you would see the hand of God at work in the life of someone that absolutely does NOT deserve God's love, but was blessed ten-fold from my relationship with Him.

I'd like to leave off with asking that you'd share this book with a loved one, with family, friends, and people in your life that this may benefit, would find interesting, may learn from, are interested in alternative holistic health, that may be blessed by hearing my story. I'm don't want to pressure you into something you'd rather not do. Please do tell others of this book if you feel lead. Thank you, and God bless.

30

Blessings

Amy

There are simply no human words to explain WHY God allows suffering in this life, but I have some ideas that were impressed upon me years ago that I can see as possibilities as to WHY God allows suffering. What we see with human eyes is surly a tiny speck compared to what He sees in even one of our circumstances, be it good, bad, or otherwise. I trust that God knows best when He allows suffering, and when He gives and takes away.

Concerning Kelly's state of health, especially during the fall of 2014 into the summer of 2015, we acted upon our faith during the entire process from illness (2010) to clean bill of health (2017). What did act upon our faith look like? Lots of prayers, and unwavering trust—faith. Sometimes, it was a cry for "help". Other times, praises in the storms, or tears knowing He was listening to our hearts breaking and us knowing He was in complete control. Some days we would ask for Him to reveal Himself in some way that we would know His hand was working in the details. But most often, we were asking for His healing touch to deliver Kelly out of this painful health situation, and for His will to be done, meaning: not praying for my will, Kelly's, Darren's, or Troy's will, nor any human being's will for Kelly, just His will, whatever that might be in this awful chronic health situation. There was way too much suffering on Kelly's part, daily.

Healing comes in multiple forms, through medicine being one. Kelly was using "food as medicine" and nutritional supplements from her health practitioners as optimal nutritional aids. Both food and supplements were medicinal. She was adamant about not taking prescription medications, so our standard American medical doctoring system for healing was out of the picture and already in some other country at this point.

Doctoring is another avenue of healing. Doctor means "teacher". Many people think Dr. means ''healer'', but that is just not so, although God does heal THROUGH people's knowledge and guidance. We were learning from various doctors up to this point, through both alternative doctors on health summits online, and those that she was working with. Putting into action what we were learning was not getting to the deeper issue going on concerning the pain she experienced daily, but we believed that what she was doing thus far WAS helping heal her intestinal permeability--leaky gut.

Healing also comes through death. When a loved one is suffering on a daily basis, it's trying to know how to help them. To just be with Kelly and be silent was welcomed, I think. Hearing Kelly's thoughts in her journal entries as I've combed through these chapters here, she writes about being at peace--going home to Papa God, was not shocking to me. She and I are very open in our communication, being bluntly honest in our conversations and discussions on topics. We'd had that discussion on death. I knew where she was at, or should I say I trusted her where she was at. I knew she was depressed. I TRUSTED her to be honest with me, which she has been since her change of heart not so very long ago. One thing about Kelly, and I guess about myself too, is she despises being lied to. Once caught in a lie, her respect for a person plumets— like a fishing line going down with sinker on end leading. Honesty is always the best policy with us. Even if we don't agree, being honest is vital in having integrity. Let's just say, if a person is brave enough to be honest in telling the truth, even if we don't agree what they are saying, they get our respect for BEING BRAVE and HONEST!

During this particular time of doctoring, early 2014 into 2015, I too had come to terms with the real possibility that Papa God, as Kelly calls Him, may take my baby from this life. God gives. God takes away. I know and believe this from reading the Christian Bible and because of how He speaks to me in daily life. Dying doesn't scare me. I have a lot of peace about death, trusting and believing it's the end of life here as we know it, but a beginning to eternity with our Savior… and a large clan of family. I knew that if Kelly were to pass on, that I would be with her in eternity. That gives me great comfort and peace of mind. Thankfully, my husband and I haven't experienced the death of a child, putting our faith to an immeasurably difficult test as other people we know who have lost a child. I believe "loss" is a grief that never goes away, but changes as one goes through the rest of their life. The mourning may pass, but the heart that has lost a great loved one will forever hold the grief of missing their loved one when they think of them. That grief can change over time, allowing the heart to expand on memories without the mourning, but still feeling loss with perhaps a smidgen of gratitude for having had the person in their life for such a time as they had them. Maybe I think too much, but those as some of my beliefs on death and loss.

I fully believed we were doing the best we could in finding help and searching for help and answers with Kelly. We were seeking God's direction for who to reach out to for alternative helps. I was present at most all of her appointments--discussions with doctors. I talked with her daily about her symptoms or whatever she wanted to talk about, supporting her however I could. My role was challenging during jacked-up pain episodes while she was detoxing, she having die-off effects--toxins needing to be eliminated from her body. I couldn't do a single physical "help" at these times. But I could pray. And I did.

Since I was the closest person in Kelly's life, I knew that my daughter, being strong-willed and determined to follow through with her choices, was not going to give up the fight for her life. Anyone could've asked me, "Why didn't you just take her to the ER?' Or, "Why don't you make an appointment with a medical doctor?" And, "You knew she was depressed. She could've taken her own life! Had you thought of that?" Believe me, I did want to take her somewhere, especially at crisis times. And, yes, I had thought of all the possibilities of what could had happened. During those times my heart became anxious FOR her. I'd panic in my mind with thoughts of *will she make it through this one*, *what if*, and *what will people think if ...*? But then, I'd be reminded of a scriptural promise and simply gain back peace of mind, and ask God to do His will... and making it known to us would be much appreciated.

Was Kelly reckless in her choice to not go to a medical doctor? It all depends on what a person believes is right. I know what it is like to be depressed. I know what it's like to be depressed and NOT go to a medical doctor for help. I also know that when a person is depressed that they have to want to have change in their life in order for change to happen, and then act on making any change happen. I know that for me, I had to make that same choice to want to find answers to change my mental and physical health back in 2002 through to this day. That being said, I understood where she was at and I knew the possibility of deliverance. I was giving Kelly that same respect to want change and make decisions for herself. When she asked for any kind of help from us, we were there for her, to listen, give advice, to listen more, and give her room to grow in her choices.

As a parent of an adult child living in our home making her own choices, we were leaving the results of those healthcare choices in God's hands, doing all we could to make Kelly's life as good as it could be, but not imposing our will on her. Reckless? Or trusting? Honestly, as hard as it was to stand by and respect her choices, we trusted that God would act for healing on Kelly's behalf, whatever that looked like day to day, stringing out into years.

Many nights I awoke with a strong urge to pray for Kelly during the 2014-2015 season of induced detoxing. I'd stayed lying in bed, making my requests known to God. Sometimes I'd have a sense that Kelly was not going to make it through the night. I'd stay awake for hours, sometimes going to her room to make sure she was still with us. Her breathing was so shallow I'd bend right over her, awkwardly with my head next to hers, feeling her breath on my ear. I recall three specific nights waking up IN prayer, having an undoubtable urgency in my heart to lay hands on her and pray. So, I would. Going downstairs to her room, listening for her shallow breaths, I'd put my hands on her back while kneeling next to her, praying, each time ending in "…but Thy will be done, not mine". And I meant it. His will, not mine. It was His choice to heal her how He saw fit. I'd laid her at the foot of the cross.

"Be anxious for nothing, but in everything by prayer and supplication,
with thanksgiving let your requests be make known to God; and the
peace of God, which surpasses all understanding will
guard your hearts and minds through Christ Jesus."
-Philippians 4:6-8

There will be those who read this who may say I'm "crazy, negligent, gullible or fool-hearted". I'm pretty okay with that at this point in my life. If anyone said that to my face, it wouldn't be the first or the last time I heard it. Faith is trusting the outcomes to God, having done your part in faith to the best of your ability, then leaving the results to Him. I was at peace with what He would do in Kelly's health situation. That doesn't mean it was an easy thing to do, or that I never panicked. There were battles in my mind, as you can imagine. Words will just not convey my heart, in this, to you. Maybe the song **"Blessings"** will. May I suggest the reader do an internet search and listen to the song, **"Blessings"**, by **Laura Story**[4]. The song is truly a blessing.

Sometime before the worst-of-worst times in Kelly's health battle, she made the decision during a discussion I had with her privately, to not openly discuss her health with people outside of her inner circle, her tribe. I had my tribe of women, too, that often over-lapped as Kelly's tribe, that were, are, supportive. Those women listened if I called, prayed for our family, and loved on us whether they were geographically close or afar. I would give them random updates in group emails on Kelly's health so as not to have to explain to each one individually. I'm thankful for their supportive friendship in our lives. Kelly and I agreed that there were those people who we wanted them to know what was happening, those we knew would be praying for her. Other people, who didn't actually need to know, were spared any dependence we may had put on them in their learning of her health battle.

Our major concern was that Kelly needed to focus her energy on getting well, not worrying about what others thought of her choices, and her feeling she had to defend her choice. It seemed to us, too, that the more people who'd know that she was sick could possibly be worse for her in the case of people sharing their "helpful tips" to "try working with so and so", or outright tell her, "You need to see a qualified medical doctor", which could cause her to second guess her choice of alternative doctors and healing modalities, all of which are "qualified". The more voices speaking into her life could take her attention away, instead of focusing on her present daily health needs and trusting the guidance she was seeking and following. Bottom line, she needed her energy focused, not divided.

[4] Christian Music singer and songwriter Laura Story, from her 2011 album "Blessings" https://www.youtube.com/watch?v= XQan9L3yXjc

With all the bodily energy one uses in a given day, Kelly amazingly put forth the energy of a person being well in health most days. How could that be? I think a part of it was that she was not putting medications into her body to treat symptoms. Also, she was eating clean, untainted food, had fresh air and exercise daily, and so many other positive daily doings to uplift her instead of drain her. She was drinking lots of water and bone broth. Also, the supplements from her alternative health-care providers were fully natural (with no additives that would set-off her gluten sensitivity or some other negative response), boosting her body with nutrients and minerals that she'd been deficient of from probably the beginning of her lifetime in the womb as a fetus--that's a subject for an entirely different day.

Since Kelly was putting good things into her body, and because she wanted to work and be of use, I believe those were big reasons as to why she was able to keep physically working during her illness. And thank God for that being possible, because she'd had probably gone into a deeper depression without a work to do. Putting her focus on someone else, helping them, was a blessing.

We are thankful for every blessing, and friends' and families' love.

31

A Hot Mess

Kelly

JE December 8th, 2014

My gut is bad today, again. It's continuously getting worse. It's getting harder and harder to hold my bowel movements in. This is getting very... I'm at a loss for words, I don't know what to say. Lord, please, I need some direction, insight, or even answers. Help me Papa God, please? I woke up this morning with stabbing left-side pain. I had hot and cold sweats, along with the need to vomit. It lasted a good half an hour and has gone into today. I'm not feeling good. In all reality, it sucks. Each day I go to bed and wake up utterly exhausted. I still "seize the day by the reigns" and get through it. I wake up every night feeling sick. The pain and symptoms can last minutes to hours. There is no rhyme or reason to how long it will last. I have constant burning and stabbing pain in my left side. I battle bloating, nausea, headaches, total body aches, low back pain and much more daily. I continue to do all my "helps" in different ways of selfcare. Papa, I need Your help.

It was the week of Christmas, 2014. Work was very busy and I was putting in longer hours, being the holiday season. Tired, worn out, and not getting enough sleep meant I was past exhausted by the time we locked our doors on Christmas Eve. My health had been slowly and steadily declining.

Christmas day we spent with relatives, which meant we drove three or more hours to get to any holiday gathering. I spent the majority of that day laying on the floor due to abdominal pain. Grandma was concerned about me. She, and my aunt Lori, whose house we were at, knew more about my health than the other relatives. I felt Grandma's love and concern. It was a long day traveling there and back home.

New Year's Eve 2015 was coming up. I worked late again that week, into the night on New Year's Eve. After work, I finished up everything I had to do despite just wanting to go home and sleep. I arrived home and took a hot shower, letting the steaming water penetrate deep into my back and abdomen. Soon I was in bed. My abdominal pain was intense. I felt like puking. This was common, battling nausea numerous times daily. Unsuccessfully, I rolled around attempting to find a comfortable position for pain relief.

Eventually, I drifted into sleep only to be awakened with electrifying abdominal pain. Hot and cold sweats racked my body. I couldn't breathe deep as the abdominal pain ripped inside me in every direction. I muffled a cry into my comforter. My abdomen was bloated. I couldn't touch it, due to it hurting so severely. The slightest touch brought searing pain. My head was spinning from dizziness. I felt like I was going to faint even though I was lying down in bed. I was laying on my back as the pain ripped through my abdomen. My back hurt so bad that it pained me to lay on it. I slowly attempted to roll onto my left side. Like a knife, pain speared through my abdomen into my back. I cried out at the intensity of the pain. I knew I couldn't finish rolling onto my left side. I needed to lay on my back again. My stomach felt like it was in my throat. My head was pounding. It hurt to open my eyes. I thought my head might explode. *That actually might be okay,* I thought. I knew I couldn't move because of all this pain, so I was going to have to let it take its course. I tried to breathe, making myself as comfortable as I could. No position brought any relief. I prayed, crying ever so softly because, like always, it hurt my abdomen to cry. I threw back the covers as the hot sweats came again. Not long after that I was cold again, so I wrapped the covers around me.

After some time passed, I got an acidic taste in my mouth, and again I felt like I was going to puke. I knew I had to get out of bed and into the bathroom. I slowly got my legs to the side of the bed. I groaned in pain. Both of my cats raised their heads, four eyes glowing in the dark watching me. "Hey you two. I think I'm going to puke."

120

"God help me!" I muttered as pain ripped through my abdomen while trying to sit up. There was a garbage can near the end of my bed. Reaching for it, I was light headed, dizzy, and almost fell to the floor. I caught myself as one of the cats moved to get out of the way. I had the can but couldn't move. I hurt and was battling another hot sweat. I then laid with half my body in bed and half falling off the side of the bed, head in the garbage can. I felt even more nauseous, then the cold sweats hit again. The pain in my abdomen quit, momentarily. I took as deep of a breath as I could and exhaled. I knew this was my chance to get to the bathroom.

I stood up holding onto the closet door, getting my balance. My abdominal and back pain were flaming hot as it seared like electricity through me. The intensity of it doubled me over. I grimaced, unable to speak. Suddenly I felt the urge to have a BM (bowel movement). One hand on the wall for balance and the other attempting to cradle my abdomen, I limped the short distance through the hallway to the bathroom. I was sweating profusely. At rest on the toilet, my urge to have a BM still present, I couldn't push or strain because the abdominal pain prevented it. Frustrated and hurting, I patiently waited. I was still dripping with sweat and my head was pounding. Abdominal pain electrocuted through me again, leaving my head spinning. I grabbed the walls on both sides of me to help me stay balanced, even though I was sitting on the toilet. The pain again decreased momentarily, and the urge to have a BM lessened. It hurt to sit, and since I didn't have the urge to go anymore, I NEEDED to move. Sitting hurt so badly at this point in time I avoided it at ALL costs. I decided to try to cool down by laying on the cold granite bathroom floor. Once down, I realized I was absolutely exhausted and just wanted to lay there and sleep.

I started to drool as I lay there. "I'm a hot mess" I muttered to myself. Another searing pain ripped through my abdomen into my back. The intensity of it left me in the fetal position. It felt like my stomach was in my throat. Slowly, I attempted to push, then pull myself up using the walls and the shower door to grasp. Sitting up, I leaned over the toilet and within a few seconds I was puking my guts out. This was not a case of having a flu bug. The same scenario had happened a couple other times during the last few months, although not to that severity.

The waves of puking ended. The electrifying abdominal pain vanished. My stomach was empty and feeling raw. I cleaned the toilet thoroughly, and then washed my face and hands, and brushed my teeth. It felt like a train had run me over a few times, then backed up again over me. Walking out of the bathroom I tenderly held my abdomen, walked into my bedroom and turned on my bedside lamp. I slowly changed clothes and then crawled into bed while both of my cats looked at me, curiously. One of them started purring and nudged me ever so gently. "It's okay you two, I feel better. Let's go back to sleep." I shut off the lamp and laid on my left side and soon fell asleep. When I awoke hours later, I felt like I'd just slept for the first time in months! My body still hurt but the pain was back to a constant dull and achy state, although at any given time, day or night, the pain could take a turn for the worse.

A few things to note:
1) Yes, it probably sounded like I needed to go to the emergency room (ER). BUT I was certain that I would be observed for days and they'd want to do testing, which was just not what I wanted. Nor did I want to be put on any kind of medication. I'd be utilizing their restroom, only to be going home with no answers, no results, and a lot of bills to pay. Going to the ER wasn't something I was willing to do. And YES, my parents asked many times if I needed to go. My answer was always the same, "NO."

2) There are a couple things in life that are really hard for me, one of which is vomiting. There's just something about it that is really difficult for me. That being said, when I puke, it is NOT easy and is always a last resort.

3) The nights weren't easy. I kept my phone in my room in the case that I needed help. Mom ALWAYS kept her cell phone's ringtone on low beside her bedside when she slept, in case I needed her. She was only a text or phone call away. "NEVER hesitate if you need me. I don't care if you wake me up, Kelly." She meant it. And I knew it, and agreed to if need be.

The next weeks went by. Taking life one day at a time, I would daily go outside for a walk and do a small workout. It didn't matter if I had energy or not, I'd do this remembering Dr. Ann's words, "It is important to get your body moving. When you exercise and move your body you are promoting circulation. It is important that you sweat, Kelly. Sweating will help get toxins out of your body and heat up your core body temperature. I don't care if you do a 15-minute workout or an hour, you just need to get your body moving." I knew that Dr. Ann was right, so with sheer determination I would work out to some degree every day. It wasn't easy, believe me, especially on really bad days. But, on a not so bad day I loved my little exercise routine! Going for walks always helped lessen my headaches. The fresh air in my lungs was always what I needed. It was enjoyable, therapeutic, and healing to me.

With the year of 2014 now over, it had ended with me becoming humbler as my health was at an all-time low. Ringing in the New Year, well, life could only get better, right?

32

Spinning Out of Control

Kelly

February 2015. While working with a client doing massage therapy, my body was literally roasting from the inside out with illness. Symptoms had me spinning out of control. My stomach was deeply upset. My left side, underneath my ribs, burned deep inside like it was on fire. I'd battled upset stomachs daily, but this day felt very different.

I knew that I was going to have explosive diarrhea. The problem was, I was only a half an hour into a one-and-a-half-hour session. Hot sweats started, then rotated with cold sweats. Within minutes I felt like I was going to vomit. Pain ripped through my abdomen into my back. My abdomen was bloated and hurt from the pressure, making the left-side and back pain more intense. I prayed silently, grimacing, while breathing through waves of the ripping pain.

My client was face-up as I worked. Eyes closed, oblivious to my immediate state of illness, this client would normally converse with me. Today, I was very thankful there was no conversation. I worked all the front and side muscles thoroughly, focusing on the client's need for healing, as waves of pain ripped through me. At times I would have to lean against the massage table to keep from doubling over in unbearable pain. I was dizzy, the room having started spinning. Spinning room had happened a number of times throughout the session. While taking a few steps for more massage oil I nearly lost my balance, grabbing the wall to keep myself from falling over. I was feeling out of control. The urge to have a bowel movement was a battle throughout the session. It was horrible. At times I crossed my legs and bent at my waist to refrain from "letting loose". The thought of filling my pants was terrifying. (I

124

apologize if this is too much information. Just being real. Writing is therapeutic too, remember.) We were halfway through the client's massage session, having turned laying on the stomach. I still needed to work the back of the legs and the back. I checked in with my client, making sure the pressure being applied to the muscles was tolerable.

As I worked, the pressure from my abdomen was pushing into my back, making it throb with excruciating pain. My low back to the middle of my left side of my back felt like it was going to burst. I continued battling the pain that seared through my body three-dimensionally. All the while, trying to stay focused on my client, a pounding headache accommodated nausea, dizziness, hot and cold sweats, along with one very bloated abdomen kept me challenged. I crossed my legs, knowing I wasn't going to be able to hold this in for another 45 minutes. Hot and colds sweats were taking a toll, sweat dripping down my back and chest. We were one hour into the massage session with a half an hour to go. *Time just couldn't go fast enough.*

My client was feeling well when I checked in at the one hour 15-minute mark, so mutually we ended the session short. The client was glad that I'd told them, "If you want to shorten the session you can". They'd felt better and were happy to had saved some money!

I quickly washed my hands and exited the room. After I shut the therapy room door, I swept toward the bathroom in the next empty therapy room, saying to Mom over my shoulder, "She had a 75-minute session instead of a 90."

Mom checked my client out. After the client left, Mom came knocking on the door asking, "Are you okay, Kelly? You were really pale when you came out from that session."

"No," I responded weakly. "I'm not okay. I feel terrible. I will be out in a while." Minutes later, I returned to the main office area where Mom was waiting with concern written all over her face.

"You came out of the therapy room as white as a ghost, Kelly. The way you moved into the bathroom I knew something wrong." Mom said, softly.

"It was terrible, Mom…" I explained, telling her what'd just happened during the seemingly long session.

125

My stomach was still upset, but not as upset as during my client's massage session. I still had a fully-scheduled day of work ahead, which was my choice. However, I had one and-a-half hours before my next client would be coming in, so I laid down on a portable massage table in my second therapy room for some needed rest. Mom had gone to switch linens on my table in the other therapy room while I rested. While resting, stomach cramps started again. I cried in pain. Mom soon came in and held my hand. She stayed at my side for a few minutes talking to me, and then walked back to the reception desk. A few minutes later, I knew I had to get into the bathroom again. I made it to the garbage can, but not quiet in time to vomit. This time it was not "normal" vomit, but black colored. It was bile. The smell was horrendous. Upon hearing what was happening, Mom came into the bathroom. I had a couple breaks between waves of vomit, so I was able to get to the toilet after the first wave finished. I continued vomiting. The smell of bile penetrated into my nostrils, igniting the need to wretch more.

After it was all done, I looked at the mess in disgust. I reached out and Mom gently told me, "I'll clean it up, Kelly. You go lay down." I stood, weakly, walking to the sink, washing my hands and face, cleaning myself up and then brushed my teeth. Afterwards, we talked briefly in the reception area. "If you want me to cancel your clients for the rest of the day, I will. It's 12:30pm now. You are booked solid the rest of the day into tonight. I think it would be wise if you rest today instead of work." Mom said kindly. She paused for a response then said, "I will call your clients and reschedule them, okay?"

"Please just call and reschedule my next client. I'll see how I feel after I lay down for a short while." Mom just looked at me, shocked. I left the room to go lay down again. I didn't like the bright light coming through the window in the room so I pulled a blanket over my head instead of getting up to close the shade. My left side, deep underneath my ribs, had a dull achy pain. It was no longer a ripping pain, so I was thankful. My whole abdomen hurt though. I was still bloated and had a pounding headache.

Fifteen minutes passed, then Mom came into the room, whispering, "How are you feeling, Kelly?" She stood next to me feeling my forehead. "Your head is warm."

"Not much better." I replied.

126

"I'm canceling the rest of today's appointments then." Mom stated. I wasn't happy about that, but knew if I didn't feel better, I wouldn't be able to make it through the rest of my work day. So, I agreed that she could call the rest of my clients. However, twenty minutes later I was feeling better. I didn't have any pain except for my "normal" dull, achy, left-side pain that went straight through into my back. My stomach was raw from vomiting, but otherwise I felt better. I knew it wasn't the flu or a gluten exposure, and that I'd not be exposing anyone to a virus.

I slid myself up on the table, put my hair back in a pony tail and got up. Walking out into the reception area, Mom looked up from the computer where she was working. "I'm all better Mom!" I spoke. That was a statement I used to say to her when I was a little girl after being sick, then feeling better, and my face would break out in an all-tooth grin.

"Oh my! You LOOK better! You're not pale, and your cheeks are rosy again. Your eyes even look better!" Mom blurted out with a big ole' smile.

"I feel much better. My stomach is a little raw, but that's it. I'm hungry but I don't dare eat anything!" Mom gave me an approving look, then we looked puzzled at one another. Since I had given her the approval to cancel my clients for the rest of the day, I now had an empty schedule.

I called my clients back. They all agreed to come to their original appointment times. My work schedule was then full again. I felt well the rest of that day. I drank a lot of water. I didn't eat until 8pm that evening, before my last client (just in case). I ate a small bowl of chicken vegetable soup, and still felt all right.

Three things to note:
1) This was the one and only time I ever had to cut a session short throughout the whole duration of being ill, from opening the business in 2013-2017 when I got a clean bill of health. Although, other sessions challenged me and I'd just make it to the end of the session. There were some "close calls".

2) I knew the reason that I had vomited up bile was because of one (or more) of the supplements that I was taking from my FMD were detoxing me, heavily. What I didn't know at the time, was that the toxins weren't getting out of my body QUICK enough. Vomiting was my body's way of getting the toxins out FAST! I didn't have the flu. Mom and I both knew that. I had been experiencing the various symptoms from the **die-off,** a reaction that happens when cellular toxins, bad pathogens of fungus, mold, viruses, parasites, candida, etc. are dying. The fast die-off was overwhelming my body's ability to clean out in a timely manner through the skin, liver, kidneys, and final elimination through the colon. The dying pathogens caused symptoms just like I had: fever, muscle aches, headaches, ignited gut issues, hot and cold sweats, diarrhea, nausea, dizziness, and more.

3) Die-off doesn't "just happen" by itself. There has to be substantial change being made for a die-off effect to happen. For me, the numerous detox supplements that I was taking were the igniters causing this effect. Die-off is a VERY important component in the detoxification process in order to eradicate the toxins that have been built up in one's body. The die-off symptoms can be unpleasant to rigorously forgo for a person, but in the end the rewards of restoring one's health are incredibly worth it!

The majority of days during this long season of illness, I was glad to be alive. On other days, like the one I just shared, I wasn't so compelled to be on this earth much longer. To live your life in pain, every single day to some degree higher than my "new normal," I knew wasn't what I wanted, nor found any enjoyment in. Life wasn't easy, to say the very least. I didn't have a social life. I couldn't go out to eat with friends because of my very restricted diet, nor did I get invited out (or would I have wanted to go out with how I felt). My life consisted of running my business, working, dealing with my health, trying to eat and sleep, doing a small workout, taking care of my pets, and going through the days of just trying to make it through with one foot in front of the other.

What was God trying to teach me? I was in a valley, virtually feeling completely alone, but yet not alone. Mom was with me through it all. My dad and brother were there if I needed something also. I had my few select individuals that knew of my health. And, I had my biggest love, my Papa God. I knew my Papa was in control, but yet I still felt like my life was *spinning out of control.* And maybe that was just it… maybe that's what my Papa God wanted for ME to give Him COMPLETE control of my health

128

situation. That would mean handing Him, God, the reigns, TRUSTING Him COMPLETELY. Was I really ready for that?

33

Spring 2015

Kelly
JE March 2nd, 2015
*Mom, Troy, and I drove the long drive to Colorado. We packed all our food,
supplies, and ski equipment to spend the week here. Today, Troy and I are
skiing in Breckenridge, Colorado. I've been sick all day long. Despite feeling
ill and being sick, it's been enjoyable to ski some fresh powder in the
mountains. Troy and I love to ski through the trees, off small clefts, and any of
the back country terrain. We love it. It's quiet, peaceful, and serene.*

I was learning to find JOY in the simple things in life during this season of
illness. I was also becoming more of a minimalist than I already was thus far
in my life. Seeing things from a different perspective while being so sick was
teaching me lessons, like appreciating things and people instead of taking
things and people for granted. Being appreciative took on an entirely new level
of thankfulness in this journey, but more on that later.

The days after the horrendous accelerated "die-off effect" scene at work in
February, I tried to take a couple of the supplements, once again starting at a
quarter of dose. The low dose was suggested by the FMD that we'd contacted
after the horrid experience. My heart wasn't in it, to taking the supplements. I
was sick and tired of taking supplements, symptoms being jacked-up, and
getting violently sick. I was taking them in order to pacify Mom at this point,
who was encouraging me to not quit. Taking the reduced number of
supplements, the symptoms still got worse again.

I weighed 135 pounds at this time. I'd rarely weighed myself, not feeling the need to do so on any regular basis. However, I was too thin and looked malnourished, so Mom and I wanted to know where I was at for weight that spring. Mom was watching me spiral downwards in slow-motion. After about a week and a half of taking the supplements, Mom said, "Kelly, why don't you try stopping the supplements for a few days and see what happens with your symptoms."

It only took two days and I was back to my "normal". This was tolerable. Again, I will restate: Ultimately, it was MY LIFE and it was MY CHOICE. Mom and I both knew that. There was a mutual respect between us despite Mom's grave concern for me.

The first day of spring, March 20th, 2015 brought in my 23rd birthday. I had an eye examination scheduled. I arrived to my appointment early in order to fill out paperwork. In the paperwork I was asked if I was allergic to anything. I wrote in BIG letters that I was allergic to gluten. Gluten is in a lot of things, not just foods. It's in medications, skin care products, ointments, toothpastes, etc. Upon finishing the paperwork, I gave the completed forms to the receptionist and sat back down.

In a matter of minutes, the eye doctor came out shaking my hand in greeting. He took me back to his office and read through my paperwork, asking me a few questions. "You are allergic to gluten, is that correct?"

"Yes. I'm VERY allergic to gluten." I told him.

"Good to know. I will use 'gluten free' eye drops when we dilate your pupils." He stated. "Are you currently wearing contacts or glasses?"

"I've been wearing both since the summer of 2008." I replied.

Toward the end of the eye examination, he informed me, "You don't need a prescription at all, Kelly."

"Really? That's awesome," I stated with a smile on my face! Not having to put contacts in or wear glasses was going to be a GOOD change! It was time

131

to dilate my eyes. The doctor used the "gluten free" eye drops to dilate my eyes, then left the room. Almost immediately I started getting a headache. *Probably from these stupid eye drops making my vision blurry,* I thought to myself.

A few more minutes passed and the doctor came in to finish the examination. While he worked, he told me, "I will fill out a form so that you can have the eye glass restriction taken off your driver's license." I smiled, thanking him.

One may wonder, *I thought people's vision gets worse over time, not better!* Why didn't I need to continue to wear contacts or glasses? Looking back, I'm convinced improving my diet and not eating processed unreal foods that are scientifically made in a laboratory, designed to make the buyers get addicted to them--making it very difficult to resist the urge to eat them. By eating whole, simple, real foods, this was the biggest and most influential change impacting my improved vision! I'd made many other healthy changes in my life style. However, the organic diet I BELIEVE was the KEY to my eye sight improving. There is such a thing as "all-natural eye doctors" who actually DO have their client's cleanup their diets, eating "clean" and changing their eye health for the better. For REAL!

After my eye examination I drove home. I was having a hard time seeing, as the headache was getting worse. I rolled the window down for some fresh air. Arriving home, I walked into the house being greeted with, "Happy Birthday!" A friend and her sweet little toddler had come to visit our family. We all had supper together and talked into the evening. It was becoming rarer that'd we'd have company over, simply for the food aspect. Also, I never knew how I'd feel, so that just complicated making plans to have people over.

The next morning, I awoke with the pounding headache I'd gone to bed with. My left side, deep underneath my ribs extending down to just below my belly button, was more intense than my "normal" pain. I tried not to think about it, but I knew I didn't feel right. Nevertheless, I was going to the cities 4 hours away to get my monthly scheduled massage from my friend, Hallie.

Many hours later, Hallie and I greeted each other with a big hug, only I held back my tummy so it wouldn't be touched. We made small talk while we walked back to the therapy room. "How have you been feeling, Kelly?" she inquired. We always had lots of things to discuss.

"Well, I have good days, and not so good days. I have a pounding headache today. My abdomen and back don't feel very good either," I told her. She then started her work on my back side.

"Your left side is penetrating a lot of heat out of it," Hallie commented as she worked my abdomen.

"It has felt like a furnace all day, Hallie. Something is heating up deep inside." I replied.

"Yes, I'd agree. Your abdominal muscles are very tight. It's as if they are protecting something. They don't want to let go or loosen up." She spoke.

"I agree. My iliopsoas muscles are always tight. I use my 'Thera Cane' every night in an attempt to loosen the muscles. And it helps, but I can never seem to loosen them completely." I whispered back.

We continued our visit until the session came to an end, all too soon as usual. She'd put a hand on my abdomen before she left the room. The heat from the left side of my abdomen continued to penetrate outward. We both took deep breaths and exhaled.

As I walked into the reception area after my massage, Hallie asked me, "How are you feeling, Kelly?"

"I feel a lot better. My muscles are looser, and my headache is no longer pounding. Thank you, Hallie. You always know exactly what spots to work." I said smiling while I paid her. After more chatter, we hugged and said good-bye.

I started off on my long drive home drinking a lot of water. After a half an hour of letting the water settle, I decided to eat my supper. I always brought snacks and meals with me when traveling. I was only halfway through my meal when my stomach started churning.

Oh boy. Here I go again, I thought.

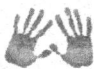

There were times when I had gone to my monthly massage therapist when I was really sick. At those times, I can honestly say the two hours of relief that I got from the massage felt like a vacation. After receiving a massage, I would be able to sleep deeply through the night, waking refreshed the next morning. For two years, sleep had been a constant battle. Receiving a massage helped me to sleep better for one awesome night!

34

Gluten Exposure

Kelly

I was on the drive home from my monthly massage, eating my supper I'd brought with from home. Halfway through eating, my stomach started feeling bad. I quit eating. My upset stomach grew worse as the drive continued.

Once home at 9:30pm, I unpacked the fresh store boughten groceries, and then showered. Afterwards, I stretched downstairs on the floor very briefly, and crawled into bed. The left side of my abdomen hurt deep inside, so I laid on my left side with my legs stretched out. I hoped that my abdomen would feel better with my legs stretched out in order to loosen my abdominal muscles. It didn't feel better though, so after a while I shifted between laying on my left side being stretched out, to curled into the fetal position. I drifted off into a restless sleep.

I awakened in the wee midnight hours throwing the covers off my burning hot body. I was drenched in sweat. My abdomen felt like it was going to explode. I whimpered in pain. My head was pounding again. I could literally feel the "thudding" in my head. I was still in the fetal position, laying on my left side. I was nauseated, dizzy, feeling very ill. I attempted to straighten out one leg. Pain ripped through my abdomen and I cried out. I didn't sob, as to not make the pain any worse, but instead let tears flow down my face, freely. After a length of time my abdomen calmed, seemingly feeling a little better.

Suddenly, I felt the urge to have a bowel movement. I knew I needed to get out of bed and into the bathroom, quickly. I gently turned from my left side onto my back. I got my feet over the side of the bed while Bun-Bun, my cat, readjusted his position. I had nudged him while moving my foot. He looked at me and started purring. I had sweat dripping down my back, chest, and forehead, my skin moist from perspiring. I sat up in bed. My head was spinning. I was dizzy. I sat on the side of the bed a few minutes. I could feel the pain increasing. I needed to get to the bathroom because if I didn't go now, the pain would only intensify and leave me immobile in bed. I pushed myself from bed, grabbing the walls to keep myself from falling. Limping along, I grabbed my abdomen as red-hot electrifying pain dropped me to my knees. I nearly vomited.

After the pain passed, I made it to the bathroom just in time. Having explosive diarrhea, and lots of it, I felt better after the release. However, I then felt like I was going to vomit. Then, another wave of diarrhea. I flushed the toilet. Knowing I was going to vomit, I grabbed the garbage can that was sitting beside me and stuck my head in it. I vomited in a couple waves. As the stench penetrate my nostrils, my stomach continued to wretch until there was nothing left. Immediately, though, I'd felt relief. I still had abdominal pain, but no more nausea. I was no longer sweating. Instead, I was ice cold and physically exhausted. My body felt beaten. I was weak, and tired. I cleaned the toilet and garbage can. The smell made my stomach wretch again, but nothing came up.

I washed my hands and face, brushed my teeth, walked back to my bedroom and changed clothes, then crawled into bed again. I laid on my left side in the fetal position trying to stay warm. Soon, I got out of bed and put a pair of socks on, then turned on my heating blanket. I had a few more abdominal pains as I laid back down. I prayed while the pain ripped through my abdomen into my back. I reached for the dull, achy, burning spot in my back that I could also feel deep underneath my ribs. I tried to reach into it, to access it to bring relief. I couldn't reach deep enough into my body to reach the firey-hot burning spot. Exhausted, I just laid there enduring the painful jabs through my abdomen and back. The pain lasted another hour and a half. I was totally worn out and couldn't keep my eyes open. As the jabs faded, I drifted off into another restless sleep.

The next morning, I felt terrible. The headache was back and thudding again. My abdomen was still having some ripping pain, but was otherwise my

136

"normal" dull, achy, burning pain. I was pale and felt like someone had ran me over with a truck and then backed over me, again. I had no energy. My torso was sore, my stomach was raw from the early morning vomiting and severe pain, and I was still dizzy and nauseated. This was a classic reaction for me to a gluten exposure.

I laid in bed thinking *I must have been exposed to gluten.* I knew that I hadn't eaten anything on Friday or Saturday that had come in contact with gluten. *What could it have been, I thought?* Then it hit me, *the "gluten free" eye drops at my eye examination on Friday.*

"You have GOT to be kidding me!" I murmured aloud.

Troy, my brother, was stirring in his bedroom next to mine. When I heard him walk by my door a few minutes later, I weakly asked him, "Please, go get Mom?"

"Sure. Are you not feeling okay?" He questioned. His voice full of concern.

"I feel absolutely horrible. Thank you for asking." I said while attempting a smile so he would know I was "okay" in my not feeling well.

Within minutes Mom was downstairs in my room. "What's going on Kelly?" She inquired.

"I feel terrible," and filled her in on the early morning hours' pain and vomiting. Also, about the questionable "gluten exposure". We talked a little while and then I weakly got out of bed. The room spun, so it took me a while to change clothes. I was able to walk up the stairs, greeting the friend and her sweet little toddler whom had been staying with us that weekend. They were going to be leaving in a couple hours. I felt miserable from my pain. I felt for them, wishing they didn't have to watch me struggle in my continued health battle.

Mom had already told Troy, Dad, and our friend what had happened. I sat on the floor and tried to enjoy their company, watching the toddler play. She giggled and laughed, warming my heart.

After our guests left, I got back down on the floor, immediately laying onto the hardwood surface. I was still having severe abdominal pain. Within a half an hour the pain reduced some, so I went downstairs to lay on the carpet. It took me a couple more hours before the pain went back to my "normal." My normal dull, achy pain in my left side deep underneath my ribs was tolerable. The headache still present was bothered by the brightness of sunlight coming through the glass doors. I pulled the hood of my sweatshirt over my head. My low back hurt bad, but over-all I was much better. Mom said color was starting to come back onto my face.

When I'm exposed to gluten, I get sick like just described. At this time in my health journey, it took anywhere from 7-10 days to fully recover from a gluten exposure. I'd have low-back pain and a constant headache during all those days. My abdomen and gut would be in severe pain for a few days, and then the last 5-7 days it slowly would improve. It's hard for me to eat or drink during this time without symptoms jacking-up. My gut reacts to anything I eat after a gluten exposure. From that one exposure, it actually took a full month in order for me to be able to eat without my body reacting harshly to whatever was being put into it, but more on that later. Times like this always set me back in my journey toward healing.

After that weekend of gluten exposure symptoms, Monday I called the eye doctor's office and spoke with the receptionist there, telling her what had happened.

"I will ask if he used the 'gluten free' eye drops, Kelly." The receptionist stated. "I will call you back." She called back within the hour. "He used the 'gluten free' eye drops. Are you sure you didn't just eat something bad?"

"I'm positive." I stated.

"You must have a little flu bug." She informed me.

"When I've been exposed to gluten in the past, I've gotten this same reaction," I said, shaking my head. "I don't have a flu bug. I didn't eat anything bad. Please give me the name of the eye drops that he used," I replied with evident irritation in my voice. I was frustrated. She provided me with the names of the two eye drops used there and we ended the call. I looked up the products, investigating the ingredients. Sure enough, even though one of the two products were labeled as "gluten free," it had gluten IN it. How could that be?

What does "gluten free" really mean? To be labeled "gluten free", a product has to have zero or less than twenty-parts per million of gluten in it. This DOES NOT MEAN that it doesn't contain gluten, but only that a minimal part of the whole product has gluten in it. The twenty-parts per million rule is the magical number, determined by the FDA, for an ingredient to not have to be included on the products ingredient labeling list (of ANY food or drug product). It is such a small amount, twenty-parts per million, that who'd notice? For someone who has celiac disease or non-celiac gluten sensitivity, we will have an adverse reaction from twenty-parts per million, or even less, of gluten! My body did notice!

Here's an example of living with others in your household that eat gluten regularly. You, who is gluten intolerant or have celiac disease or non-celiac gluten sensitivity, are exposed to the gluten to some degree, whether it be flour particles in the air used for baking, toasted bread crumbs on the counter, or even fragrant products being used that are floating around in the air, or products put on the body. As for the food part, particles can be left behind for you, the person who is gluten intolerant, to possibly pickup and ultimately be ingested by mistake. For me, even breathing air that has particles of flour floating in it gets a reaction started!

These days the reaction is not as severe, but there's still a reaction. I don't want to come into contact with particles of gluten, but these particles can fall onto my plate, or touch my fingertips, both of which can eventually end up in my mouth. You may think it's not a big deal. When your health is put at risk because of gluten, it IS a big deal. Getting sick for days after coming into contact with a trace of gluten in "gluten free" eye drops was upsetting to say the least. So much for quality assurance from the FDA.

For the first years of my illness, with a restricted diet, breads and baked goods (all containing gluten) aroma's and flour particles floated throughout the air in our home, although I was not eating the bread or baked items, caused headaches most days. At that point in my life I didn't know any better. Once I learned more about how my health was at risk because of gluten, I knew I would have to take precautions. It was important for me to clean an area in the kitchen before I started food prep, since there was always a possibility of gluten crumbs remaining there. My family, who live in the same household as I do, also learned the value of cleaning countertops regularly once they realized the seriousness of cross-contamination and gluten exposure for me.

People whom are allergic to gluten, having celiac disease or non-celiac gluten sensitivity, can't get a cross-contamination exposure or they will get sick. That, in and of itself, makes it almost impossible to eat out--the cross-contamination, or eating at another's house. Gluten can take days, up to months, to get out of a person's body. Each person reacts differently, some of whom will get seriously ill like me. It is important to be aware of individual's sensitivity to gluten, so I let people know when the need arises. That's not often, though, so I usually take my food with me where ever I go. Eating out gets really tricky.

"Gluten free" labeling now pertains to not only foods, but almost all products. "Gluten free" food labeling is VERY misunderstood. Also, a gluten free diet is not a fad diet, it's a necessary lifestyle for people like me. It's for real, and gluten exposure is a reality that can be dangerous.

35

A Special Guy

Kelly

In an earlier chapter, "Blessings", Mom talked about how she, my dad, my brother, and other people were praying for me, and how they wanted to help when I was sick. As you well know from reading thus far, my mom was with me every step of the way, of which I'm SO grateful. Today, it's time to look a little more behind the scenes and talk about a special guy that has made a HUGE impact in my life. He captured my attention from day one. Who is this special guy? My brother, Troy.

What are the first words that come to mind when I say "big brother"? Everyone's answer to this question is going to be different. For me, a number of words come to mind including: friend, protector, compassionate, big-heart, loving, REAL, honest, funny, kind, caring, and thoughtful.

Troy's a bit different than most young men that I personally know. He's full of love and compassion that's only grown stronger through his years. "He has always been that way," Mom says, "even when he was a little boy." She also says, "He came up to me once, when he was only two years old, sensing that something was wrong then gave me a big ole' hug." His caring concern, compassion, doesn't just stop there though.

Once, Troy stuck one of his fingers in my mouth to keep me from fussing as Mom was warming a bottle of formula for me when I was just short of being a new born. When the bottle was ready, guess who wanted to help feed me? Yep, you guessed right, Troy. Mom let him feed me. I think I must have liked the bonding time with him!

Troy and I are two years and three months apart in age. Growing up, we literally did everything together. We liked each other and got along well--the vast majority of time. We worked hard on family outdoor projects, did our chores together, played together, and were partners in business too. At young ages we were entrepreneurs, having our own vegetable stand (special thanks to Dad and Mom's handiwork, overseeing, and guidance)! We grew a variety of produce… planning, ordering seeds, planting, weeding, harvesting, cleaning and then selling our produce. It was a seemingly never-ending process, since it started during the winter when ordering seeds, to ending in the fall when cleaning out the garden of vines and plants for a clean sweep the next spring.

We had a system during harvest, mid-June through late September. Troy was the official "harvester", and then I'd wash and clean everything that was picked, preparing it for our clients who were happy to purchase. Mom over-saw and helped with the entire process. Alas, when finished, we were ready to pedal our produce! Mom would drive the little 20ft fishing boat with a 25hp motor, often fully loaded by mid-July, with produce and her two kiddos, driving us from dock to dock to our prospective buyers' homes on the lake we lived on.

Upon arriving at a potential buyer's dock, Troy was the salesman (whether he liked it or not), and we would walk up to the homeowner's door. And where was I? Well, Mom said I was the "cute little girl that stood there and smiled, winning over our customers with my big brown eyes and white-toothed smile." No offense, Troy--you were a good little business man, but I held the key with sealing the deal! Honestly though, who could've resisted us two, starting our vegetable sales at the ages of 5 and 7, standing in oversized tee-shirts that said, "T & K's Home-Grown Vegetables"? We were quite the pair! We became known by many for our vegetables over the course of seven seasons.

As we entered our teens, we hit the awkward years, but that didn't set us apart or affect us adversely as siblings. When friends came over, the other just blended right into the group of his or her friends as usual. Whether it was all males and I was the only female, or just the opposite—all girls and Troy being the only boy, it didn't matter. We shared our friends and had endless amounts of fun on the lake, in the yard, or in the house playing games. Our friends would even ask if the other sibling wasn't present, "Where's Troy?" or, "Where's Kelly? Is she coming to play with us?"

When Mom found out that she was pregnant with me, in her heart she had hoped that Troy and I would be best friends. She never voiced this to anyone, besides to my dad, only MANY years later in our high school years. Later, after those years, she shared her heart longing about us being best friends to close friends, who thought it was a blessing.

Now, you may be thinking that Mom MADE Troy and I like each other and had us spend so much time together. Well, that may be partly true because we were her kids. She could make us do many things. But the truth is, Troy and I really LIKED and ENJOYED spending time together. So, how'd that happen?

Well, my parents had raised us in a way that was different than that of social ways we often see. Mom spent a lot of time with us, being a stay-at-home mom, instilling a firm foundation in our little beings that she, they, would be there for us. My parents loved us, encouraged us, challenged us, and taught us a lot. We worked, played, and lived life with our family unit of four most often, but always welcomed friends to join in, and extended family too. We really did like to be together.

When we got old enough, we could choose to turn away from some, or all of, the concepts, life lessons, and foundational pillars we were taught. That being said, Troy and I are now both grown adults, making our own choices, changing dysfunctional traits we don't like, living our own lives, and running our own businesses: Troy, "Shores Edge Excavating", and I, "Helping Hands Therapeutic Massage & Body Work". I guess "T & K's Home-Grown Vegetables" helped guide us to become entrepreneurs! Thanks Mom and Dad!

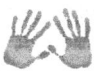

During the long season while I was sick as a young adult, Troy's and my relationship didn't change, except for the fact that I didn't have as much energy to partake in our crazy adventures. I remember some dark days of laying in our downstairs living room on the floor, in the fetal position curled up as tight as I could, laying on my left side. Troy would come down stairs, round the corner and see me lying there. I could literally feel his compassion and love before he even made it over to me. He'd walk over asking, "How you doing, Kel?" Other times, he didn't have to say a word. He'd simply get down to my level and wrap his arms around me in a big embrace. Sometimes, I'd cry into his shirtsleeve and he'd just be there for me, full of love, compassion, and support.

There were other times when I was sick that Troy knew that I was pretty down in my mood. Troy would bring out his best attempt of dry, simple humor to make me laugh. Since we don't share a lot of the same humor at all, it's comical that he'd actually got me to laugh, or at the very least bring a grin onto my face. He had a way of easing the burden and lighting up life.

Throughout our life, our friendship--a deep bond, has grown deeper. We've had seasons of growing apart with stuff going on in each of our lives, but that has only helped our relationship grow all the stronger once we made it past obstacles that separated us. People say, "Oh, you get older and then you get along better with your siblings." Well, that may be true, but we've always been close. We act a lot alike, except for our humor! We look more alike too, now that we are older! And we finish each other's sentences. Kind of sounds like were married, eh? Well, we both actually get told that we are married regularly by customers, "I just met your husband (or wife) the other day." We both respond the same way with, "Oh? Is that right? Well, I'm actually not married. You must be talking about my sister (or brother)."

These days my brother and I still do a lot together. We enjoy hanging out with each other and our parents, family, and friends--and we still share our friends! We still go on crazy adventures, although they aren't as wild. And, our conversations are deeper and more enriching for both of us these days. We can talk about anything and everything with each other, which is truly a blessing. Speaking for myself, I don't know many guys that are willing to be REAL, honest, open, and truthful, but Troy is willing to.

Troy isn't just my brother, he's my best friend. Guess Mom's prayer as I was forming in her womb came true, because her kids ARE best friends!

144

Troy, I thank God for you and am SO blessed to have you as my brother! I LOVE YOU!!!

36

Sick and Tired

Kelly

I had a scheduled appointment, one last phone consult, coming up with the FMD. I had told Mom prior to the phone consult, "I have no desire to talk to him. I want to cancel the appointment. He's just going to tell me, again, to take the stupid supplements. Then the same thing will happen that has happened EVERY time before; I'm going to feel horrible when I take them." I stated. "You see where taking the supplements has gotten me. NO WHERE! If anything, I'm more ill! I'm done talking with him, Mom. It isn't worth my time or money," I exclaimed angrily.

I had moments of anger and frustration while working with the FMD--his advice and remedies. I was definitely learning how to better DEAL with my anger and frustrations, majorly due to the "new heart" experience. My patience was much improved, but I still had moments like this last one just described. And, like most times, Mom got the brunt of hearing me spew my frustration out.

"Well, if you don't want to talk with him that's your choice. But I do want to talk to him. You aren't going to cancel this appointment. We both can be on the phone consult with speaker phone on. I think you can answer the few questions he asks you. I will talk to him the rest of the time and ask him the questions I want to know." Mom replied back. Again, despite our difference of opinions, we had a mutual love and respect for one another.

"If that's what you think you need to do." I replied. *Why did I think I needed to have the last biting remark? I still needed to work on NOT doing this.*

March 31, 2015. "How have you been feeling Kelly? Have any of your symptoms changed for the better, or worse, since we last spoke?" the functional medicine doctor asked.

"I'm not doing well at all. My symptoms are still pretty much all the same since I first came to you. I tried doing what you said, taking a smaller dosage of the supplements. I quit taking the supplements after I vomited up bile. Since I quit taking the supplements my symptoms have gotten better, especially the bloating and gas. This is exactly what happened last time when I discontinued the supplements. Now, my symptoms are at least tolerable. When I'm on the supplements I feel absolutely miserable." I replied, curtly. The FMD was very concerned about how I had vomited up bile. Bile, an important digestive juice, is produced in the liver and stored in the gallbladder. The liver is one of multiple filtering systems for the body. It detoxifies harmful substances from the blood, metabolizes nutrients, and makes blood-clotting proteins. No one can live without this organ, the liver.

The doctor asked specific questions, and I answered them honestly. After he finished, Mom talked with him. While they talked, I thought to myself, *I'm living with terrible pain, twenty-four hours a day, every day, and he wants me to keep taking these supplements? They escalate my symptoms so much that it is hard for me to function throughout the day. Are you not listening to what I'm telling you, man?* "Kelly was taking the supplements you recommended. She just stopped taking them again a couple days prior to this appointment. They're only making her symptoms worse." Mom told him, "She is frustrated. She's done everything you've recommended. She's tried the supplements at a lower dose. We looked at the ingredients in the bottles. Some have ingredients that she's intolerant to that cause her to have symptoms. Would this be a reason why the supplements aren't working for her? She's been feeling really sick. She isn't sure if you're able to help. I don't know if you can help her or not, either. At this point, I think it's in Kelly's hands to make that decision. I've watched her slowly become sicker over the last few years. It's SO hard to watch." Mom stated. That being said, Mom asked him a few more specific questions.

The FMD didn't recommend any new supplements. He said he wanted to talk to me again in a month, but I didn't respond. I wasn't getting the healing results I wanted. "Kelly, when you're ready for my help I will be willing to work with

147

you again. I'm sorry that you feel you aren't getting the results you are looking for." And with that said, we were soon off the phone. My time with the FMD had come to an end and I was happy about that. However, since I wasn't getting any better the question would again be *"What's next?"*

"That went really well." I said sarcastically. Mom started talking about all the good things that were discussed in the phone consult. I rolled my eyes, something I rarely did because it was not respectful, and then laid down on the floor, on my stomach, in an attempt to get some pain relief. "I'm sick and tired of being sick and tired!" I frustratedly reminded her.

"I know you are." Mom replied, seriously disturbed.

"No. You don't know. You aren't me. You're not living in pain every minute of every day. You don't wake up every night in pain, or wake up to your own audible cries because of it." I angrily exclaimed. "I tried everything he recommended. The only help he has been was confirming that I don't have anything 'serious' going on based upon the results of those three tests he recommended!" I was mad, letting my anger spew out on her. My words cut like hot swords flying through the air, landing on her.

Looking right at me she said, "You're right, Kelly. I'm not you, and I don't have your pain. I've watched you in excruciating pain. Do you know how hard it is for me to watch and not be able to stop or relieve your pain?" Tears pooled, then dripped like a leaking faucet from her eyes as she spoke. "You have no idea how hard it is to helplessly watch your own child become even more sick instead of getting better, Kelly."

Had my harsh words hurt Mom? I knew that her watching me hurt, and being sick for so long caused her to feel helpless. "I know it hurts you to have to watch, Mom. I'm sorry. I didn't mean to lash out at you. I was wrong. I know that. I'm really sorry." I'd sincerely and gently apologized.

"I forgive you. I'm sorry too. I didn't mean to upset you." She spoke.

Amends being made, we smiled at one another. "I still don't think the FMD has been a lot of help for me. I'm sick of wasting money on supplements and phone consults." We spoke more, then I headed outside for some fresh air to clear my head.

148

I prayed and cried while I walked outside. *Why am I having to endure all this pain with no end results in sight?* Every day I was battling for my life. I was doing everything I knew to help my body heal. *Why am I not getting results? What is God trying to teach me?* It had been four-and-a-half years of this left-side pain. I was ready to be done with this long battle. I was sick of life just existing and not truly living.

Was I really ready to give up and throw in the towel? The answer was a strong "NO"! In my heart of hearts, I knew I was going through this for a reason. I **did** believe that. Sound crazy? Maybe, but it's the truth. I DID trust my Papa God, but my trust needed to become deeper, even more REAL. And in order to do that, my faith was about to grow deeper as I walked with my Papa God through this low, low valley.

Bob Goff, an author, lawyer, motivational speaker, etc. says, **"I think God does miracles in stages, not just always one at a time."**

I agree with Bob Goff. It was a miracle that I was still alive with how sick I really was. However, my Papa God was in complete control and that gave me peace of mind. Papa had some miracles that He was up to. We'd just have to wait and see as they presented themselves. In due time.

37

Gods in Complete Control

Kelly

For the next month after discontinuing doctoring with the FMD, Mom and I didn't talk about who I would go to next for help with my left-side abdominal pain, or if we should continue to research and try to do my own methods of healing. We had no answers to our unspoken questions, but we both had our thoughts on what the pain really was. We just hadn't spoken it to one another.

After I quit having phone consults with the FMD, I continued to take three different supplements. I knew these ones weren't making me sick. I continued my all-organic diet and eating foods that digested with less burden: bone broth, boiled or baked chicken, veggie soup, and steamed dark leafy greens. Also, I ate steamed: carrots, cauliflower, broccoli, snow peas, brussel sprouts, green beans, and ate some dried fruits, raisins and mulberries. That was the extent of my diet.

Getting fresh air and exercise were an everyday doing in order to help keep my body warm, have better circulation and keeping the detox going through the skin with sweat. I was doing all the "right" things, putting in nourishing foods, water, bone broth, and incorporating healing modalities in my life. It had been five years since I started my journey towards good health. *Why wasn't I seeing more positive results?*

Mom and I continued to do our own research for my left-side pain and my gut health. We listened to health speakers that spoke on nutrition, healing (physically, mentally, emotionally, and spiritually), foods that killed diseases and illnesses, the importance of gut health, gluten issues, and some other topics that would come up on our emails from doctors we followed. At times, we each had to stop listening and researching because we were bombarded with so much information. We needed to process what we were hearing, in addition to working, juggling everyday life with cooking, food prep, chores, and keeping a routine. Life was chaotic at times, yet it was mostly enriching.

Part of my healing process meant that I needed to heal in ALL aspects of my life: physically, mentally, emotionally, and spiritually. In "A New Heart", you read of my spiritual healing, and that was a continual daily investment to have peace, even during storms that came up unexpectedly.

Physically
I was doing all I could physically to stay focused, to reverse my health and stay alive.

Mentally
I was eating foods and taking some supplements that were all working to reverse the depression. I may have felt helpless at times, but I was not suicidal, EVER. I constantly had to work to be optimistic to change the negativity of what I was going through to help myself. And with time, that optimism helped bring change through the years. I still had progress to make, but I was improving my mindset despite the challenges in life.

Emotionally
Well, let's get into that. When I was a little girl, I rarely voiced my thoughts and emotions, even when people wronged me. I didn't like to stir up trouble, or be confrontational. I went through nearly 18 years of my life that way. When my emotions had built up to the point of erupting, I was like a time-bomb going off, growing up. It wasn't a healthy way to express myself. I didn't voice my thoughts, saying, "That's wrong. I don't agree. Or, that wasn't nice." at times that I should had. I didn't correct someone with "That isn't what happened." If I was accused. Instead, I would choose to be silent, saying nothing. Being silent eats at you from the inside out. It's just like a disease. It quietly festers from the inside, and slowly kills you piece by piece, situation after situation. That doesn't help a person's physical health, but rather it grows illness.

As I said, my silence would be built up like a time-bomb awaiting the final countdown to explode. When I finally would explode, I could barely speak because I had so much that I needed to say! My words were angry, and jumbled. I couldn't think or speak clearly. I didn't know how to say what I needed to because I didn't know how to voice my emotions and frustrations into sensible words. I didn't know how to deal with my anger, hurt, and bitterness from the mean things that were said or done to me. Individual's words had cut deep into my heart. I didn't want the words that came out of my mouth, when I was exploding in anger, to hurt a person like they'd hurt me.

All of these ideas about being "respectful" that I had, staying silent instead of speaking up, were wrong. I had watched and learned what to say, or not say, from the people who were closest to me while I was growing up; family, friends, and various others who influenced my life. I had learned to be like a mouse in the corner of a room, noticeably quiet and nearly invisible.

When my health started to crash in 2010 at 18 years old and continued to decline in the next years, I needed to reexamine my life and my choices. At these times, I knew that I needed to welcome some big changes, much of it in my communication. It didn't matter how hard it was going to be, I needed to do this for myself. As for my mental, emotional, physical and spiritual health as a whole, that became clearer to me while seeing Dr. Ann, although I'd known it in a "sensing" kind of way. I had some of uncomfortable things that I needed to work through. I knew that this dysfunctional trait, or learned behavior, needed to stop with me.

I started talking with the people that I loved most, my family. My family was where I spent most of my time. This was where, many times, the pain and hurt had happened. I was the youngest child and I got picked on a lot. I got blamed for things I didn't do, received harsh verbal reprimands, and was the brunt of jokes, which they had thought were fun or loving, but they weren't. I am very sensitive. I just wanted to be loved. Due to that desire to be loved, I would go along with what my family did or said to me, most often not speaking out when my feelings were being hurt. I know they did not intentionally try to hurt me.

As a young adult, the end of 2011 and the beginning of 2012, I started to voice my thoughts and emotions. In doing so, I found freedom. As tough as it was, and is at times, I don't regret my decision to start using my voice. I learned I had only been holding myself back by not being willing to be real, truthful, and transparent with people. By being more real, truthful, and transparent, my spirit and personality were freer to come through me so that I could be expressive, and be the person that I was created to be. I no longer would knowingly or unknowingly carry an oppressive spirit. I laughed, loved, smiled, cried for emotional relief, when need be, and enjoyed living my life the way I wanted to. The atmosphere of our household lightened, and the relationships with members of my family were more freeing. We all communicated easier with one another as I started to use my voice with them. I wasn't the only one who was learning to find my voice. Many of us were. We were all in this together.

A relationship takes two people. One person can't do all the communicating and changing in the relationship. True relationship change doesn't happen with just one person doing the work. Our family is proof of that. As a family, we have gone through A LOT together. Living together as adults in a family isn't easy. Loving each other isn't always easy. Agreeing to disagree isn't easy, but it is becoming easier. Through all of the changes, I, we have grown as individuals and as a whole.

I have found freedom in using my voice to speak my heart with words. I've also found the freedom through forgiveness of past pains and hurts. I have learned that if I really love people, and want to be real with them, I will go to these hard places of being REAL with them in communication.

Life is precious and should be lived to its fullest each day. I learned I had only been holding myself back by not being willing to be real, truthful, and transparent with others. Working through my past wasn't something that I could do all at once. It took years and is still a work in progress. Once I started to deal with past negative memories of happenings, understanding myself better, and letting these all go along with the negative conversations or events, I was becoming freer. My heart felt lighter and I had more energy. My mood lightened. I felt a new freedom in my life. I was processing, learning that healing comes in these different forms.

The body is an amazing, intricate being. In order for the body to function optimally, we need to look at a variety of aspects of feeding it to attain optimal health to be whole. Our body remembers and holds onto conversations, situations, injuries, harsh words, actions, abuses, and even smells. I didn't know that during my younger years. My body had retained a lot of memories, some that I did know and other memories I didn't know about—the body protecting me in a way, shielding me until I would be ready for the memory and to deal with it. When I'd worked with Dr. Ann, she spoke to my inner heart longing for peace, and I began to work through these layers of junk for needed healing in my body. In turn, my body started a process of unlocking itself.

Acknowledging ALL aspects of healing during my entire health journey, and still to this day (and forever I plan to), have helped change and set me free at a whole new level. It's not all been easy. Some has been really tough and trying, but I'm healthier in ALL areas of my life because of it.

As Bob Goff (BG) says, **"What is simple often isn't easy. What is easy often doesn't last."**

I want lasting results, so I'm willing to go to those hard places and heal as fully as possible in this life. Gods in complete control, but we have the choice in daily life to how we live and learn through each day's happenings!

38

This Feels Right

Kelly

Spring was in the air! The snow had begun to melt as April 2015 came around. Spring is a season of change and new life. I was ready for a season of change! Warmer weather was welcomed!

Warmth, in those last years while becoming more ill, had proven to be essential in healing for me, so much so that I had thoughts about moving to a warmer state. But realistically, moving to a warmer state was not going to happen anytime soon.

My health was teetering on the edge. I was in constant severe pain. Death was lurking. I had done everything recommended to me by natural health professionals. Since I'd quit working with my former FMD, I currently wasn't going to any specific health professional for my left-side pain. I was completely on my own. I was incorporating all the information that I had learned in the last five years. I was eating an all-organic diet that was feeding my body nourishing nutrients. That was important and I felt good about eating in this way. However, diarrhea was a constant battle, going to bathroom 7–15 times per day. I battled hot and cold sweats daily. I was malnourished and pale, even though I ate healthy. Nausea and dizziness were present the majority of the time. I had no energy and was fatigued, desiring to sleep all the time, although that too was unrealistic since lying down was very uncomfortable for sleeping. The left-side pain deep underneath my ribs was severe the majority of time. My abdomen was always bloated after I ate or drank anything. The bloating pressure increased the severity of the left-side abdominal and back pain. My whole abdomen hurt and would cramp. The left side of my back hurt

155

all the time too. It felt like someone was stabbing me with a knife. It was a searing hot, jabbing pain that grabbed me deep inside, working outward. The pain was 3D, starting from deep underneath my abdomen, going straight through to my back. The pain in my back was about an inch or two from my spine, on the left side. In my abdomen, the intense pain was just off the center of my body, to the left side about an inch to two. No matter how much I tried to reach in and touch that constantly burning spot, I couldn't reach it. Try as I might, I couldn't access it. I would lean against the corner of a table, or use a "Thera Cane", a self-massaging tool, in an attempt to reach it. Sometimes I would lie on a racket-ball and put all of my weight into the ball. In one last attempt, I would use my fingers reaching under my ribs, attempting to access that deep, burning spot. Finally, I would give up, enduring the hot, searing pain within the deepest part of my being. It was so exhausting.

There were times when I couldn't touch the left side of my abdomen. That was mostly when I was really bloated, and my abdomen hurt because of the bloating pressure. Sometimes Mom would put a hand on my abdomen when I was in pain, only to have me grab her hand to take it off because even her very gentle touch hurt.

Headaches had been constant for a couple years now. They'd gotten so bad that at times I just wanted to be in a dimly-lit therapy room. Given my line of work, this worked out conveniently well, because I worked in a dimly lit therapy room. However, I knew that I needed sunlight too, so I opted not to spend time in a dark room except while at work. Every day I would go outside. Sometimes I'd close my eyes, letting the sunshine warm my entire being.

My breathing was shallow and my frame was small and slender. I had been able to maintain some of my muscle tone by doing a very simple workout. Some of my symptoms had been getting better, subtly in the last couple years. Other symptoms had only gotten worse. I was gassier and more bloated than ever. Together, the two made all my abdominal and back pain worse. My body was exhausted from the fight that was going on deep within.

I still felt like I was existing, not really living my life. At times when the pain got so bad, it took all my energy to bear through it. I was having a hard time handling the pain. There were nights I would go to bed praying; *God, if it's*

156

Your will, I'm ready to come home. If it isn't Your will, help me Lord, because this pain is more than I can tolerate anymore. It hurts Papa, really bad. Help me, heal me, and show me what I need to do. Lead me in the right direction, Lord. Let this be Your will, not mine. Give me the patience to endure this fight. I trust You and have peace knowing You know what's best for me. Thank You for hearing my prayers, Papa. You know my heart. Help me, please!

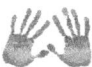

Toward the end of April, 2015, while Mom and I were at work, I was working with a client and Mom was doing computer research on the internet between clients coming in and leaving. We'd done a lot of research on natural health remedies in recent years, so we both received emails and articles from various organizations, holistic doctors, and a few chiropractors. Mom had checked her email while at work on this particular day, deciding to read an email from a doctor who specialized in "gluten". In that email, he shared how a friend was launching a second group for a gut healing program, starting in June of 2015. Both he and the friend had a short video they'd done together about the program.

Mom, more curious about the program, watched the video since there was a link to it on the email. That video gave broader information about the program. She then googled and researched more about the founder of the program. In doing so, a different short video about the gut healing program was there to view, with only the founder talking in it. Mom learned that the program had been able to help a large group of people with gut problems through eliminating inflammation, addressing leaky gut and pathogenic overloads on the body that cause chronic illnesses, pathogens like parasites, yeast, fungus, protozoa, bad bacteria, viruses, heavy metals, and other toxins. This program was said to be transformative for people with chronic autoimmune or digestive diseases like Hashimoto's, lupus, Crohn's, colitis, IBS/IBD, fibromyalgia, and also crucial for those with skin conditions like eczema and psoriasis. The first video Mom had watched initially, talking about "If the gut healing program is right for you", had attracted Mom's attention. While she'd watched that initial video, deep inside her heart she knew the program was what I'd needed for my abdominal pain and digestive issues. She couldn't explain WHY, later, but she just knew.

When I'd come out of my therapy room after working with a client, Mom looked up from the computer, her eyes twinkling. Curious, I walked around to her side of the desk. She stopped the video, turned and looked me in the eyes, then said, "You'll never guess what I just found! It was a link in an email." Mom's eyes twinkled with hope!

"If I'll never guess, why don't you just tell me then." I chuckled.

"I don't always open emails from this doctor, but for some reason I opened today's email." She then proceeded to tell me about the gut healing program. "I've already watched an informational video with him talking with the founder who designed the program."

"Okay…" I replied, listening intently.

"Kelly, I want you to watch the very first video that I watched. It's about 'IF the program is right for you'. I know the information will resonate with you."

"I can do that but not until late tonight, or tomorrow night after work." I replied.

"Kelly? Please, make time to watch it within the next 24 hours. Enrollment for the program ends the middle of May, unless it fills up before that." Mom stated. "I think this program is exactly what you need, Kelly. With all your digestive issues and abdominal pain, you are a perfect candidate for it. Watch the video and find out for yourself." She smiled, encouraging me.

"Okay. I will Mom. Thank you!" I smiled and hugged her as my client came out of the therapy room. *My heart didn't know whether to believe that there was actually something out there to be able to aid in healing my digestive issues and abdominal pain. I had tried so many different avenues of healing that didn't bring the results that I had hoped for. Could this possibly be something that could help me?* From what little Mom had told me, the program sounded too good to be true.

Later that evening I watched the video. Mom was right. The program sounded like a perfect fit for me in my ill state of health!

158

That weekend, Mom and I together looked through more information on the founder of the program's website. I was beginning to see the reality of possibly healing through this gut healing program! *This could really be an influential factor in helping me be free from all my digestive and abdomen pain. THIS FEELS RIGHT.* We read people's testimonials who'd gone the program, all of those people who have struggled for years with autoimmune disorders, infertility, SIBO, constipation, bloating, brain fog, and endless other symptoms, and people who could not find a diagnosis or solution and the program was the key for their healing. After our research session, we both left the room with our own thoughts for a time.

I had to make a decision within a few days. Mom and I talked in great detail about the program days later, how it could help me. We shared our opinions and thoughts we'd been thinking about the last few days.

The program was an on-line program. We learned that there was a specific diet to follow depending on what specific group you were put in based on a lengthy digestive health assessment, to figure out the root cause of an individual's gut microbiome imbalances. The program included eating an all-organic diet with weekly meal plans--including grocery lists, recipes, required supplements to purchase, lots of material to read and food preparation to do, and much more information! These aspects of the program weren't all new ideas, so I knew it wouldn't be a huge problem for me. However, I would definitely need some help from other people. *I can't do all of the things required here completely on my own,* I thought.

Mom had been thinking about doing the program with me (which I didn't know) since the day she'd found the information. It wasn't until she voiced her thoughts before I would sign up for the program saying, "Kelly I'm going to do this program with you."

"You don't have to do that, Mom. Really. I'll be fine. You don't have to."

"No, I don't HAVE to. I WANT to. Yes, I'm doing it for you… but I'm also doing it for me."

"Are you sure you really want to do this?"

"Yes, I'm sure. I've been thinking about this for a couple of days. I've made my decision and I'm doing the program too." This is another example of Mom's willingness to walk alongside of me so I didn't go through this alone. In all my years of having to change my diet, no one besides my mom (until this past year, my brother did for himself) had ever been willing to change their diet, even if it was only to help me. Mom, whom had gone to Dr. Ann many years before I had, knew how hard it was to not only CHANGE your diet, but in addition, to being around other people eating foods right in your own home that I couldn't eat. We'd both dealt with that already! Mom would be very helpful in grocery shopping, cooking, and helping me to learn how to make meals in a healthier way.

I was thankful that Mom wanted to do the gut healing program with me. It is easier when someone does something WITH you, not just cheering you on. I was glad we decided to both do it together! At that point, I literally had nothing to lose in regard to my health. In my eyes, *this was my last chance. Whatever is going on deep inside my body is slowly killing me. If this program doesn't work, it will only be a matter of time.* Mom and I both knew that.

It may sound like I was suicidal when I say "It would only have been a matter of time," but truly, there was NO chance at all I was going to kill myself. NONE at all! I was respectfully, and responsibly, having to face the reality that death was a REAL possibility. And if my health didn't change soon, it would have been only a matter of time. So, this online program? Well, for the first time in many, many months, something just felt RIGHT in my heart. I truly had HOPE! REAL HOPE!

39

REAL HOPE!

Kelly

Mom and I had a week-and-a-half to sign up for the online gut healing program before enrollment closed in mid-May. Mom wanted to check a few more details before we signed up. A couple more days passed, then we both separately paid online to purchase the program. I didn't receive an email receipt that day. *Weird*, we both thought, as Mom and I both voiced our concerns to one another regarding my not receiving a receipt that day. We waited to see if they would send a receipt the next day. They didn't. A couple more days passed, and STILL no receipt.

The day before registration was going to close, Mom called the customer service line. "Hi, I'm calling to see if my daughter and I are signed up for your spring enrollment program? The enrollment closes tomorrow and we had signed up last week. My daughter, Kelly Lang, never received a receipt via email. I'm wondering if you can tell us if we are signed up on your end or not?"

It turned out that the online registration had been having a few glitches. That happens. Turns out that we both hadn't actually been signed up for the program. Thankfully, Mom had called to make sure we were signed up and then got us signed up for REAL!

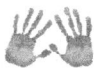

Prior to the first gut healing program webinar, the founder had sent out an informative email saying, "If you have any questions about the program that we haven't already answered elsewhere, please send your questions in via email. We will answer the questions you send in during the webinar."

The following week the founder did a live webinar with all of us enrolled in the program, to answer any questions. I had sent in one question. I wanted to know if she thought the program could truly help someone as sick as me, and I had written up a very brief history telling how sick I'd been, including the pain that leaves me immobile, to vomiting up bile while taking supplements to detox.

Wow! They read my question during the webinar, then talked directly to me saying, "Kelly, this program is PERFECT for someone like you. Vomiting up your own bile gives me chills. You are the perfect candidate for this program since your body, and gut, are very sensitive. You haven't done well with supplements in the past which is good to know. You will want to take the supplements in the program, but starting at a very low dose. I recommend that you start taking the supplements at a quarter or half of the regular dosage that we recommend. Be extra good to yourself, Kelly. Please feel free to take an extra week, or a couple weeks, on this program, that way you get the full benefit of the program to help heal your gut."

What the founder of the program said was all I'd needed to hear to confirm that this was right for me. Deep inside my heart (even prior to those spoken words, a confirmation) I knew that this was going to change my life for the better. I had REAL HOPE!

The program was going to take a lot of time and energy, both of which I had little of, especially the latter--energy. Mom and I started the program in June, 2015. It did not take me very long to realize I was VERY grateful that she was doing it with me. I thanked her periodically throughout the program, for her willingness to do to the program WITH me.

We prepared our mind and body through reading the information and cleaning up all our diets of any sugar and junk. We also got accustomed to using the online links and looking through our individual "Group Plan". Each individual in the program was placed into one plan according to the lengthy health assessment we'd completed online. Mom and I were both in the same group, fortunately, which emphasized Small Intestinal Bacteria Overgrowth. The first

162

week was not difficult for either of us. We read a whole lot of information and watched many videos prepping us for the next ten weeks. Cleaning up our diets of sugar and junk was easy for me, as I didn't have to change anything!

The first week flew by, then the second week was upon us. We'd started taking multiple supplements in this part of the program. Just like in all my prior experiences with taking supplements in the last few years, I got more ill upon taking them. Deep down in my heart I knew that I HAD to take these supplements, even if they made me feel worse. I was now fully determined. I was ALL IN. That sheer determination, along with hope for healing results, kept me going each time I swallowed the supplements at meal times, or in between meals, or upon waking up, or going to bed!

Diet is important and was very emphasized in the program. We used foods, along with herbs and supplements, to decrease and eliminate inflammation in our bodies. People in Mom's and my group have more digestive issues because of bacterial overgrowths. Diet was limited, but for me I hadn't eaten this much of a variety of foods in the last two-and-a-half years! At first, when Mom and I started the program, I had to overlook the fact that all these foods were going to make me feel more ill. I knew we were using these foods as medicine to heal the body, so I needed to respect that and be open to this new, and beautiful but difficult change.

"Let thy food be thy medicine and thy medicine be thy food."
-Hippocrates

I loved this new change of diet and my body loved it too, although at times it was hard on my gut. The program was designed so that we ate foods to help detoxify, cleanse, and improve our gut health. These foods were also aiding in better digestion, encouraging gut healing and optimal gut health. We made our meals according to what we wanted to eat each day within the limits of the weekly meal plan. We had the option to follow daily meal plan strictly or loosely. That being said, Mom and I spent a LOT of time doing food prep. Truthfully, Mom more so than me because I was still struggling to get by each day. Many of those hours spent doing food prep included cleaning vegetables, preparing a variety of meals, trying new recipes each day, to begin with, then a few more new recipes each week that followed. We were also making condiments and our homemade bone broth. Together, we made sure we had enough leftovers in our meals to help make it through our work week. The portion sizes in this program were perfect. We ate three meals daily, and we virtually never felt too full or ever hungry afterward! On the rare occasion that we ate a big meal where we did walk away feeling full, we never felt bloated or uncomfortable! How awesome is that? This was unlike what would happen in the past! We were getting lots of nutrients and energy out of our meals! We felt very satisfied and healthy! We didn't crave food between meals! If either of us got hungry we could have a small snack, but otherwise we would just drink water and wait 15 minutes to see if we were really hungry.

Our bellies were satisfied doing this online gut healing program. I definitely had REAL HOPE in reversing my gut health!

40

What am I Drinking?

Kelly

In the last chapter, "REAL HOPE!", I said we would drink water to see if we were really hungry.

So how does a person know if they are truly hungry? To truly know if I was hungry, I would drink a cup of water 15 minutes before eating anything. After waiting 15-30 minutes, if I was still hungry, then I was most likely not thirsty, but actually hungry.

Here's an interesting fact I hadn't known until I was informed by Dr. Ann. Drinking a significant amount of water, or any beverage while eating a meal, disrupts digestion. It's "okay" to drink NO MORE than a half a cup of water during a meal. It's BEST to drink water 15-30 minutes before a meal. When the meal is over it is wise to wait 30 minutes before drinking any beverage. This is a great way to aid in smooth digestion so it will not be interrupted or have to work harder.

Over 70% of the human body is made up of water. This means every person needs to be drinking water daily to help their body function properly. A goal to strive towards when drinking water each day consists of drinking half of one's body weight in ounces of water. For example, say a person weighs 100lbs. This means they'd drink 50-ounces of water each day. However, there are a lot of variables that play a role in how much water a person drinks each day. If we have a very physical job, if we sweat, if we exercise, if we are detoxing, or we are just plain thirsty, then we NEED to be drinking more water!

Our bodies NEED clean and pure, plain water to function! Clean, pure, plain water. **What do I mean when I say clean, pure, plain water?** Well, we live in a society that puts additives, preservatives, flavorings--a majority of which are fake, and sometimes minerals into drinking water. Many years ago, I drank Gatorade, soda pop, flavored water (Propel, Aquafina, etc.), and Kool Aid. What is the common theme going on here? These are ALL fake drinks with nothing healthy added to the water in these products, which means there is nothing nutritious or healthful in these products for our bodies.

I came to a point in my life when I had to ask myself a serious question, *"What am I drinking?"* and *"Why am I even drinking this?"* Drinking clean and pure, PLAIN water is the BEST thing we each can do to help our bodies function optimally. **What water do I drink?** I drink water that comes in 5-gallon jugs from a local water company that delivers to our house once a month. They filter the water to take all the contaminants out, and then safely add back in minerals, giving the water a distinct and better taste. Not every company does this. Finding a company or a place to purchase water that is TRULY providing us with healthy drinking water is an important key to living a cleaner life and becoming healthier. Water is vital to our existence. So, these days when I ask myself, *"What am I drinking?"* I know what I am drinking.

How do I know if my water is clean and pure? Well, this is where it can get tricky. We hear about chlorine and fluoride being added back into piped-in water to homes from city water plants in communities all over the United States. Speaking on just one of these, fluoride[5]; is fluoride good for me? The FDA has told our society fluoride is good for us. Do I agree? No. Why? Too much evidence goes against this being true. Fluoride is one of the worst "top 10 toxins" to the human body! There is nothing good going into the body from consuming fluoride, even for our teeth. Fluoride in toothpaste isn't good for us, plain and simple. Unfortunately, this labeling is printed on packaged containers of toothpaste found on store shelves all over the United States, "If more toothpaste than the size of a pea is swallowed, contact your local Poison Control Center". If this were actually read by the consumer, then why on earth would one buy it and use it on their teeth?

---

[5] The American Cancer Society, July 2015, https://www.cancer.org/cancer/cancer-causes/water-fluoridation-and-cancer-risk.html

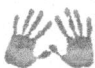

I was told by the public school system, the dental offices I've went to--including their assistants, the dentist, and dental hygienists, all while growing up that I needed to have fluoride to better the health of my teeth. Well, through my research I've found out that fluoride actually enhances the chances of getting cavities.

Growing up I had my share of cavities. And with that, that meant something had to be done about it--fillings. Oh, joy. Back in my day, amalgam fillings--known as silver fillings, were still the standard. The amalgam fillings are made up of 50% mercury! The pretty white fillings that were "safe" of mercury cost extra on my parent's dental insurance. I came to find out as an adult that amalgam fillings have the ability to release their toxic chemicals into our bodies every time we eat, drink, brush our teeth, or, stimulate the teeth in anyway simply by breathing. It seems we are constantly putting food or water into our mouths each day, so what was I really swallowing? Mercury vapors? Yes, mercy vapors. Long story short, after learning this as an adult, I knew that if I wanted to truly help myself detox and become healthier in ALL aspects, I needed to take the steps to initiate the change(s) I wanted for myself. And I did.

By going to an all-natural, holistic dental clinic and working with them, I had all of my amalgam fillings removed with specialty equipment, safety measures and precautions in place, and had the "pretty white fillings" put in instead, all at my own expense. And guess what? My mouth FELT better. Call me crazy, but it's the truth. I'll restate, research for yourself, don't take my word for things. Do your own research!

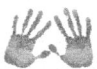

I kick start my day drinking water. Do you? I've taken to starting my day off with drinking a few water-based concoctions both of which are a good way to kick start and help to cleanse my organs for the day's work ahead of it! I'll share the recipes with you. If you decide to try them, I would recommend starting with the second concoction, so as to acclimate your body to drinking water first thing in the morning, causing a gentle and subtle detox. If you don't want to try them, that's okay too. Just sharing information!

The **first concoction** I drink right away once I wake up on an empty stomach. It includes: Take a 16-ounce drinking glass and put 2 tablespoons of pure, organic lemon juice in it. Add 1 tsp. aluminum-free baking soda. It will fizz. Then add 12-14 oz. of water, but don't fill to the top because it continues to fizz. Once the fizzing slows down, add 2 tablespoons organic, apple-cider vinegar. Once that is added you can stir it (it may fizz again a little), then drink it! I drink this one first because this one is important to drink on a COMPLETELY empty stomach. This concoction is good for breaking up and reducing the growth of inflammation in the body.

The **second concoction** I drink (reminder, start with this one to acclimate your body before trying the first concoction just spoke of) is a 16-ounce glass of pure drinking water with 2 tablespoons of lemon juice added to it. It dilutes well, so it's not sour to swallow. By drinking lemon water initially upon rising, we're helping our body's organs to detox, helping our cells to prepare and function optimally for the day, and it boosts our PH to be more alkaline!

A person's PH balance should IDEALLY be 7.4. This is true alkaline, 7.4PH. An over-alkaline 7 or above PH is KEY to having good gut health. Acidic, 6.9 or below, is "concerning" or may be even "bad", as it promotes illness in our bodies. An acidic PH has been linked to pathogens, parasites, and the formation of many illnesses like cancer, diabetes, heart disease, auto-immune diseases and many more.

Low body temperature correlates directly with PH balance as well, being acidic verses alkaline. Remember how I said, earlier in this health journey, that I was ALWAYS cold, especially my hands and feet, but now my core was too? Yes, I was acidic, my PH being just under 7 regularly. The immune system, AKA the core of our being, helps control our body temperature. If a person is ill or has disease, our immune system isn't working optimally, so it is vital to look specifically at our gut health!

I had a deeper underlying issue going on that NEEDED to be addressed, sooner rather than later. However, I was doing daily helps to aid in changing my digestive health. Drinking good water, and staying away from premade beverages found on store shelves all across the world were one of my best offerings to myself.

41

Getting in Deep

Kelly

On June 22nd, 2015 we started the online gut healing program. During the first week I thought it went fairly well! My abdomen was less bloated and I had less gas. Headaches weren't as severe and I was having less of them. Even though I was still very tired, I had more energy to get through the day.

> **"The natural healing force within each one of us is the greatest
> force in getting well. Our food should be our medicine.
> Our medicine should be our food." -Hippocrates**

My body, especially my gut, wasn't resisting the new additions of foods that we were eating from the meal plans! In the past, I had reacted to so many foods negatively, which in turn set me up for more inflammation and an intestinal candida overgrowth. Symptoms of inflammation include: bloating, gas, food allergies and sensitivities, painful joints, headaches, stressed organs, and abdominal and back pain. The foods and supplements we were taking was getting inflammation under control, but it wasn't going to go away that easy for me. I still had battles, daily.

With this new specific diet, I was relearning the simple joy of eating a variety of foods! These weren't little changes for me! They were big changes! For instance, not having a severe headache for as long as all day and night was a true delight. Given I'd had headaches to some degree constantly in those last couple years, to not have a headache for part or all of a day felt amazing! I didn't even remember what it was like to not have a headache until one day, I didn't have one at all! Furthermore, I could be outside for longer periods of time in the sunshine and it didn't aid in the formation of a pounding headache! It is important to get outside in the fresh air and sunlight for natural vitamin D and fresh oxygen!

Sunshine is ESSENTIAL to our health! It's a great way to easily get vitamin D3. Sunshine can aid in relieving depression, regulates hormones, decreases stress, aids in healing of skin conditions, decreases rheumatoid arthritis and IBS, lessens menstrual pain and cramps, increases bone density health, naturally improves the immune system, and aids in preventing and fighting cancer.

Too much sun at once can damage our skin. I'd learned years prior to this time that conventional sunscreens aren't actually preventing us from getting skin cancer. The chemicals in many sunscreens are actually CAUSING skin cancer. When the sun's rays shine onto our skin while wearing conventional toxic sunscreens, our bodies are actually MORE at risk of skin cancer growth than if we weren't wearing sunscreen at all. If you want to know more about sunscreen safety, check out the sunscreen article on Dr. Josh Axe's website, "Best Sunscreens and Toxic Ones to Avoid"[6] by Leah Zurbe. Great information there.

So, what are some simple and safe alternatives to getting Vitamin D3 and not wearing sunscreen? Limit sun exposure, and cover up your skin if you'll be outside for longer periods of time. If a person can't get outside in the sun for 15 minutes every day, then they can get vitamin D3 in the way of supplementing by taking an omega-3 fatty acid, or via foods loaded with vitamin E, such as: pumpkin seeds, asparagus, almonds, beta-carotene (carrots), blueberries and red grapes, and drinking green or black tea. Food knowledge is easy to find, but making sure the information is ACCURATE can be tricky with so many opinions out there on the internet. Educating ourselves through safe sources is the key to better health.

Back to the online gut healing program. Mom was doing really well on the program. She felt less inflamed, less bloated throughout her entire body, and

---

[6] Dr. Axe Co-founder of Ancient Nutrition, Leah Zurbe, "Best Sunscreens & Toxic Ones to Avoid" May 4, 2021 https://draxe.com/beauty/best-sunscreens/

her joints didn't ache. She had more energy and didn't have as much brain-fog, she said. She was very happy with the results so soon in the program, even though we were only one week into it. Despite only being a week into the program and having many positive changes myself, I struggled. It wasn't easy, and I wasn't giving up on this program.

JE June 28th, 2015
Very painful and hard day for me. Physically in a lot of pain. I had a huge lack of oxygen due to the intensity of the pain. I had headaches, low-back pain, left-side (three dimensional) pain, bloating, gas, belching, nausea, dizziness, and the burning fire feeling deep inside of me. My sinuses are stuffed up and I feel like vomiting. Major gut pain in my left side, neck, and back. Uffdah. Please Lord, I pray that this gut healing program would help me to begin to heal. The pain that I am in DAILY, like today, is so close to unbearable. I hurt so very bad physically all the time… I'm in miserable pain.

The next weeks of the program aided in taking toxins out of our bodies and lasted for two weeks, or longer for those who had increased symptoms. We extended this part beyond two weeks and into three. Mom thought I should extend it even longer, but I wanted to trudge through.

This part of the program was a lot harder, more intense, than I thought it was going to be. In addition to supplements that were taken daily (3-5 times per day), there were more food preparations and additional daily food plans with some new recipes. We chose to do daily coffee enemas and oil pulling, 3-5 detox baths and castor oil packs weekly, and a variety of self-care helps including exercise, quiet-time for reflection and healing in ALL aspects of our lives. These were all "optional methods" of cleansing. My days were so filled up with taking care of myself that I didn't have any extra time in a day, and actually having less time for sleeping at night. *This is INTENSE!* I'd thought to myself. There was a lot of information to read, along with live webinars to attend weekly throughout the entire program. Mom did a lot of the reading to keep us on task, and I followed her lead at those times. The supplements we were taking were specifically designed to promote the body to detoxify itself, so it worked well to incorporate the optional cleansing methods mentioned above to aid in the detoxification process. We were learning a LOT. These detoxing methods, many of which were new to us, really made me feel awkward, vulnerable, and uncomfortable… ESPECIALLY the coffee enemas.

If you don't already know what an enema is, here's what it is and how it works. An enema is a procedure where liquid in a hot water bottle bag or small enema pail is inserted through the rectum via a tube which is connected to the bottle or pail which holds the liquid--in our case holds coffee, and flows directly into one's body. Without further details of doing an enema correctly, a person lays on the bathroom floor while they "relax", allowing the liquid inserted into the rectum to flow directly into the colon/large intestine. Once the liquid has been held for (working up to) 10-20 minutes while in the fetal position, the person gets up from the floor and releases the liquids into the toilet. The procedure cleanses the colon of pathogens--die-off from the foods, supplements, and cleansing techniques we were doing in the three weeks. We did coffee enemas for three straight weeks, every day.

Some of my vulnerable and uncomfortable thoughts were, *who does enemas? I have to stick that tube up my rear? Coffee in my rear, are you kidding me? Am I dreaming or is this REALLY happening? There's got to be something else I can do instead of this. I've already been through the wringer the last five years. Can it get any more interesting than this?* Well, little did I know, coffee enemas were going to be MY BEST FRIEND that I'd be spending time with daily for the next almost two years.

Whether I liked this or not, I was in this for the long haul, completely unbeknownst to me at the time. And that is probably a good thing that I didn't know I'd be doing coffee enemas up to 2-3 times a day for the next year-plus. Had I known, who knows for sure if I'd chosen to keep going on that regimen. Coffee enemas were going to be THE KEY in moving toxins from my body, and moving out cancer from my pancreas in a future time coming near.

JE June 29th, 2015
I woke up to SEARING, RIPPING pain in my left side and abdomen. It continually got worse and I went through 3-4 waves of the pain. The left-side pain was truly maxed out this time. The nausea, dizziness, bloating, hot and cold sweats, fire feeling, cramps, searing pain, and headaches... it's so painful that I can't begin to explain. I have never had pain this bad. I nearly passed out numerous times, and was crying. Crying however, made the pain only worse so I was unable to REALLY do that. I tried to do an enema, but could literally only hold if for about two minutes. It gave me a little relief, enough so

172

that I could function through the day. Lord, how am I going to get through this gut healing program?

Trust me, God reassured me in my heart. My mind needed peace.

Tears trickled down my face. I knew that this process was not over yet, it had only just begun! "Okay, Lord. I trust You." I said out loud as a sense of peace engulfed my entire being.

42

Detoxing Isn't Easy

Kelly

During this time of doing an online gut healing program, I was implementing additional ways of healing into my life, of which I hadn't done before. For example, I tried doing a salt-water flush.

The first time I did a salt-water flush I had already been constipated for a few days. I felt like I needed to have a bowel movement but I couldn't move anything out. I was VERYmiserable. I was bloated, which only made the situation worse. My abdomen and back were in severe pain because of extra pressure in my gut.

A salt-water flush consists of drinking 32oz. of pure water and two tablespoons of Himalayan Sea salt mixed in. I chugged the mixture down and waited for the "whoosh" effect. The "whoosh" was supposed to take toxins out of my body, and in turn clean my intestines, aiding in the detoxification process. Within 15-30 minutes, I was supposed to feel the "whoosh" effect, and proceed to the bathroom to detoxify—eliminate the concoction I'd drank and taking out with it the toxins from inside my gut. I waited two hours, never getting the "whoosh"! This made my bloating, abdominal pain, and back pain even worse! *My gut felt like it was going to explode!* I couldn't touch my abdomen it hurt so bad, let alone put any kind of pressure on it. My head was pounding with an explosive headache. I felt absolutely miserable and sick, not to mention super constipated!

Since the salt-water flush did not work, I needed to try something else. *What's next?* I thought.

At my age, then 23 years old, like I already said in the last chapter, I learned how to do a coffee enema. Mom taught me how to do the enema. When I first started doing coffee enemas, I had no idea that I would end up doing enemas as often as I did. Coffee enemas were my best friend throughout the whole gut healing program! As the program got more intense, I was doing coffee enemas daily, because I ended up constipated through the entire program. *What's going on?* I thought. If you recall, prior to this program I had diarrhea 5–15 times daily.

Enemas helped to eliminate toxins quickly, detoxifying my body. They cleansed and hydrated my colon (depending on the type of enema), and killed bad bacteria's such as fungus, bad pathogens, parasites, bacterial overgrowths, and who knows for sure what else in my opinion!

Enemas are a good way for all people to detoxify. Why? Because when a person's body builds up with toxicity, their organs become stressed. When organs are stressed, they can't function optimally. Over time, the organs grow weaker and can't maintain their function. This is very hard on not only organs, but the entire body. This welcomes illness into our lives.

Depending on a person's state of health, the detoxification process can be easy or hard. For me, detoxing wasn't easy. My body was so built up with toxins that I needed to detoxify more than a normal "healthy" person. I was doing daily enemas because I was constipated. Since I was constipated, that meant that the toxins weren't getting out of my body. In turn, I had more abdominal and back pain, and many other increased symptoms. There were times that I needed to do a second, or even a third enema in a single day.

So how did I know that I needed to do another enema? I could tell by the signs and symptoms my body was giving me. I had learned to listen and become in-tune with my body over the past few years. When I knew that I needed to do a second enema, my symptoms were exacerbated. The low back, which was normally a dull ache, was painfully increased. It hurt to bend over or move. I could only stand or lay down flat on the floor when my low back hurt. It felt like my back was going to burst at these times. My entire abdomen would bloat and hurt. I was no longer as gassy, which was awesome! The left side in my upper abdomen, directly underneath the ribs, just to the left of center of my body, felt like it was on fire deep inside my body. The heat would penetrate outward throughout my entire left abdomen. The heat extended from under the ribs to just below my belly button. At times it felt like a knife was puncturing through my abdomen going straight through into my back. That searing hot, electrifying, painful spot in my abdomen was the same spot that went into my back, just to the left of the spine. It was that deep inside my body.

Other symptoms that I had when I needed to do an enema included feeling like I needed to have a bowel movement, but couldn't physically have one. I would get abdominal cramps along with searing, red hot, fiery pain under my ribs. Headaches would make my head feel like it was going to explode. I was nauseated and dizzy. I'd feel like vomiting. Hot and cold sweats were intense, often leaving me feeling weak. Over all I felt very ill, plain sick and tired.

By listening and being in-tune with my body I was able to learn these signs and symptoms in order to help my detoxification process. All the things that I had learned while working with prior health professionals the last few years were still being applied. I especially thought of all the important aspects of healthy living Dr. Ann had taught me, which I was continually reminded of. Everything had happened for a reason, and I had been prepared during the last few years to be where I was at during this time.

There was a specific routine that I needed to accomplish each day, for my own mental well-being. I was determined to execute that routine, to give my best offering to regain my health. As Mom said, "Kelly is devoted to clean living. She's totally 100% on this." And I was. I wasn't able to travel or stay overnight anywhere--I had daily coffee enemas to do each morning! In addition, I wanted to help make all our meals, which took coordinated time. I was eating ALL organic, whole, nourishing foods that would aid in the healing of my body. For the past five years I had made the decision that I would feed my body what it needed to bring healing. I continue to do that. I wasn't going to cheat just because it was inconvenient or I was traveling.

"If you fail to plan, you plan to fail." -Benjamin Franklin

I wasn't going to put myself in a position to fail. If failure came, it wasn't going to be on my part. I'd have NO REGRETS with my choice because my health and life were at stake. I couldn't afford that risk.

43

Plans and Goals

Amy

Does a person need to have a plan in place, or goals set, to keep them putting one foot in front of the other toward accomplishing something or to have success? What is success, really? Good questions, I think.

During the summer of 2015, we set out planning a winter 2016 trip to Hawaii for a family vacation combined with Kelly doing a class for her work-related "Continuing Education" requirements. Kelly had been talking of going to Hawaii for a number of years before this time. Hawaii was a place she was considering she would like to live, but definitely a visit there would be necessary. Kelly was really stepping out, putting it into action, by telling me she was going to GO there for a work-related reason, some sun, and fun. She also said she "was determined to be well (in health) by then." She had set a goal on a semi-vague timeline.

My response, on this particular day of her talking about not just someday going to Hawaii, but actually GOING there was, "What a great idea, Kelly, to take your class, see Hawaii, and get some sun! That would be fun! I think you should definitely look into this! Do you have anybody else that you think might like to join you taking the class you're looking into?"

Kelly set the goal in her mind to go to Hawaii AND stated aloud, "to be well in health" by the time the trip would take place, and she was determined. She was ALL IN for going somewhere warm!

We talked to my husband, Darren, and Kelly's brother, Troy, to see what they thought of going to Hawaii. Not only were those two in, but so was one of my sisters, Lori, and her husband Brad, when I told them about the possibility of Kelly taking a class there and seeing if they'd like to go, too! Kelly also asked around if anyone wanted to take the class with her, then she herself signed up for the class. The six of us, for sure, would be going to Hawaii the next winter!

Gone were the days of out-of-state alpine skiing trips with her brother to chilly winter climates. Kelly's body couldn't take the cold outdoor winter activity all day outside anymore, especially with the symptoms she'd been experiencing the last year. She was seriously considering the idea of moving to a warmer climate, once she was well again. "Hawaii is a place I may like to live. I should really check it out," she'd stated months before, "...and learn how to surf, too!"

For real? I'd thought, when she'd stated that moving to Hawaii part! I should have seen this coming. I was thinking maybe she'd want to live in a location south central in the United States on the mainland, a drive up to 10-16 hours away. I'd not imagined her wanting to live in Hawaii! But it was her life and her choice, so who was I or anyone else to sway her otherwise if that was her dream and goal. And learning to surf? That, I knew, was something she had wanted to do for REAL, on REAL ocean waves, not just behind our wakeboarding boat "wake-setter" she and her brother played in the lake on a wake surf-board...which she was really good at--having great balance!

It wasn't long before I got to looking on-line for where, on the island of Oahu, HI, we would stay for next year's adventure! Honolulu, the capital of HI, was on the island, as well as "Pearl Harbor" and multiple other interactive, fun attractions to ocean water activities that we were all interested in for one reason or another, and of course, Kelly's class was there.

We talked back and forth with my sister over accommodations to stay at. We needed to be somewhere that we could make our own meals. Eating out would not be an option for Kelly, although in the future something could change and then maybe she could eat out again! Who knew for sure? We looked at bungalows and villas, but ultimately, we agreed to renting a 4-bedroom house along the "North Shore" of the island. Pictures of the rental house on-line showed the imagery to perk my own imagination. "Oh, joy!" I imagined that this place would be therapeutic every morning and night, to sit out on the lanai watching and listening to the ocean waves crashing onto the beach for eight full days! Perhaps Troy and Kelly would go surfing right out front on the ocean from our rental house and we could watch from the lanai, or from on the beach in front of the house.

I'm not going to jump ahead and tell you about the ups, and more ups, of that trip because we're just not there in the unfolding story yet! The point is, we made our plans, and Kelly set her goal to be well in health by that midwinter trip coming up in 7.5 months or so! *This goal is doable*, I'd thought to myself. *I sure hope that she will be well by then.*

During the summer of 2015, we had so much hope for healing going into the online gut healing program. The week of preparing for the program I had to get off of sugar. Truth be told, I had a red "Twizzlers" addiction. There was nothing good for me in those plastic pieces of artificial food. *I know, what was I thinking?* The craving for them never totally went away during the program, and I gave into the cravings at times. I was not eating dairy and grains before the program, for the most part, so it could had been worse. I didn't crave bread or cheese. But "Twizzlers", seriously? Yes, seriously. I longed for them.

After three days, the sugar cravings (but not specifically for red "Twizzlers") left. I was onboard for the program. It was good for both Kelly and me. The next weeks would be challenging with "to do's", but we both pitched in and helped one another, making a way for healing to begin for Kelly.

And that, our friends, is what happened. Healing began by starting to detox pathogens out from inside of her body (and mine too). It was not an easy road, but it was worth every effort she put into it.

During the program, I saw the need for us to extend detoxing to further eliminate toxins from our bodies, as we were mid into the initial week of the detoxing. Kelly agreed to taking an extra week. We would be a week behind in the program, but that wouldn't "set us back" per say. We had a change of plan, but would still accomplish our goal to complete the program. Which brings me to my original question: Does a person need to have a plan in place and goals set to keep them putting one foot in front of the other toward accomplishing success? And really, what is success?

First of all, everyone has their own definition of what success looks like. So, what may look like success to me may look like failure to you. The definition of success is very personal and individualized. I don't think I need to explain that any further. We all get it, right?

Secondly, I personally believe that plans and goals can be great, but they can also become a burden, troublesome, limiting further "growth" or walking a "better road". Here's an example: Say I set my mind to a project and having it done by a certain date. As the project moves along, new ideas about the project make way and I choose to flow with them. Great, the project became a better project that I really like more-so than the original plan. As the planned date to be done with the project nears, I am obviously going to miss the mark to attain that first set goal of a date to be done. Is this a problem? No, not really. But, depending on if my mind HAD been set to meet that deadline date, then it would have been a problem. Being the plan changed, becoming a better project, more time will be needed to execute the plan. That is not a problem for me. But it might be a problem for the next person. See what I mean?

Another example: Let's say I have a goal to make so much money in a year, and plan for in multiple years of making so much money each year so I could attain a goal of making a set number of dollars in a set number of years. I start my first year meeting my goal for the larger goal in place. Great. During the second year, some issues occur that throw me off to meeting my larger goal. No problem, I'll work harder the next year. So, I do. During the years I've committed to attain each year's goal for the greater plan, I see how I've missed out on many opportunities that I hadn't foreseen. Was it worth sticking to my plan to accomplish my goals? The answer to that is also very individualized. One person may say, "Yes, I attained my goal by executing my plan!" without hesitation. Yet, another person may look back and think, *I wish I would have… blah, blah, blah.* In that case it wasn't worth it. The person had regrets, having lost out on other opportunities.

The bottom line is that we each have to find out for ourselves what's right for us, to set goals and make plans, to stick with them no matter what, to be lenient in allowing the plans or goals to shift, change or discontinue, or to not have any plans and just see what happens along the journey. That last one may sound really scary. I'll be the first to say it: YES, it is scary not having a plan and seeing what happens on the journey.

I believe we have opportunities of faith presented to us during our lives. Opportunities to trust in something we cannot see with our physical eyes "to be" or "to happen". Trusting in an idea, a dream, or a knowing, to present itself to us at a future time that we have no control over… is that scary? Yes! Is it exciting? Maybe, for some! For me, not everything in my life has to have a plan in place. As for goals? Yes, they are great. But I don't stay the course when everything in me is telling me to change something, to take a turn in the road, or flat-out stop reaching for a set goal when seeing that the road has changed before me and that I may need to change my plans. That's really okay with me. But maybe not for another person.

And so it goes, we all live our lives. Roads traveled, lessons learned, plans executed, or plans changed, goals set, goals disrupted, faith put into action, dreams fulfilled… you get the drift. I hope the plans we are making, the goals being set, and the lives lived by faith, are working out for everyone's personal destiny and best possible life scenarios. That said, I'm not saying I wish everyone be happy and free of any kind of adversity, cause gosh, if nothing hard had ever happened in our lives it sure would give us less character-building opportunities and reasons to change for the better.

44

A Typical Day

Kelly

July 2015. What did a typical day look like at this point in life? I would get up between 6:30-8am, go upstairs and start my coffee. No, my coffee wasn't your usual morning cup of coffee that you sit back and relax, sipping on while reading the paper. No, it was made for the purpose of doing a coffee enema. Nothing like a little coffee to kick start a person's day, right?

While the coffee brewed, I would do my morning facial skincare and cleaning my teeth routines, then prepare food and feed Mr. Rabbi. It took me exactly 13 minutes to get Mr. Rabbi's food ready for the day, feed and pet him, and let him out of his hutch so he could go play with Goofy (who would accompany me out the door every morning to feed Mr. Rabbi). I'd make sure my two furry amigos were "okay" and "safe" before I'd come back in, 13 minutes later.

When I'd get back inside, the coffee would be done brewing. I'd cool the coffee to a reasonable temp with some ice cubes, load the enema bag with coffee, then head to the bathroom for the enema, which typically took 40 minutes. Morning coffee. Check.

Following morning coffee, I would help Mom cook our breakfast. Breakfast always filled us up. We also took the program supplements at breakfast time. By the time my morning routine and breakfast were completed, it would be anywhere between 8:30-10am, depending on if it was a work day or be at home day.

After breakfast I would get some exercise by going for a brisk walk. I kept my muscles toned by walks and by doing some simple resistance strengthening

182

with the "Bow-Flex" machine for about 10-15 minutes. I'd sweat during my workout, so that was an additional way to aid in detoxing. Workout completed. Check. After morning exercise, I would shower and either go to work, or be on my days off at home.

Mom and I chose to drink a variety of healing teas daily. Each day we would drink these in addition to LOTS of water. I consumed between 1.5-2 gallons of water per day. Remember, our bodies NEED water, daily!

Time flew by quickly during the given hours of a day. We ate very well on the program! Our lunches usually consisted of our own homemade-soups with boiled chicken added to it. We might have a small side of a specific salad from the program. We'd add ghee, chunks of baked squash, or a handful of parsley on the side. Parsley is a great detoxifier, a cancer preventer, promoting better bone health, and is alkalizing to our PH balance, BTW. Homemade ghee--is organic butter baked at a low temp to separate the dairy from the butter-oil, then the dairy is sieved from the oil. The oil is then cooled and stored. YUM! We LOVE ghee! Home made ghee, in my opinion, is much better than store bought ghee.

By mid-afternoon I usually felt tired. I'd want to stop and take a nap. However, that wasn't an option when working. Rarely did I ever take time for a real nap, but there were days that I could lay out in the sun and rest for a while soaking in the rays of warmth!

Some days I would have an afternoon snack. And for supper we had a variety of foods. We cooked our meals according to what we wanted to eat daily that fit into the dietary plan of our online program's group specifications.

During this time, I worked at my business in town from 11am -5pm, and as late as 9pm two nights a week. A typical work day could average anywhere from 4-8 hours of massage per workday. A majority of the time it averaged to five hours of massage daily. This amount was perfect during this season of the gut healing program. I would be at work a full day, four days a week, so whatever number of massages that ended up scheduling each day always worked out fine. A full-time massage therapist usually looks to have 20 hours of massages per week. I'd spend 35-40 hours per week at work, but on average half that time is hands-on work.

I liked going to work! It's a 20-minute drive both to and from work. Upon returning home after work, I would alternate days of either taking a detox bath or applying a castor oil pack to my liver. Each of those averaged 25 minutes up to an hour of time, daily. If I was feeling really ill in the evening after coming home from work, I would do a coffee enema again. I also showered again each night. The hot water was refreshing to my abdominal and back. It helped to loosen the muscles and for me to forget my pain, momentarily.

Each night before bed, I would do 15-30 minutes of stretching to help relax my body. After accomplishing a day's tasks, I would tuck myself into bed between 9pm and midnight, depending if it was a workday or not. Bedtime was usually always closer to 11pm-midnight on workdays.

Days were LONG, and it took a lot of energy to get through them. There were lots of days that I didn't have energy. Those days, I had to focus on getting through each hour. The days were full, focusing on my own healing, detoxifying, and working, not to mention regular tasks anyone of us has in a day!

At the end of the day, I would crawl into bed, often times in the fetal position, being so exhausted that I couldn't get to sleep. I also journaled every night: the foods I'd eaten, symptoms that I'd experienced, remembrances of the day, thoughts I'd had, and sometimes the prayers I prayed. I'd journaled since I'd went to the acupuncturist, and I'm glad I journaled because it let me express myself and be free in so many ways. It also aided in looking back to help in this book writing!

So, you see, I had my daily routine. Truth be told, bedtime was my life saver. I loved my rest. Sleep is important, so take your sleep seriously! Your body LOVES routine, especially when it comes to the subject of sleep. It is best if we can be consistent with sleep, getting 7-9 hours a night. I was not getting that much sleep yet at this time, but in a future time, good rest did return. I had a long way to go to gain my health back. But healing is a process and I had now come to accept that in fullness.

I was changing, from the inside out. And with each day, my health was too. It had taken years for me to become this way, ill, and it would take time to reverse my ill health--step by step, one foot in front of the other, hour to hour, day to day. I was totally committed. I was ALL IN. My mindset was good (for the most part) and I had truly changed my mindset. Depression was now virtually gone due to using food as medicine and nutritional supplements. I was optimistic and was now looking at seeing the good in every circumstance, especially my health. I knew this illness was happening for a reason, and now I was truly embracing it in FULLNESS.

45

Finding Freedom

Kelly

During the detoxing part of the program, we were doing online, the days were literally hit-and-miss with no rhyme or reason as to WHY I felt good, felt really good, felt bad, or felt really bad. However, throughout the entire program I can honestly say that I was beginning to feel better daily, better than I ever had in the two years prior to starting this program.

I was disciplined and determined, knowing what I had to accomplish in order to improve my health. I stayed focused on this. It was hard for many reasons, one being that I didn't have the time or energy to do any extra "fun activities". Opportunities came up from friends to get together for the weekend, which I chose to say, "Thanks, but that just isn't going to work." Events were declined. Gatherings for holidays came up, which always revolved around food, and so I easily backed out of at that season of life by simply saying, "I'm sorry but I can't."

I also gave up activities I loved to do because I didn't have extra energy to do them. One example was hunting. I had been duck hunting since I was eleven years old. I had hunted for eleven years, which was half of my life at the time. I choose to give up all hunting: deer, turkey, and duck, the fall of 2015, for three main reasons. The **first** reason was the most important, the deer ate genetically modified grains in local farm fields where I'd hunted on our property which was in close proximity to the farm crops. Crops of corn, wheat, and soy beans are grown in the midwestern United States in large production, but where I live it surrounds us and is everywhere. I wasn't going to eat meat that was contaminated by GMOs. Also, there were chemicals sprayed on the crops the deer grazed on, which also contaminates the meat. As for waterfowl, they were exposed to these GMO's and chemicals through watersheds in the area, whether the waterfowl grew here or came in from elsewhere, and then having no idea what they'd been eating.

To those that may think that wild game is the cleanest meat, or wild game is organic, I'm sorry to say that this is not ALWAYS and accurate belief. Just because wild game is out in the "wild" doesn't mean that it is organic. GMOs are not organic. Hence, if wild game is eating GMO crops or are feeding in contaminated water, the wild game is not organic, nor is it "clean meat", but rather contaminated GMO meat. Where I live, we have mostly all GMO grown crops. Our game meat is not organic, and this is what I've learned. I am just stating what I've come to believe. We each are entitled to our own opinion, and our choice of what we eat.

The **second** reason I gave up hunting was that I wasn't going to shoot an animal that I wasn't going to eat. I believe there is no reason to shoot an animal just for "the thrill" of it. That belief was based on a respect for myself and for the animal.

The **third** reason for laying my gun down and stepping back from hunting played the *least* role in matter of importance. The reason being, I didn't have the energy. On days that I worked doing massage I exerted extra energy. My energy reserves were depleted, which made sleep very important for me. I couldn't afford to lose precious sleep; therefore, no more lost hours getting up early to go hunting.

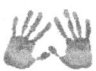

Giving up hunting was easy, but yet it wasn't because of one big factor; my dad. My dad taught me how to duck hunt. He'd sat with me through my "Firearm Safety Course", was the one whom first taught me the basics of how to hold and shoot a gun, and later how to hold and shoot a bow and arrow, which came in handy when I started deer hunting in my late teen years with a bow and arrow. In addition, Dad taught me safety for myself and those around me when hunting.

187

My dad grew up duck hunting. It is precious to him because HE grew up duck hunting with HIS dad. Dad loved to hunt and gave me the opportunity to learn to hunt, too, if I choose. It was my choice, kind of as a little kid. That being said, if I wanted to go hunting that meant I had to get up really early in the morning.

Dad, my brother, Troy, and I would arrive at a slough or field early in the morning, unload all our gear and set up all the decoys, get tucked into the weeds or hunting blind all before the sun would rise. Shortly after sunrise we could legally shoot. If we were going hunting in a slough, this meant all of us would have to wear waterproof waders. Wearing waders made it possible to trudge through thick muck in order to get to our destination. At times the muck would be up to our knees. One time in my early years, Dad had to come and lift me out of the muck because I was stuck, unable to move or lift my muck-sunk boots! It was always a tough walk going through muck to shoot ducks! Duck hunting exerted a lot of energy.

I have a lot of special hunting memories made with my guys growing up. To give up hunting meant giving up time spent with those two. The three of us hunted together virtually every weekend during duck season in the fall. It wasn't easy to tell them, "I'm not going to hunt anymore." Furthermore, "I can't. This is a decision that I'm making for myself and my health. I hope that you each can respect this decision. It has nothing to do with either of you. I love you both." And then I explained myself more in depth with reasons one and two, stated earlier.

"I respect your decision, Kelly. I'm sure going to miss my hunting partner though. What am I going to do without you?" Troy had told me.

"You do what you need to do, Kelly. If you change your mind, you're always welcome to join us." Dad had said. I knew it was going to be hard for Dad to understand that I was giving up hunting, forever. He, like myself, loves nature and wildlife. Hunting was a time my dad and I shared together watching beautiful birds fly around us and land in the decoys. Instead of shooting them, at times we would sit in awestruck wonder, enamored by their simple elegant beauty and gracefulness in flight. My choosing to not hunt wasn't easy for him to accept. It felt like a death for him, I'm sure. Who ever said change is easy? It's not.

Change isn't always easy, or comfortable! Sometimes change is uncomfortable, stressful, and frustrating! We have our need-to-do list, want-to-do list, and our general go-to to-do list, making us pressed for time. Seems there's never enough time. We have deadlines to make, meetings to attend, and are on time frames due to our hectic schedules. We are stressed, and our bodies are stressed due to our hectic lives! Our lives have the ability to become so hectic that when we are introduced to something new, change, how do we react? For example, when we try a new food, meet a stranger who could turn into a new friend, walk into a room with two people arguing or making out, a devastating or surprise event occurs, or we move to a new area. ALL of these new changes can be hard, uncomfortable, new, frightening, or exciting! Our reaction to any change is life absorbing. Meaning, change affects us at all times.

We can choose to embrace change in our lives or we can choose to reject change. Rejection, often times, will only leave us bitter and unhappy. Choosing to "reject" in general, in many circumstances, means we aren't being open to change in our life. It means we are running away from our problems and fears instead of engaging, figuring out a situation, and embracing change.

Giving up hunting didn't just affect my life; it affected the lives of those around me too. But I can honestly say that giving up hunting was a great decision for me. How each individual choses to let my choice of giving up hunting affect them was their choice, just like it was my choice to give it up. Laying my gun down opened up new opportunities for healing in my life.

Throughout the online gut healing program and those past five years combined, I learned that I needed to embrace change. Until the age of eighteen, for the most part, I had rejected change. I liked my "comfortable" life. I didn't want any new, drastic, uncomfortable changes. Bottom line was, I was afraid of change. I grew up with relatives who had these same traits. I don't think this was a genetic trait, but a learned trait being passed down from generation to generation. I learned from these relatives to not be open to, or accepting of change. When a new change or opportunity had come into my life, I chose to reject it just like I saw them doing. They, too, were scared of change! People can blame it on "genetics" saying this trait was in my blood. However, I say it is a CHOICE. I didn't have to follow their choices, letting it take control of my life. I no longer was living in fear, in the past, or letting choices I made in the past define me and my life. When this happened, I embracing change, I started taking big strides in my personal growth.

Life is precious and should be lived to its fullest. I had been holding myself back all of these years of growing up by not being willing to be REAL and transparent with people, and stepping out of my comfort zone. My life from being sick--dis-ease, to being well again--ease, was continually changing for the better. And with that my life got harder, too. Freedom doesn't come free of some kind of cost.

46

A Close Call

Kelly

During the start of detoxing while doing the online gut healing program, I started all the supplements at the full dosages. I knew I was going to feel miserable whether I started them at a quarter, or half-dosage, or full-strength. This was MY CHOICE to start at the full dosage. I'd been told before the program started that "a person with my specific severe gut health should start all supplements at a low dosage." I need to be clear on this, because it was not the programs' fault for my choosing to do what I did at this time in taking the full dose. I am responsible for my choices and the results of those choices.

The supplements had an immediate and direct impact on my gut. The first few days were miserable for me. My symptoms were all exacerbated. My abdomen was very bloated, making it difficult to breathe deep. Headaches were constant and intense, especially immediately after taking the supplements. My left, upper abdomen, underneath my ribs, hurt deep inside the core of my being, going straight through my body into my back. I was waking up in the wee hours of the morning, although not consistently every night. And, I was still constipated since the start of the program.

One morning about a week into detoxing, I had a close call. I got up from bed not feeling well. I hadn't slept sound that night, feeling like I'd not slept at all. I got up, glanced into a mirror looking very pale. I had a pounding headache, was nauseated, had an upset stomach and a bloated, hurting abdomen. By the time I had managed to change from my pajamas into clothes, and walked upstairs into the living room, I'd laid back down on the couch feeling as though I'd had used up all my energy. I laid there for a while, then the hot and cold sweats started. *Dang it.* I thought. I was on my left side, holding my abdomen and back, in utter pain. I was nauseated during the night of sleeplessness, and it had only continued getting worse. My head felt like it was going to explode. I closed my eyes, praying it would all get better.

Mom had come into the kitchen, which is just off the living room where I was laying on the couch, the two areas having no wall between the two. She didn't know I was laying there. She started doing a task and then stopped. In the silence, I moaned to get her attention. She came over to me immediately, looking at me with grave concern.

"What's going on? You're in pain." She stated knowingly. At the same time, stomach cramps ripped through my abdomen. I had been laying on my left side with my legs extended straight out, but as the searing pain ripped into me like an electrical current, my legs immediately drew up to my chest into the fetal position. "Do you need to go to the emergency room?" She asked. I shook my head "no" in response. Over the course of the next 15 minutes the pain increased. "Where is your pain, Kelly? What can I do to help you? Do you want some water?" I pointed to where the pain was and she reached out, touching my abdomen. Her gentle touch hurt, so I grabbed her hand and threw it off my abdomen. I have a very high pain tolerance but this pain was off my pain chart, making it unbearable. The cramps continued, each growing worse than the last. My breathing was very shallow as I couldn't take deep breaths. I held my bloated abdomen. The heat pouring off of my abdomen was hot. It felt like it was on fire! It hurt to touch it, so I moved my hands towards my chest, withering in pain. The electrical bolts of pain continued, sporadic as a switch going on and off, I never knowing when they would flip on or off. My headache got so intense that I couldn't open my eyes. Alternating hot and cold sweats turned to just hot sweats pouring off my body. I was nauseated and completely miserable. I was reacting harshly to the supplements I'd taken full doses of.

Mom got a cool, wet, wash cloth, attempting to cool me down. She brought a glass of water with, helping me to get a small drink down before another bolt of pain ripped through me. For another 20 minutes I battled the striking pains. It felt like an eternity had passed before the pain subsided. I would have loved to let sobs out from deep inside my soul, but I couldn't. Instead, I did what I had learned over the course of the last few years. Ever so quietly and softly, tears flooded down my face. I didn't stop them. The damn had broken loose. Mom cried with me. Slightly begging, she asked, "Kelly, are you SURE you don't need to go to the emergency room?"

Mom had asked me this same question dozens of times in the last few years. My answer was still the same. "No. We'd just be paying for me to use their bathroom. I don't need to throw up all over their floor when I can do it 'comfortably' right here at home. Doctors would try putting me on medications, making me sicker." Pain grabbed my abdomen, searing through me again. I cried out, withering in pain. It finally passed and I finished my thoughts. "The doctors would want to run thousands of dollars of tests. As before, they'd all come back 'normal'. I would then get labeled IBS (irritable bowel syndrome) again. So, do I want to go to the emergency room? NO!"

"Kelly, I can't handle seeing you in all this pain. I feel absolutely helpless. There is nothing I can do." Mom softly cried. That said, another pain started deep inside my abdomen. I was completely immobile. My mom put her hand ever so gently onto my low back as I unsuccessfully attempted to muffle a shout in agonizing pain. I was drenched in sweat. I thought, *my head is going to explode, and my gut is too.* I could do absolutely nothing to stop the pain. My gut burned like FIRE. My abdomen, going into my back three-dimensionally, felt like a furnace. The burn started from deep inside the inner most part of my body.

I finally responded to her, "Pray Mom. That's what you can do for me." The fire was ragging intensely.

During the last few years, I had times that I was immobile because of this same kind of pain. However, it usually lasted between a half-an-hour up to 2-3 hours. More often than not I'd been successful to limp through it. This time, however, I couldn't wither away from the pain. It hurt so bad that I couldn't move when I tried. *If the pain gets any worse, I'm not sure I will be able to handle it.* I had been immobile over the entire course of this time on the couch. My whole body hurt from the trauma it was enduring. I put my head over the side of the couch into the garbage can beside me. My stomach wretched. Nothing came out except acid. I spit, feeling helpless. My body was in shock. *God help me,* I prayed deep inside my heart. After one more wave ripped through me, the pain slowly got less intense. Mom, seeing my pain had diminished to a bearable state, decided to contact the program's customer service team. She labeled the email URGENT, hoping that they would read her important message. In the email she described my pain, telling them details of the shock and how I had been immobile from the current pain. She asked them questions, trying to get help for me. Mom prayed the customer service team would read her urgent email and get back with answers.

A half-an-hour had passed. I felt better. I attempted moving from the fetal position. *Success!* My legs shook, hesitantly. The hot sweats had ended. The cold sweats started. After a few minutes of laying straight with my legs fully stretched out, I wanted to get up and change clothes. I was drenched in sweat. I also wanted water. I reached for my glass of water unsteadily, as my head was spinning. As my head started to fall towards the floor, I put my arm out catching myself as Mom grabbed my upper body. She helped push me back onto the couch, while grabbing the glass of water. I slowly sat up from the couch, managing a few cool sips of water from the glass. After, I tried to stand hanging onto the couch, feeling exhausted. My abdomen was so woozy, I sat back down.

Mom and I discussed what we both thought my abdominal pain was from. I knew deep in my heart it was a result of the full dosage of supplements, they were doing their job in my body, trying to extract the toxins built-up inside of me. As I shared my thoughts with Mom, she smiled, agreeing with me. "I can't stop taking the supplements, Mom. I know they are doing exactly what I need them to be doing to detoxify the pathogens from inside of me. I'm going to continue taking them." I stated softly.

"I agree. Those are my thoughts exactly, Kelly. I love you!" Mom said and we shared a smile.

"Thanks, Mom. I love you too!" After a few more minutes of talking, the pain started again. I was absolutely exhausted from the last rounds. *How was I going to endure yet another excruciating escapade?*

47

Fading In - Fading Out

Kelly

I'd like to take a moment to say, PLEASE read this chapter with an open mind of "there is a bigger picture going on here" than just reading about the pain and suffering. What I mean, is that God was using this all to bring about so many amazing things, and in the midst of this pain going on, I knew and trusted that. So please, bear with me while I tell my story more specifically about the bigger picture throughout this and the next chapters to come.

Picking up from "A Close Call". *How was I going to endure another excruciating round of pain?* I resumed the fetal position on my left side, laying back down on the couch in the living room. Pain seared through my abdomen with an intensity that was worse than earlier. *I would have welcomed death at this point if I truly WANTED to die.* My whole body burned with hot pain, especially my abdomen and back. It was a FIRE that seared from the deepest most inner part of my core, *it took my breath away.* I attempted to breathe but at times I couldn't. I couldn't move. Any movement was like a lightning bolt. All of a sudden, the pain stopped. My stomach had an upset feeling. I realized *I need to get to the bathroom.* Then came another pain in my abdomen that burned. *I have to get to the bathroom right now!* I was NOT going to mess myself! "I need to get to the bathroom, Mom." I candidly told her.

Mom helped me upright on the couch and up to my feet on the floor. We hobbled to the bathroom. I stooped over, favoring my left side, attempting to bring relief. The pain grabbed me with such a vengeance I doubled over onto the floor, crying out, but stopped because that made the pain worse. Mom cried for me, holding my head in her lap and trying to touch my abdomen. Again,

195

like before, I threw her hand away. "NO! It hurts." I muttered. Exhausted, I tried to concentrate. *The pain. I hurt. Help, Papa.*

"I'm sorry, Kelly." Mom said, sobbing. For the next one-half-of-an hour I struggled through searing bolts of red-hot abdominal pains and hot and cold sweats, all leaving me weak.

During this time, I was so nauseated. At times the bathroom would spin. My eyes closed because the light hurt them. And then, my eyes rolled to the back of my head through closed eye lids. I fought for control. Pains continued ripping through my abdomen. I tried to move in an attempt to escape it all. I'd arch my back trying to get relief, unsuccessfully. Moving made the pain worse. I realized, thinking *my energy is fading.*

I couldn't breathe when the pain raked through me. My head felt like it was going to explode. Sweat dripped off my forehead, my chest, and down my back. My stomach felt like it was in my throat. I was fading in and out of consciousness. I lifted my abdomen in a feeble attempt to get away from the pain. I didn't have any energy to move. I tried to hold my gut. I COULDN'T hold it due to the raging fire going on inside.

At times I could hear, and then it would be dead silent. I fought for control to stay conscious. It took all of my focus to be present. I reeled trying to squirm from myself. *Help!* was my only prayer. I had no energy. "Exhausted" didn't begin to define what I felt. My abdomen hurt like never before in my life. I fought to stay present and focused. *I'm spinning. The room is spinning. I just want to be done with all this pain.*

While fading in and out of consciousness, I'd been completely unaware that Mom was praying out loud. The only thing I remember were my eyes rolling to the back of my head. I was oblivious to what was happening around me. I was fading fast.

One last red-hot electrical shock of pain seared through me. I yelled out, arching my body trying to free myself. *My head is going to burst.* I tried to open my eyes in a last attempt to stay conscious. I opened them, but all I saw was the color gray. I closed my eyes. And then I couldn't hear a single thing.

196

Peace. Quiet. I had no oxygen left in me. There was utter silence. I felt, heard, and saw nothing. I was present in the gray. I'd lost consciousness, for a brief time. Somewhere deep inside my brain, I was still fighting for life and I was somehow aware of that. My body knew, even in my unconscious state, that I wasn't giving in to death. Then there was light, and I was moving towards the light while hearing Papa God's voice. "My daughter, you can come home to me now. Or, you can go back and finish the work I've set for you to do."

Without hesitation I responded in my thought, *"I'm not finished yet."* And just like that, suddenly, I could hear around me. I was alive again. Papa had more in store for me, and I was ready to be His hands and feet here on earth. Sobs were coming from Mom, who was still praying and holding my head in her lap. I took a BIG breath. *I can BREATHE!* The intense pain had stopped. In its place, a very achy abdomen. My low back felt like it was going to burst, and a few small cramps grabbed at my abdomen, but I was able to breathe through them while letting them pass.

Twenty minutes later, all the cramps and surging hot pains were gone. I could breathe normal again. I could see clearly! A headache was still present. I could hear it pound. My clothes were wet. My body was drenched in sweat. The abdominal pain was back to its normal dull ache deep inside the inner most part of my being. My low back pain was terrible, so I tried cracking my back, which helped release some of the pain when it did crack. I was thirsty. *I need water!* My whole being was totally exhausted. I was ready to sleep. I felt like I could sleep on the rug right there on the bathroom floor.

I need to get up and drink some water. Slowly I sat up, which caused the bathroom to spin as I leaned against the vanity. It took a few minutes before I was unsteadily standing, then took a few steps, paused, and walked out of the bathroom into the kitchen. I sat at the kitchen counter drinking the glass of water Mom gave me. She sat down next to me. "Do you still think you got sick from the supplements, Kelly?" she inquired.

"Yes, without a doubt in my mind. The supplements ARE doing their job, which is a GOOD thing."

"I think your body is detoxing too fast." Mom said. "The supplements are grabbing the toxins, causing the die-off effects. Your body can't keep up quickly enough to move them out. Those toxins REALLY need to get out of your body."

"I agree. My body couldn't keep up with it. I'm not going to take any of the supplements the rest of today or tomorrow, but I will the next day. That way my body can have a little break to recover." I said matter-of-factly.

"I'm so glad to hear that. I was hoping that you weren't going to quit taking them altogether." Mom smiled.

"No. I'm going to keep taking them. I need to get this body detoxified so I can heal and move forward with my life." I knowingly spoke. I continued to sip my water and think. *I was gone. Like, really gone. God, you brought me back. You have bigger and better things in store for my life. You have brought me out from the deepest, hardest, and most painful experience. You are and have always been paving the way for me. I get it. I DO trust You, Papa. You have not only saved me once, but You've saved me twice. My life is truly in Your hands, and I'm eternally grateful. I'm a living miracle.*

I opened my mouth, telling Mom all of what had just happened. She listened, intently, in wonder as tears continued swelling in her eyes, freely flowing down her face. We embraced in a long, long hug as I felt gratitude swelling inside of my heart. *It is good to be here. I am forever thankful, Papa God.*

48

Keeping It REAL

Kelly

Mom and I sat in the kitchen continuing our talk right after the painful morning I'd had on the bathroom floor. We were keeping it real, talking frankly again. My body had felt like a freight train traveled over me, then stopped and backed up over me again, then changed direction back and forth a few more times all while in motion. I was completely drained of energy. *Thankfully, it's my day off work* today, I thought.

I took it easy the rest of that day, resting and re-cooperating. The abdominal pain was back to its normal, feeling dull and achy deep in the inner-most part of my abdomen, under my ribs. The low-back pain continued though. I used a lot of peppermint essential oil in an attempt to take the low-back pain away. The oil helped immensely. The coolness of the peppermint stopped the burning sensation. I used the oil many times throughout the rest of the day.

Mom received an email response from customer service team later that afternoon. Their email confirmed both of our thoughts as to why I had gotten so sick; the supplements were causing the die-off of toxins, detoxing my body, and that it was detoxing TOO FAST, hence why I had gotten so ill! They'd instructed, "Stop taking the supplements for a couple days. Slowly start them again at a smaller dose in a few days. Work your way back up to a full dose." I smiled at Mom as she read the response to me.

"We, ourselves, are our best doctors!" I said as I laughed. Deep down in my heart, I knew that things had to get worse before they would get better. Today was a prime example of that. My life had been teetering on the edge of destruction and I needed to keep detoxing. If I didn't continue to take the supplements and detoxify, what else was there FOR ME TO DO?

I'm certain that had I chose to take the conventional Western medicine route of doctoring, putting any kind of drug in me to kill the pathogens, that it would have killed me, simply because I could not handle any type of drug that may contain gluten, and many prescription drugs do contain gluten. And not to mention the many other menacing side effects of taking medications. The detoxification route I chose was a process that would cleanse my body of disease without doing further damage to my vital organs, mostly my liver but also my kidneys and intestines, nor would this route compromise my immune system.

I was choosing to heal in all aspects of my life: physically, spiritually, mentally, and emotionally, detoxing in all these areas. I was balancing my body's energy and relieving stress where it was possible. I was using these ways of healing to turn my life around. This was ALL MY CHOICE, not my parent's choice, friend's choice, or anyone else's choice. It was my choice. I chose to use alternative healing methods to turn my health around.

What I didn't know at this time was that the major illness deep inside my body was just STARTING to be addressed as I was beginning to detox through the online gut healing program.

As you've read, I had put my trust fully, completely, in my Papa God. I was not doubting the course of Him having me here at this time for a reason. Someone may be reading and thinking, *"God wanted to almost kill you, but instead let you suffer through some 'living hell' and then come back to endure a few more years of suffering? You think God actually wanted that for you?"* I'm not here to say WHAT God wanted, because I'm not God and can't answer for Him. But there is something I do know, and that is, when I put my COMPLETE trust and faith in my Papa God, I gave up all of my control and my plans. I let God be in the driver's seat. In doing so, I've found that I am a different person than who I used to be. I'm definitely more patient, more calm, more considerate, more kind, and definitely more care free. This is what God has done in my life, from the adversity I'd faced. Something tells me, He wants to do that with all of us, if we let Him have His way with us.

In Mom's writing in, "Plans and Goals", she asked some thought provoking questions; "Are goals good to have? Can goals actually hinder us if we are set on them; our heels dug in?" Personally, I think goals CAN be great, but here's what I was learning when I gave up MY control and gave God COMPLETE control. What plans and goals that I had pre-determined and set in my mind, on MY time frame, were NOT God's plans for me. In Mom's writing she'd talked about me wanting to "keep on keeping on" with the program. However, she thought we should extend the detox even longer. I was determined to forge ahead. Should I have extended that part of the program another week, or even a few weeks? YES. Would that have ultimately fixed my issues? No, but it would have helped. The point is, here I was trying to control my life and my health by forging ahead with my ideas that worked for MY plan. Taking full dosages of detoxifying supplements from the gut healing program was my idea. The founder of the program had instructed me to start a quarter of the dosage just days before we'd started the program, and had said to give myself extra time AND care on the program. But I wanted to be healthy and well ASAP...being healthy in time for leaving for Hawaii. Would I meet that plan and goal? Time will tell.

Goals. Plans. Success. I believe these are all great concepts. Wise counsel is important too, in setting and attaining these. But, if we are controlling our goals, plans and successes, and God isn't in the structure of these being set, we are running a race that may have never been meant for us to run. We may run ourselves weary, being disappointed and frustrated in our efforts because success is often just not enough. The stakes keep getting higher.

On the other hand, with God in the driver's seat (it might not always be easy or comfortable in the passenger seat) we are in the best hands. I can't explain this as well as my heart knows this, but let me try. While I was ill, I was learning to put my complete trust in God. I was FREER than I had ever been--from stress, worry, doubts, and fear all the while walking so much closer with my Papa. And you know what? I was communicating and hearing from my Papa more regularly than I was in year's past. How so? Through feeling His presence, His voice speaking to the inner most part of my being, in visions, and speaking to me in some very distinct dreams. God was speaking to me in what some would say "profound ways". The most important aspect that I was learning at this time is that it wasn't about "my goal of being healthy and well". Yes, that was important. What God was teaching me was that I was on this journey for a reason--which I already knew in my head, but was embracing it with my heart. And, I was being refined by Papa to be the person that He desired me to be, being fuller of His goodness and love. It was the WHO and WHAT kind of person that I was to be and become more of on this whole journey that was important, way more important than "good health" and focusing on meeting my goals, my plans, and ultimately achieving my success.

God had bigger and better things in store for me than I knew or even dreamt possible. How do I know? Well, what I thought were GOOD plans and solid goals to reach health success by a certain date was futile compared to when I let God have control, because living allowing Papa's control was life changing. This isn't just a concept that a person does once in their lifetime, either. I find this to be a continuous life process, a flow if you will.

Another huge concept that I was accepting in FULLNESS was that any kind of healing is a process that most often doesn't happen overnight. God was making ABSOLUTE beauty out of what looked to be "ashes" daily in my life. I am not lying when I say that even through these hellish days shared openly here, God was making beauty out of what most people would view as ashes. I'm so thankful this happened to me. Why? Because I came to a place of ABSOLUTE peace and acceptance of my health, actually having gratitude for this illness, looking forward to a future that was in His hands.

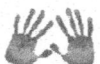

I knew that I was fighting for my life at this time. With God, I knew the best was yet to come in whatever form that would be, death or continuance of life here on earth as I continued to detox. After nearly dying, I felt I knew in my heart of hearts that this was the last close call that I would have. Was it? Yes, it was. Were there other awful days after that one? Yes, but nothing ever compared to that morning on the bathroom floor fading in and fading out. I came to know that God had me in this place for many teachable moments and reasons. I was being prepared for what was to come, unbeknownst to me during my future daily coffee enemas. My hellish nightmare was just starting.

"With God all things are possible." -Matthew 19:26

202

49

What is Detoxing?

Amy

What is detoxing? Hop on the internet and search "detoxing". You'll find endless results including "Teas", "Diets", "Body Cleanses", "Treatment Programs" of all sorts, and many articles including, "How to 'Quickly Detox' Then Pass a Drug & Alcohol Test".

I freely admit that for a long time in my younger life, the word "detox" meant that a person had to go to a treatment center to get off of drugs and, or, alcohol. Why did I think that? That's all I'd ever heard of. I came from family trees that indulge in alcohol. In my teens through mid-early 20's I'd had a span of almost ten years of binging on alcohol and experimenting with recreational drugs. I'm certainly not bragging, but I'm also not embarrassed to state these facts. Once, again in my early 20's, I drank way too much alcohol, which landed me in a hospital emergency room. Fortunately, the ER team knew how to detox my body quickly, as I was told the next day once I surprisingly awoke in a hospital room. I was told that if my friends had not brought me to the hospital when they did, that I would have been a goner if only up to ten minutes later arrival time to the ER. *Woe.*

The counselor that came to see me that next day in my hospital room asked me if I had a drinking problem. Hmm… "I don't think so," was my answer. Denial? Or ignorance, on my behalf? Probably both. This would have been a prime example of someone who needed therapy, and perhaps go to a treatment center to detox and get needed help. It seems God had a "plan B" or even "plan C" for me.

I'd quit smoking cigarettes (and marijuana) and stopped drinking before turning 25 years old. My new boyfriend at that time, who is now my husband, inspired me to leave these vices behind, but it was totally my decision. I happily did so, never craving a cigarette again. However, the alcohol having been set aside for nine years from that point was picked back up again, but more conservatively. Now, in my 40's and beyond, I do not drink much other than clean, pure water, kombucha (a ferment), and various teas. That is about it for my consumption of drinks!

Back to detoxing. Another idea of detoxing came to me in my mid 30's. My health was failing me. I thought I had fibromyalgia, possibly cancer (breast or lymph, or both), and a host of symptoms and ailments that all aided in my being sick and tired. While doctoring with a nurse practitioner in late 2002, we discussed my options and a possible plan to execute tests to see what my ailments were stemming from. The plan was devised in the way that insurance companies (and health clinics, and medical doctors of the American Medical Association, AMA, are all affiliated with doing business amongst) would pay for.

After that discussion, while still siting in her office, I made a mentally hard decision, then told the nurse practitioner that I was going to seek an all-natural route to deal with my health issues instead. Surprisingly, she praised my decision and we had a real authentic discussion! Yes! FOR REAL! I also reminded her that if the AMA knew she was having this discussion with me that her license to practice medicine within the walls of the AMA would be pulled. Lovely. She simply smiled, looked me directly in the eyes and said, "I've known you long enough to know that you would not do that. Now…" And we continued our discussion, ending with me leaving the clinic I'd been doctoring at since our second child, Kelly, had been two years old, never to return.

I was 38 years old when I made that decision to take control over my health, seeking an alternative solution to aid in making me feel better and be well in health. Kelly was ten years old when I walked away from the Western medical system, the medical system who prescribed drugs for chronic-illness treatment instead of all-natural approaches to change the direction of one's health. It was during that time which I learned a new definition to the word "detox", once I started doctoring with a holistic healthcare doctor named Dr. Ann shortly after leaving Western medicine behind.

Dr. Ann was a bright, brown-eyed gal with dark hair, olive skin, a joyful spirit, a jolly laugh, and a matter-of-fact no-nonsense personality when talking about health. And this is where I learned a portion of positive changes, ones I started to live daily, from my weekly, then semi-weekly to finally monthly visits to her office. Dr. Ann walked what she talked, which was why I chose to follow her instructions to regain my health. I've spoken about her in a former chapter, "Doors Open, Implementing Change". Dr. Ann was the picture of health. The word "vibrant" comes to mind when I think of a word that would accurately describe her.

While doctoring with Dr. Ann in my mid-to-late 30's, she addressed my organs that were failing to thrive: my kidneys, liver, heart, reproductive system, and my lungs, having me build them back up with nutritional supplements, teas, food as medicine, tinctures, and other healing modalities like chiropractic and massage therapy. Once we got my body strong enough to go through a detoxification and cleansing process that supporting my liver and kidneys, she said a series of "colonics" would cleanse my colon and upper and lower intestines to clear pathogens from my gut. If she hadn't helped me to build-up my digestive system and organs before the cleanse, the "die-off" effect of pathogens from the supplements and cleansing concoctions I'd be taking during the fast would have over-loaded my system and made me worse off, feeling sicker and possibly causing further damage to these organs. I understood that we were working to build me up to being strong enough TO detox during the time, spring of 2003-fall of 2003.

Having turned 39 years old and after nine months of building strong organs, I went on an 8-day fast that fall of 2003, which included taking supplements and drinking lip-smacking concoctions to prepare me for my 40's and beyond! I'd made a week's worth of appointments for a series of colonics during the fast as well. I prepared my mind and heart for continued elimination of negatives in my life during the 18-20 hours daily I'd be awake, potential opportunities to continue dealing with my garbage mentally and emotionally.

Physically, having learned how to do enemas during the months prior to that, colonics were an upgrade that I was ready for in mind and body. The system

205

of putting pressurized water in through where the sun does not shine, called a colonic, was just what I'd needed to improve my over-all health, cleansing the colon and cleaning the walls of my intestines. Granted, I had felt much better before those colonics with clean eating--eliminating dairy, grains and sugar from my diet and supplementing with various vitamins, minerals, and good fats. However, the colonics would flush away pathogens causing symptoms I'd had for many years of life, those being: allergies, sinus headaches, mental fog, sleeplessness, anxiety, and mental (brain) illnesses, such as depression-- undiagnosed by medical doctors, which I never complained to any doctor about, ever.

Swoosh. By reversing the water pressure during a colonic, the suction pulls the water back out from the intestines through a contained clear-see-through tubing system that we could view from the table I was laying on, watching the elimination pass by towards elsewhere to be destroyed. That was simply amazing, seeing built-up garbage that had stuck to the walls of my intestines floating through the tubing. I asked the hydro-therapist, Gloria, LOTS of questions. She was not asked anything she hadn't been asked before. She'd been doing this for 35-plus years, having started the colonic service with a friend in her basement back in the late 60's! At the time I met her, she was working out of Dr. Ann's office in the metropolitan area the time.

Anyone I talk to these days in this line of business, hydrotherapy, knows or has heard of this woman, Gloria the hydro-therapist. She's a legend, I guess! Since none of these young hydro-therapists have ever met her in person, and I had, I felt almost like a "groupie" for having gotten to work with her as her client!

Like I said, Gloria knew the answers to all my questions and got me further up- to-speed on the importance of, "...cleansing our bodies twice a year to eliminate toxic built-up wastes such as chemicals, pharmaceuticals, heavy metals, and also parasites, fungus, and other bad pathogens that live in our guts, thus wreaking havoc on our health." She had used a term, "ropes" when answering my question to "What was that?" during the first colonic, in which I'd asked about some lengthy, long-and-loaded, specimen traveling through the see-through tubing. It looked like a dark colored, damaged rope, to be honest. She said the "ropes" live on our intestinal walls, collecting the garbage in our gut. And that we needed to cleanse our gut environment periodically of the bad pathogens that build-up within our gut. Hmm, didn't think much about those "ropes" then, but I sure did years later during Kelly's health ordeal.

I'm very grateful to have met and worked with Gloria. During that short season, having great teachers like Dr. Ann and Gloria, I also read books that I could refer back to, learning and reminding myself how to take care of my body. The internet was not what it is today, a universe of information to be had. I was learning through people, books, and through experimenting.

Our kiddos saw changes in me, as did my husband and extended family during this time of detoxing. I'd had a spiritual revolution the year before, so I had literally become a new woman in a year's time! What changed was that I was happier, less intense, willing to change and be challenged, and over-all I became more loving, trusting, and accepting of others. Good changes all due to detoxing, and spiritual helps as well--a personal relationship with God.

Dr. Ann had told me one day in her office while I was pulling the trigger on her with lots of questions, "People fail to thrive because since the turn of the century, about 100 years ago, our ancestors stopped passing down information on cleansing our bodies with herbs and roots, sharing aged recipes and tinctures, cooking methods, and the like. Also, before the industrial revolution brought new ideas and new technology that changed farming, towards growing food in mass production, we had a much cleaner food system. Now days, there are chemicals in our food, and food companies creating "foods" with non-food ingredients, along with chemical companies having their hands in virtually every part of our lives, including growing our food. These and other reasons are why people fail to thrive." Wow! At the time, I was amazed at this new knowledge. Now, I'm not surprised by how unhealthy our world has become.

Back to Kelly's health situation. Kelly was doing the same kind of process in the gut healing program like I'd done with Dr. Ann, but the time frame Kelly was working within on the program was too fast for her toxic-overloaded body. Since Kelly, too, had worked with Dr. Ann, she had a number of positives that were in her favor already, like strengthened organs, vitamin and mineral support, clean eating, and lots of water going into her to aid in her detox process.

50

Everything Happens
for a Reason

Kelly

In the case that you were confused with the last chapter, "What is Detoxing?", it was written by my mom, who shared about some of her experiences in life. A quick reminder, that the chapter's "writer" at the beginning of each chapter, will be who is writing the particular chapter you are reading. Always check that for clarity, as Mom and I are two different writers contributing to this book. Obviously, our life stories are different.

I believe it's true that everything happens for a reason.

Mom and I were still on the detoxing segment of the program. When a person is detoxing, many different symptoms can surface such as: bloating, dizziness, gas, headaches, nausea, skin rashes, constipation, diarrhea, a dormant virus emerging, and a host of even more symptoms. Most of what we both experienced is listed here, above.

During the seven years while I was sick, I never got a cold, the flu, or any type of virus. Actually, the last cold I had gotten was when I was still in high school. That being said, when Mom and I started detoxing toxins out of our bodies, some "ickies" began to surface. We both got skin rashes that lasted the duration of the program, plus even longer for Mom. Her rash was scattered throughout her torso onto her limbs and was itchy, sometimes more prominent because of the heat of summer. And my rash? It was localized to only a couple places, and thankful not too itchy for the most part, but I had my moments.

In the online program, many times the three health professionals informed us that we were probably going to be detoxing some latent viruses out of our bodies that may have been laying low for an extended amount of time. Honestly, I didn't think anything of it when they'd foretold us about that. I figured I just had "gut issues" to deal with, so that probably wouldn't happen to me. Ha!

As well as a skin rash, another virus had surfaced for me a week into July that summer of 2015. I had strep-throat symptoms. *Great.* I thought. I'd had strep throat 2-3 times in high school. And now, the detoxing supplements that we were taking in addition to the other "helps" we partook of, were purging out this latent virus. I endured the symptoms, hoping that it would pass quickly. It did go away for a time, but re-surfaced once more before we finished the entire program. These were GOOD happenings though! Mom and I weren't just getting a surface level cleanse, we were getting a deep cleaning that addressed various ailments we each had no idea were going on inside of us!

As Mom and I tuned into our weekly online webinars, the leaders would have a time of questions-and-answers AFTER they talked about the coming week's information. They'd inform us of what was presently happening or was to come with possible symptoms, issues, and problems for us during the program. They suggested ways to help ease discomfort in different situations when they arose. It was all very informative and enriching. We learned a LOT from the health professionals, some of those being doctors.

During the question-and-answer portion of our weekly meetings, we could write in our questions and then one of the three leaders would answer each individual's questions during the live gathering. It was nice to be able to get answers promptly, and for everyone to hear other's questions because so many of us were experiencing many of the same symptoms, having the same issues. We were all in this together! I recall that we, the people meeting online, were from all over the USA, Canada, and elsewhere overseas! Although we were from all over the world and each of us being uniquely different, we could come together as a health-related family! Pretty neat!

In each of our lives--yours, mine, and ours, we endure trials, tribulations, joys, pains, heartaches, traumas, loves, and so much more. Whatever each of us has endured has the ability to change us, change the quality of our character for better or for worse. All those things that each of us has experienced or "endured" has helped make us the unique individual that we are. And in the moment of these happenings, they are preparing us for our future, for our future self, and for whatever we may go through in life. We were brought into this world and have been challenged uniquely to grow into better versions of ourselves. Through all of our lives thus far, all these experiences we've had have contributed to the people that we are today. Yes, both the ugly and the beautiful experiences, planned or unplanned circumstances, joys and sorrows, we get to choose who we want to be, or become, through all that we endure and experience.

Again, I believe in my heart of hearts that everything happens for a reason—the good, the bad, and the ugly. Do I believe that it's God's WILL for us to experience EVERY good or bad THING that we do? No. I think our own free will can get in the way of us following God's will for us and other people's choices affecting us too. With that said, our choices may not be what God would want for us, but He allows our choices to play out and happen anyways because He loves us unconditionally. And with allowing those experiences to happen, I DO believe that God ALWAYS makes good of every situation happening immediately or somewhere down the road in our lives and in the lives of those who love us. We may not agree on this, and that's okay. I'm just sharing what I believe.

My Papa God made good out of EVERYTHING in my ill health. Ultimately in the end of this 7-year health battle, I do have my health restored! But during those years of illness, Papa was refining me to become more of the unique person that I was, bringing me to the individual that I am today. I wouldn't trade ANY of those experiences for anything! They grew my character and helped me to be, like I said before, more kind, compassionate, and patient. Stuff happens in life, and it's not always received as good in the eyes of every individual. People can look and judge me, my life, and my story, saying that what I went through was terrible. But I find beauty in it because I CHOSE to become a better person through it.

I'd like to leave off with reminding us that that everything happens for a reason, and we were each brought into this world for a reason. OUR uniqueness is amazing. Whatever we each have experienced, are experiencing, or will experience in the future, we can choose how it will affect us as an individual. We each are loved and cherished by God for the individuals that we are. That being said, let's lace up our sneakers and embark further on this journey called LIFE together because we are in each other's lives for a reason!

I've been blessed sharing time with you, and truly hope that you're blessed too. I know that the last half dozen chapters have been hard reads. I want to personally thank you for hanging in here with me and continuing to read. Please, don't feel sorry for me in any way for what I've went through during this health battle. I'm thankful that I went through it because it's helped me to see life in a much bigger picture, to love deeper, and to trust God deeper and see Him much more profoundly.

I hope and pray that wherever you are at in life, that you are growing, maturing, and seeing all the ways that God is working in your life, consistently making "beauty out of the ashes" with you too. That tends to happen with all of us. God bless you!

51

Eastern and Western Medicine

Kelly
The detox brought forth various types of "ickies" for us other than some of the aspects already talked about. Honestly, it was slightly disgusting hearing about some of the stuff brought up during the weekly webinars, but it was good to be aware of these issues as well.

So, what were some other people enduring? Some individuals had the feeling of their skin crawling and it wouldn't stop. Others were having a lot of mucous--biofilms, coming out of different orifices. Some individuals were having respiratory coughs, strep throat symptoms, itchy ears, sinus issues, etc. Some people had different types of parasites coming out in their stools. The point in saying all of this is that each of us had latent viruses and deeper issues going on than we had even known. We are made up of cells, living organ-isms. Everything living is a cellular expression.

In hearing of all of these symptoms forementioned, and more, I was learning that detoxing is NOT easy OR pretty. It was often difficult to listen to other people's symptoms. Mom and I each had our own stuff going on, and that was enough to keep us preoccupied and not dwell too much on what others were experiencing. The coffee enemas were actually starting to address, and therefore detox, the soon to reach pancreatic cancer out of my system unbeknownst to me, although I strongly knew in my heart I HAD pancreatic cancer—but not having been medically diagnosed. I'd had a lot of inflammation in my body, mucus--biofilms, that were coming out during coffee enemas. Although I was actually thin in human structure, inwardly I was inflamed due to the mucus--biofilms, but the detox supplements were slowly but surely addressing those biofilms, killing them, causing a die-off effect that I'd already been experiencing at times prior to this program we were on.

I'm not here to make you believe what I believe. Like I've said so many times before, I'm simply sharing my story and what I've learned. And please, know that we CAN agree to disagree. I respect that and hope you will too! So, that being said, have you ever thought about what cancer is?

Cancer is an "umbrella term" for disease and illness. What do you think of when you hear that word "cancer"? Maybe you think of scary? Surreal? Death? Illness? Disease? This may happen to me? Or denial, that this won't ever happen to me.

Each of us have "cancer" cells in our bodies. These cells develop from stored toxins inside our body, then the cells feed on toxins to continue growing. Cancer can be caused by a great number of toxins, some of which I'll list. (Note, it's usually numerous toxins together, not just one). GMOs (genetically modified organisms) in food products created in a laboratory for consumer use. Toxins of various parasites, fungus, mold, poor air quality, heavy metal poisoning, chemical exposures through the skin and lungs, all these and more impacting hormones causing cellular imbalances. Toxins of bad pathogen growths and overgrowths of various bacteria. Also causing cancer can be mineral, bacterial, and nutrient deficiencies. And as I've talked about earlier, a non-alkaline PH, meaning an acidic body is the environment for cancer to thrive in.

We are complex beings. We cannot keep throwing GMO foods--unreal engineered food, in our bodies as fuel and expect our bodies to function properly. Our bodies just don't work in the long run eating materials like that. We need the right balance of nutrients, minerals, fats, bacteria, hormones, and an alkaline PH to make our bodies function optimally. Too much or not enough of some specific thing(s) can be exactly what plummets our health, causing illness and disease. To everything in life there is a balance.

I just want to say that "cancer" isn't a death sentence, nor does the label need to scare us. But it seems that's exactly what it does these days, scares people and makes us think we have to act RIGHT NOW, quickly, in our decision making of how to illuminate it from our body. I'm not saying we shouldn't act right now, because time IS precious. But, maybe, we each need to take a little time to find out what path—Western or Eastern, if we have cancer, is best for us. We ourselves have the ability to be our own best decision makers in our health, and be our own guiding "doctors" for ourselves. And no, I'm not saying we shouldn't have doctors, because doctors are our greatest teachers and help, given what they are teaching is healthful!

Western and Eastern medicine are pretty amazing. I believe that there is a place for BOTH of them! I'm thankful for our medical doctors and surgeons, and functional medicine and holistic doctors too. They each have a job to do, and they recommend what they think is best for their patient, based upon what they've learned via their schooling, research, time tested remedies, etc. They genuinely care about the health of their patients, and they should!

I explored the Western medicine route but found out that, for me, it wasn't the right route. I'd had no solid answers from medical professionals, or just didn't feel right about how some of those doctors wanted to "address" my issues. I knew myself well enough that I walked away from Western medicine for help. But again, that's not to say I didn't think there wasn't a place for it. Eastern medicine was the right fit for me, for my whole being--mind and body. I'm not going to lie and say, "Oh, it was all peaches and cream easy." Because it wasn't. I just knew all-natural was the right path for me. I'm not judging anyone for the path that they choose to take. Please know that. We each do what is right for us.

In my practicing Eastern medicine throughout the years with Dr. Ann and others, I was being guided in addressing my gut issues all-naturally. At this point in telling my health journey, in the online gut healing program, I was still addressing the gut issues, but at a much deeper level than prior to the program. I was starting to address the cancer, which from what I've learned-- cancer is made up of bad pathogens and toxins that are overloaded in the body, NEEDING to be detoxed out of my body in a non-harmful way. Drugs,

214

burning and cutting, chemo and radiation, antibiotics, and prescriptions medications weren't going to be part of my regiment in getting to the real issue going on inside of me--cancer. Supplements, using food as medicine, coffee enemas, and so many more daily modalities of healing were "addressing the issue". This felt like the right fit for me.

Life was grueling with detoxing every day, but yet so enriching! I had SO much joy in my life despite my every day routine of working to heal my body from the inside out. It was such a beautiful learning journey, and that's the way I was seeing it. Taking one step at a time, one foot in front of the other, slowly but surely, I was feeling better and better thanks to practicing some of the numerous Eastern therapies out there, even though I was having some pretty heavy days of detoxing.

52

Overload

Kelly

Coffee enemas were my daily best friend. The daily supplements were killing biofilms, bad pathogens, and bad bacteria with each dose I took, so I needed to get those toxins moving ASAP (as soon as possible). Food, real whole foods, was medicine I ate, and teas were medicinal to drink. In turn, all the good going into me was helping to override the bad that was exiting my body with each enema. At this point, I still was unable to have bowel movements (BMs) on my own.

When a person's body is so built up with toxins it is an overload to the organs, and ultimately on the entire human body. This was exactly what was going on with me. Some of my organs still weren't working optimally, and my pancreas was not doing its job at all, so this just made it all the harder to extract the bad stuff out, hence the help of enemas.

I'd now embraced the fact that this was my "new normal". I ALWAYS felt better once the toxins were eradicated out of me via enemas. I mean, who wouldn't want to embrace something that makes you feel better, right? The toxic build-up inside of me had been growing for what I presume to be my whole prior life, prebirth up to 18 years old. It wasn't like these toxins just came in one day and planted themselves and took over my body with a vengeance at 18 years old. It was a process for the pathogens to build up and override the good inside of me, just like it was a process to get those pathogens out of me. I was in this battle for the long run to gain my health back. Whatever it took, I'd be doing it.

JE June 28th, 2015
Very painful, hard day for me. Won't lie, I was pretty irritated today because of the physical pain and lack of breath... the headaches, left-side pain, nausea, dizziness, sinuses stuffed, back pain and MAJOR stomach (left side) pain. It's time to go to bed as I write in my journal and I wonder if I will sleep? *SIGH* Please Papa, let this gut healing program HEAL me, although YOU are the one that makes it happen. Please Lord, I trust You and what You have in store for me.

The human body is truly amazing. How everything works together so intricately to function, eradicate, maintain, and work. It just amazes me.

It was around this time near the end of the program's "scheduled" detoxing that mom and I talked about extending the detox. She wanted to extend it a week. I didn't. "I don't think we need to, Mom. We'll continue to heal while moving on in this program." I'd suggested. I was ready to be done with eradicating pathogens and continue on with the rest of the program.

Mom had been battling chronic sinus issues. She'd also broken out with the skin rash which ultimately extended over much of her body at this point. Her rash was a result of detoxifying heavy metals. Her body was detoxifying via her skin, which is the bodies largest organ. She took additional supplements to help the process, and would soak in hot baths of Epsom salt and aluminum-free baking soda, which helped carry toxins out of her through her skin faster, and soothed her rash--lessoning the itch.

I had battled with strep-throat symptoms that lasted about a week-and-a-half during the first part of the detox. The symptoms had come back again towards the end of two weeks. My weakest link, my immune system, was actually detoxifying old viruses that were hanging around, dormant for who knows how long. Mom had some of those same reactions with her chronic sinus issues too, dormant viruses being active and moving out. These were just a few different ways that our bodies were detoxifying, both of us in different ways but with the same intentions of healing to our guts.

JE July 2015
Came home from work and took a HOT shower. Did lots of stretching to off-set working posture and help with my gut stuff. Now it's time for

bed. My throat is still very sore today and I've got my usual headache, plus worse with this throat and sinus stuff going on. I used essential oils tonight though, and that stopped the coughing and cold symptoms in their tracks! PROGRESS! Please Lord, help. Papa, I want my health and life back so I can live it to its fullest, the fullest YOU want me to live. I trust You Papa.

53

The Unknown

Kelly

By nature, I'm an introvert. But now I say, "I used to be an introvert!" What does that mean? It means I'm choosing to NOT be an introvert. I like alone time, but I don't always HAVE to be alone or with my "safe" others.

When I was a young child, I was the quiet, shy girl that clung to her mom... "calf at side". Wherever Mom was, I was too. I was a home-body. I loved being home in my safe place. You know, comfortable and carefree. I liked "my tribe" of people, which back then consisted of Mom, Dad and Troy. Some would say I'm still that way, and I do spend a lot of time with those three people—my family.

Well, as we each grow, we change and evolve as individuals. However, it can get easy for any person to get stuck in the comfortable, and not grow towards being the person that we were meant to be. Through the years, my tribe of people has grown. Gone are the days of "calf at side, Kelly". I've changed and grown up, facing into life's many unknowns, including finding out who I am as an individual.

Sometimes I wonder that if we, as human beings, came into the world with specific instruction manuals, would that somehow make life easier? Sound silly? Maybe. But then again, how often when we buy something do we read the instructions? If we are told to do something, would we do it, like read the instruction manual before using the product—in this case a person's body?

As humans, we can be very unreliable about caring for and unconcerned about our bodies and their functions. Sometimes we are so out of touch with ourselves that when we give someone our word, we don't follow through with what we said. I think we do that with our bodies too, telling ourselves we are going to be healthier and make plans to exercise or eat a better diet. Then, life happens, plans fail, and back we go to our everyday patterns of living, having no regard to the impact we are making on ourselves.

I think a lot. Maybe I think too much. But, what about if, based on a living instruction manual, we would know the outcome of every detail of life, would that make us excited and interested in living our life to the BEST of our ability in taking care of our human vessels?

I've come to see that life in and of itself is an unknown. We don't know our number of days here on earth. We don't know all the details of our future. We don't know anything for certain. Yet despite our not knowing, we keep putting one foot in front of the other. We are living IN the unknown. Is that scary for you, or is it an exciting adventure? What if the unknowns were the things that helped to make us the individuals that we are to become in this life? What if the unknowns are what make life interesting, a continuous adventure to be had? And, may I ask, why can it be so hard to face into the unknown for people?

Maybe life is really meant to be one great big adventure! And maybe that adventure isn't just filled with fun, laughs, silliness and excitement. Maybe, just maybe, the adventure is going to be filled with unknowns that make the adventure the BEST one yet, growing us in ways we never saw coming, as in a major health crisis, a natural disaster, losing a loved one, and so many more human situations that are life altering!

The way I see it, is that each and every last one of us is on the biggest adventure of our lives in "living our lives". The people that come into our lives--some stay for a season, and some stay forever. The job that we are at--it may be a good fit for a time, but maybe ten years from now it's not the right fit for you. The choices that we make--affecting ourselves and in turn affecting others, positively or negatively, are unknown. We just don't know what the outcome will be in any of these situations.

As I said before, I used to be an introvert, and I can still be at times, because it's in my nature. But now days, I'm choosing to not really be much of one. Is it possible that something in our past has to define our future? Another thought. Is it possible that just because we believe something for an extended amount of time means that we have to believe it for the rest of our lives? Is it possible that what is right for me or you, may not be right for the next person? Is it possible that if we came into this world with an instruction manual, that life would be predictable, comfortable and dare say even boring? Is it possible that we can change from the people we once were? Where am I going with all of these questions?

I don't think we were meant to have our whole lives planned out before us. I don't believe that any of us are to be the same people we were ten years ago. I don't believe that we weren't meant to change and evolve as individuals. I don't believe that we were meant to have the same tribe of people forever around us, tight, never letting anyone else into our tribe or never letting anyone leave from the tribe. And, I don't believe that God intended for us to know all the answers to the unknowns, because how or why would we trust Him or have faith in Him then? And gosh, would we even have a relationship with Him then?

We are meant to meet other people. We are meant to have emotions and express ourselves, and these can take a lot of practice in learning how to. We are meant to keep putting one foot in front of the other. We are meant to share our gifts with other people. We are meant to live life to the best of our ability. And, we are meant to face life's unknowns. Facing into the unknowns is really "being brave". Being brave in the unknowns CAN BE scary, but it is enriching in so many beautiful ways.

You know, I think Bob Goff is right. Maybe we need to **"quit waiting for a plan"** and face the unknowns. Maybe, we'll find out that living in life's unknowns is our best adventure yet!

In my health journey thus far, I'd faced many unknowns. Those unknowns taught me so much about alternative health choices, about myself, about life, trusting in my Papa God, and also helped me to define what wellness means to me. I learned to embrace the unknowns, although it wasn't always easy, or comfortable. I was trusting God, and leaning on Him through it all. And there came a time in which I was ready and willing to face whatever unknowns that I needed to in order to get my health back. I already was facing many unknowns, I was in the thick of it, with even more to come.

Unbeknown to me at this time in my health journey I've been writing about so far; I was facing a hellish nightmare that would forever change my life, and ultimately would change my health for the better.

54

Fasting Time

Kelly

When we first started the online gut healing program, June of 2015, I'd decided to cut some time off of my work week, working from four days a week to just three days.

I changed my schedule in order to allow more time for myself, to not only focus on the program, but to tighten up the schedule so I wouldn't be at work more than I already was. People would need to adjust to my schedule. I'm SO glad that I did this! I needed all the rest I could get at that point in time. By taking an extra day off midweek, Wednesdays, it helped me to recuperate from my long workday on Tuesdays. And, by cutting back to three days a week, I was still able to get the same amount of work done, but just make three longer days instead of working an extra day. It was a win-win.

I've talked a lot about detoxing already, during this program. Let me say, it was intense! While on this portion of the program, Mom and I did a four-day fast. This was the first fast I'd done in my life! I didn't know what to expect! Mom had fasted before, so she'd told me a little about how fasting worked.

The founder of the program had advised the entire group doing the program through our weekly webinar to "not do a lot of strenuous activities while fasting and detoxing. It's important to be extra good to yourselves by listening to your body, hearing and becoming more in-tune with your body." It was also important to get enough rest. Having an extra day off in my workweek was a good change.

"The natural healing force within each one of us is the greatest force in getting well. Our food should be our medicine. Our medicine should be our food." -Hippocrates

Mom and I started the 4-day fast on a Wednesday. I worked Thursday and Friday that week but I wasn't overly busy, so it wasn't overly-strenuous on my body. Working also helped keep my mind distracted from hunger the few times "hunger" hit me. I focused on my clients and their need for healing.

I was tired while I fasted. My body just wanted to sleep. On Friday night, though, I was beginning to feel better physically. My digestion process wasn't "working" strenuously or affecting me negatively. I felt lighter physically, mentally, emotionally and spiritually. It was a good feeling! By Saturday I was truly starting to experience what it felt like to "feel WELL!" I could truly say the words, "I feel really WELL!" compared to the last two-plus years.

The 4-day fast was a BIG help for me. My digestive system got a break from having to work so hard. I was setting up my body for healing to take place. This fast was essential to help aid in my body's ability to detoxify itself. My body was detoxifying more than I could fully understand at that time.

Fasting, and ANY kind of detoxing for that matter, is something that needs to be done respectfully, responsibly, and is best done with the guidance of a health professional. Fasting just to lose weight, or to diminish a person's appetite, are NOT good reasons to fast.

JE July 13th, 2015
I actually got more than just 6-7 and-a-half hours of sleep last night! It's been WEEKS since I've gotten that much sleep in one night! Yesterday was day three of the fast. I know that my body is trying to heal, and it is very exhausted and tired. I'll keep on keeping on, putting one foot in front of the other.

Unfortunately, like I've said already, I didn't want to stay on the detox another week, so Mom and I were soon going to the next phase of the program, but we wanted to end this portion of the program by doing a series of colonics, via our own choice. It was time to face yet another UNKNOWN—colonics!

55

Facing The Unknown

Kelly

Talk about "unknowns", a colonic's (and enema's) intention is to cleanse the colon by introducing water (or coffee, or water with essential oils) by way of the rectum. This was an unknown for me, doing colonics.

So, why do a colonic when we were doing enemas during the gut healing program? Well, enemas are a one-time entrance into the body where a person "holds" the water (in my case, coffee) until ready to eradicate its collective toxins. Enemas address mainly the lower colon. Colonics, also known as colon hydrotherapy, involves multiple infusions of water into, and out of the colon in a short period of time. The water isn't just introduced into the lower colon, but into the intestines as well. Colonics are meant to cleanse the larger portion of the bowel.

Mom had done colon hydrotherapy when she had worked with Dr. Ann, so once again, Mom helped me to understand what was going to happen during a colonic therapy session. *Thanks Mom!* I was uncomfortable, facing yet another new unknown.

An enema takes anywhere on average of 20-50 minutes of time in the bathroom. A colonic takes an average of 50 minutes to one hour just for the colonic process. I'm not going to go into too much detail about a colonic and how it works since Mom has already covered that earlier, but here's the main take away points. The client lays on a therapy table, undressed and covered with a gown, then a licensed hydro-therapist comes back in the therapy room. The hydro-therapist inserts a tube gently into the rectum. This tube will transport water into and all the "ickies" out of the colon and intestines. During the colonic, warm water is released into the colon. The pressure promotes a reflexive contraction of the colon muscles, called peristalsis, which forces waste out of the colon, back through the hose, and flows into a closed disposable system. Nothing escapes, hence no mess and no fuss. In many cases, the client may experience abdominal discomfort during his/her colonic. The hydro-therapist applies light massage to the client's abdominal area to help ease any discomfort. Once the treatment is completed, the client sits on a toilet, alone in a designated bathroom, to pass any residual water and stools. Sounds great, right? It may be a little uncomfortable, and humbles a person a bit more, but it certainly was worth doing!

Mom and I each did four colonics within seven days during the last week of detoxing. After completing the first two colonics I felt clean and actually "healthy" inside my body. "I think I can truly say that I feel GOOD today!" I told Mom as we left our very last colonic appointment. "I've never felt this good, so this is an awesome result!" However, feeling well only lasted 24 hours. *It was SO worth doing the colonics, having 24 hours of NO pain!* I thought to myself. It was like a mini-vacation, truly!

Our bodies were still continuing to detoxify when we completed the last days of that portion of the gut healing program. The intense detoxification process would be subtler from this point on in the program. Next, we would be setting up our microbiome to function optimally and get it all working in good balance. Mom and I continued to do our own methods of detoxifying and lots of self-care. I was still doing coffee enemas daily, even twice daily at this time of transition. The reason being I still was unable to have BMs on my own.

Being unable to have a BM on my own meant toxins were sitting in my body longer than they should have been, so then they became more toxic just sitting there. I spent much time in the bathroom, daily. It was a long process, doing enemas daily so often. They were taking a big amount of time and energy, but I always felt better afterwards, when the toxins were out of my body.

I continued eating according to the program. Mom was with me every step of the way and continued to help keep me on track.

JE July 18th, 2015

Nearly done with week 5 of the program. I feel SO much better and I have a true joy and love for life. So neat and awesome! It makes me want to run, dance, scream, shout, laugh, smile and love. I'm feeling yucky today from all the supplements. Pretty exhausted today too, BUT it's TOTALLY worth it to get all these toxins out of my body. And that is KEY! Thank You, Papa, for doing just that and continuing to heal me. I'm able to continually make myself do my daily exercise routine, food prep, normal daily "stuff" and do my job. Somedays it takes a big effort, I won't lie. But I KNOW this is what I have to do, daily. I find TRUE joy in the simple things, and I'm so very grateful.

56

What are Biofilms?

Amy

For illness and disease to stay out of our bodies, a person's PH needs to be alkaline. Illness grows in acidic bodies—bodies lacking oxygen.

> **"No disease, including cancer, can exist in an alkaline environment."** -Dr. Otto Warburg

Kelly and I are by nature scientific beings, getting excited about experimenting in various ways. It was through the online gut healing program that we first heard the term "biofilm". Biofilms were something we did a LOT of research on and actively experimented with by working to eliminate them from our bodies during the entirety of the program.

So, what are "biofilms", you ask? From an article titled, "Slimy Clumps of Bacteria Kill Thousands. Scientists Are Fighting Back", written by Usha Lee McFarling,[7] she writes, "Unlike free-floating bacteria that drift in fluids, biofilms consist of bacteria that settle onto surfaces and begin to aggregate into large clumps surrounded by a protective coating of DNA, proteins, and polysaccharides--slime to you and me."

We learned that biofilms are "complex 3-D structures that use various chemicals to self-organize bacteria, which in turn divide up tasks, some growing and secreting slime, some dispersing to colonize new areas, and some

---

[7] Usha Lee McFarling, "Slimy Clumps of Bacteria Kill Thousands. Scientists Are Fighting Back." June 28, 2016 https://www.statnews.com/2016/06/28/biofilms-bacteria-research/

hibernating until they are needed. The biofilm structures even contain channels to take in nutrients and expel waste. They communicate with each other and coordinate their activity." Also, "In a biofilm, you see cooperative behavior. It's a lifestyle choice." Wow! That's amazing! And wow, that is biological energy working not in human favor, in my opinion.

The article goes on to tell why are biofilms so hard to kill. "First there's the slime, which antibiotics and chemicals have difficulty penetrating. In addition, electrical charges on the slime's surface can form a barrier that keeps out antibiotics." Also, the article informed us, "Because many cells deep within a biofilm are nutrient and oxygen-starved, they grow fairly slowly--and are therefore less susceptible to antibiotics, which work best on actively dividing cells. To make matters worse, biofilms contain zombie-like 'persister' cells which lie dormant when antibiotics are present but spring into action after antibiotic treatment ends. Finally, cells within biofilms can organize themselves to pump drugs right out of cells--a kind of bulimic behavior.'"

Okay, so that's a whole lot of biochemical scary in my mind. Maybe yours too. However, we have to start somewhere in learning about biofilms in the 21st century of biowarfare we live in, and this was a very good explanation to what biofilms are and how they operate.

We have learned more about bad pathogens and biofilms, experimenting and trying to eliminate them from our bodies. By seriously looking at what we eat, staying away from "inflammatory" foods, reading ingredients labels, and making better choices of what we put into our bodies as fuel, researching how the food we purchase is grown or produced, finding safe companies and stores to purchase our food and personal care items from, and caring about what we put on our skin, etc., we have vastly reduced these crazy cellular pathogens from our bodies. To think we've totally eliminated biofilms from our bodies, though, is a far reach from reality, in my opinion.

57

Seriously?

Kelly

In the last chapter, "What Are Biofilms?", Mom shared information from an article that explained the what, how, and why's of biofilms. I'm going to take this one step further, because, well, it gets a bit more interesting! Seriously? Yes, seriously!

A biofilm is a group of cells sticking together from inside the intestinal walls. The cells latch together and form a blob of mucous. Yes, this is gross, but MAYBE kind of interesting? Anyway, remember way back when, when I told you that my PH was acidic? Well, my body's acidic, cold, damp and leaky gut was GREAT territory for producing biofilms. These biofilms are actually pretty common for individuals with small intestinal bacteria overgrowths (SIBO), candida overgrowths, leaky gut, cancer, and most all chronic auto-immune illnesses.

At this time, I weighed in at 130 pounds. I had muscle tone but was slender overall. I wasn't inflamed outwardly in my body, but inwardly I had inflammation and a lot of pathogens that were wreaking absolute havoc in my body, especially in my gut. The biofilms were BIG factors in my illness.

So how did I first find, then address these biofilms? Well, the truth is, I first saw them come out in stools brought on via enemas. Seriously? Yes, I'm a scientific type of "nerd" that wants to KNOW and see for herself WHAT was coming out of me, what I was dealing with. I cared about my health enough to face the unknown. So that being said, I carefully examined every bowel movement outputted before flushing them away, and that is how I first saw the biofilms. I'm sorry if that's just too much information.

Anyways, in natural health avenues of Eastern medicine we can determine a LOT about the state of our health based upon our stool. Again, without going into too much detail, I'll just say that my stools were "loose". I could see chunks of food along with the biofilms in my stools. I had issues going on inside my digestive system that NEEDED to be addressed. The online gut healing program wasn't going to be enough help, unbeknownst to me at that time, but since I didn't know this at the time, I was giving this program my complete effort in hopes of healing.

You may be wondering by now in the story, *"How were you not feeling better? Everything you were doing and eating was pure, organic, clean and wholesome. Why was it taking so long?"* Well, those are both good questions. I'll answer how I wasn't feeling better and why it was taking so long for me to feel better.

1. **Gluten exposure and cross contamination.** Gluten is a part of many different store bought pre-packaged food items, including supplements that are not pure/clean, "gluten free" produced food items that often times still have various kinds of gluten in them, and, as was the case in a former chapter, "Gluten Exposure" when it came in the form of eye drops through my eye examination at the eye doctor. Gluten was a "filler" in the ingredients the drops were derived from. Frustrating, for sure. Obviously, gluten can be in medications and skin care items as well.

    Living with others in your home, some of which eat gluten, opens up the possibility of cross contamination also. As hard as I tried to not let that happen, I couldn't control if others picked up after themselves. It's not as though others weren't aware of it, because through the years they'd learned the severity of gluten exposure for me, but it still did occasionally happen that crumbs were left behind. Or, with company over it's pretty easy for food crumbs to end up on my plate, unbeknownst to me at times. Getting nailed with

231

gluten cross contamination would make me severely sick for 7-10 days, ultimately taking my gut a month's time to get back to its "normal". Yes, that's a long time. At this time though, I still reacted to gluten severely.

2. **A compromised immune system.** Like I said before, I hadn't had a cold, "the flu", or any other sickness for about ten years, including up to now, today as I write. That being said, my immune system was strong enough to fight off bad pathogens at the "surface" level during the program. Deep inside, my immune system was compromised. It was partly because of GMO foods, gluten, dairy, processed foods, sugar, and other junk fillers found in processed foods and supplements I'd consumed for years while growing up. These junk foods affect the body negatively, weakening a person's immune system over time. However, my immune system had been compromised probably since pre-birth, since Mom had gut issues long before she was pregnant with me.

What is the immune system? It's the body's defense organism against pathogens; invaders, viruses, parasites, and cellular diseases. Our immune system is designed to attack pathogens and boot them out. **The immune system is our first line of defense against disease**.

Did you know that a large amount of our immune system health comes from our mothers? Yes! It comes through a vaginal delivery--being swabbed in all kinds of good bacteria, and via the umbilical cord while being fed during the nine months of incubation time, and after birth it comes through breast milk the first three days after birth.

When a child is born, one of the first and best choices a new mom can do for their child is to nurse--breastfeed, their newborn infant. NO offense to my mom, or to ANY moms or parents out there, because as mom's they LOVE their children and want to do everything in their willpower to do their best for them, but often they don't have enough time and energy to do everything they want to do to take care of themselves let alone to know and do what is the best for their infant children. Again, please don't take ANY offense to this. I'm not condemning anyone, but rather I'm giving information.

The first three days after a baby is born are the most important days to building a healthy immune system in an infant. Breast milk is filled with colostrum. Colostrum is made up of VITAL anti-bodies that protect the body and fight disease, fighting off bad bacteria in our bodies. When an infant drinks the mother's breast milk those first three days of life, the nutrients of the colostrum are setting up the baby's immune system for a GOOD, no, a GREAT start in life!

Those facts said, what about the babies that don't receive their mother's breast milk? Those babies will have a weaker immune system than their peers. In turn, their bodies are more at risk of disease and illness. If you weren't breast fed as a child, and have a weak immune system, catching most any viral infection passing through town, you may be wondering, "Can I boost my immune system?" The answer is, YES!

Immune system BOOSTERS include, but aren't limited to: oxygen (which is free so go ahead and breath deep!), vitamin C, colostrum supplementation, probiotics and prebiotics, some specific herbs and teas, and vitamin D via, 1) sunshine, or 2) nutritional supplementing. Also, immune boosters are clean air, pure water, organic meats, fruits, and vegetables, dark leafy greens, various essential oils, mineral supplements, coconut oil, bone broth, collagen, and good fats.

What are some of the things that SUPPRESS an immune system? They include but aren't limited to: medications (including antibiotics), smoking, indulging in alcohol, over-the-counter drugs, gluten, pasteurized dairy products, processed GMO foods, exposure to chemicals, chemotherapy, radiation, toxic air, chemical fumes, amalgam fillings, food coloring or dyes, stress, unhealthy relationships, and ingesting processed sugar.

Okay, so wrapping this up, again you may ask, *"How were you not feeling better? Everything you were doing was good and wholesome, and you were eating pure, organic, wholesome foods. Why was it taking so long?"*

My answer? Like I said earlier, my immune system had been compromised from since I was in Mom's womb. Then, after I was born, I'd been fed a soy-based milk formula, having not been breast fed at all. Believe me, if Mom had known better, she would have breastfed me. But, as she had said once she learned this truth, "I didn't know, just like a lot of other parents... I didn't know."

Infants grow into toddlers, to young children, into teenagers and adults. Through a majority of my growing up years, my diet wasn't "clean". I was living what I'd learned. There were also some nutritional supplements my brother and I took while growing up, but many of them had gluten fillers in them unbeknownst to any of us—not that we cared at all then, either. When supplementing with nutrients and minerals, one needs to research to make sure the chosen products are clean and overall safe, knowing exactly what is IN them and how they are produced.

The point in saying all of this, is that it took a LONG time for my health to get to this ill state. My health wasn't going to reverse overnight miraculously, let alone super quick. It'd taken 18 years to get this way. Like I've said before, "healing is a process."

I WAS taking positive steps towards healing, but it was a process. With each day being filled with many choices to make, I was one day closer in gaining health and wholeness.

58

Creative Expression

Kelly

JE August 1, 2015

THANK YOU for continued healing in Mom and myself, Lord! Please continue to heal us each mentally, emotionally, physically and spiritually. I LOVE You, Papa! Thank You for this online gut healing program, for the leaders and everyone involved, Lord. Bless them.

The foods we ate were pretty much the same throughout the duration of the program, so far. However, I was starting to get bloated again whenever I ate. I also had more headaches. I continued to have good and bad days in my health. My body was continuing to detoxify itself, so the good and bad days were "to be expected". However, deep down in my heart I thought, *I should be feeling better than I do at this point in the program.*

Mom saw that I wasn't making much progress in the first few days of this next part of the program and voiced, "Do you think maybe we should do another colonic or two, Kelly?" I didn't know what to think. My mind wandered, and then I thought, *I felt REALLY good after doing the colonics before, so why not just try it?*

I replied yes. So, Mom made us a couple of appointments and off we drove to the city, a three-and-a-half-hour drive to the hydrotherapy office on the weekend. Mom was in the driver's seat. And me? I was doing my usual semi-laying/sitting and squirming in the passenger seat, unable to really get comfortable. Sitting still hurt like crazy and I continued to avoid it at all costs.

In the city, by the time the second colonic was done that weekend, I finally felt better. My gut was back to its normal dull achy pain, which was tolerable. I was regretting MY decision to end the detox part of the program as soon as we had. *I should have listened to Mom about extending the purge two more weeks.* I later voiced those thoughts to her. We both had regrets that we hadn't listened, really listened to her voiced concern at that time.

Our bodies were both still detoxifying hard, though we were not taking supplements for that to happen. Our bodies were doing this on their own! We found various ways to help Mom ease the itching of her rash which included: Aloe vera, chlorella, oregano oil--a few drops diluted in olive oil or a carrier oil, Coriander-Cumin-Fennel tea, Boswellia lotion and a few other helps. The point wasn't to STOP the detoxification process, but to let those helpful healers soothe the severity of the itch during the detoxing process. I continued detoxifying daily with the aid of coffee enemas. I was still unable to have bowel movements on my own, so some days I was still doing two or even three enemas. Coffee enemas, at that point, were the biggest help for pain relief due to the toxic overload inside my body and getting the die-off out of me quickly. We were both fighting our battles with what each of us had going on physically from detoxing. I was sure glad we were in this together, Mom and I!

Most days I would get out of bed and seize the day, whatever it consisted of. On days I didn't want to get out of bed, my pets were BIG motivators to get me going as they needed me to take care of them! I had a daily detoxification regimen that I had to follow by choice. For me, there were no IF, AND's, or BUT's about it. It was what it was, and I accepted that. I had moments of frustration, impatience, and irritation, but in my heart of hearts I trusted my Papa God to guide me through each day and I WAS gaining patience overall. At the end of any given day when it was time for bed, my cats, Bun-Bun and Goofy, would accompany me to bed. They'd take their designated spots on the bed with their favorite blankets, or snuggle right in by my feet, the crook of my arm, or at my side. They kept an eye on me, and kept me company. Also, I'd take out my journal before crawling into bed, get comfy with my pets and write…every single night. It didn't matter what happened during the day or how I felt, I just picked up my pen and wrote, sometimes writing my inner most longings, desires, or prayers of my heart. Sometimes I'd simply write about my day, or my attitude throughout the day. Maybe what I'd gotten accomplished, or my ideas for tomorrow, etc. As I wrote, I healed in expressing myself, becoming vulnerable, and I was becoming more of a creative expression God had design me to be.

As I'd finish journaling, sometimes I'd reread what I'd written. Sometimes, tears filled my eyes as I thought about things I'd wrote. And other times, I just smiled because I was so grateful. Before I'd put my journal notebook away, I'd take up my other notebook and write five things I was thankful for. It didn't matter WHAT or WHO, just five things (minimum). This ALWAYS helped me find the good throughout all of what may have happened during the day. This helped me to see beauty in ALL things. And best of all, I always went to bed a bit lighter, happier, and more at peace.

All these years later from when I first started journaling back in 2010, I still do these same two journaling expressions before I go to bed. Doesn't matter how late it is, if I feel like it or not, I'm just drawn to that blank page at a day's end. Maybe you've encountered the same thing? Writing isn't JUST a random exercise. It's a form of creative expression! It exercises our brains, and reading does too! Writing engages us as both writers and readers to explore, express, relate, agree or disagree, and learn.

We are all creative human beings! Seriously? You don't think you are? Well, you are. Whether you like telling stories, doing do-it-yourself projects, teaching a class, writing, refurbishing old antiques or broken objects, buying clothes (our clothing expresses what we like and are artistic expressions of who we are as individuals), the food we make (what we like to prepare for food, and how we can be creative in both taste and appearance of the food), and in how we relate, communicate and interact with other people. Some of you reading this might be saying, "Those are creative? I'm not following." Well, if you might still be confused, creativity isn't just a select number of things such as art, dancing, scrap booking, and photography. Creativity is expressed in ALL we do in life daily. We are ALL creative creatures!

Elsa Gidlow says it straight, **"We consider the 'artist' a special sort of person. It is more likely that each of us is a special sort of artist."** That being said, none of us are better than the other, including in the way that we are creative, artistic. Your gifting might be in drawing. Another's might be in cooking. And yet another's might be in designing apparel, or doing other people's tax returns. Point is, we are ALL special creative expressions that have a place in this world! As individuals, I do believe we were born to express ourselves, to relate with others, and to be creative. It's not something that always come easy at first, but something we grow into, over time. No matter who we each are, we are creative. Can we be, and are we willing to share our creativity with others to bring them benefit, and maybe even help encourage them to express themselves too? The choice is ours to get creative!

Each day, we have CHOICES to make. Tonight, I'm once again drawn back to my blank journal page to express myself and to heal.

59

Food Is Medicine

Kelly

Tired of the same old tasteless, dry, and boring salads? Want to mix up the way to get some yummy greens into your diet? Try making your own salad dressing! Don't feel up to it? Well, purchase a different salad dressing to try! GOOD fat such as flax oil, omega oil, fresh avocado or avocado oil, or any nut oil is a great base to start off in making of a healthy homemade salad. Try adding some chopped nuts or some superfoods such as hemp hearts into the salad with any of the good oils mentioned above. Incorporating a 1/4 cup of grapefruit, orange, berries or finely chopped apple into your salad greens makes a delightfully colored and flavored salad! There are so many ways to mix up the foods we eat simply by changing a few ingredients in our meal!

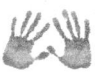

As Mom and I started the last portion of the online gut healing program, we introduced foods that we hadn't been eating for the last couple months, or for me having not eaten for years! *This is going to take time,* I thought, *to introduce more foods into my diet.* Introducing new foods was not easy for me. It was like introducing new foods to an infant. I'm NOT kidding. I had to introduce any new food ONE bite (sometimes it wasn't even a full bite, but instead being a 1/2 or 1/4 bite) in a day. Then, a few days later, I would try that same food again. *Baby steps, for sure!*

One day I tried a bite of an egg white since I could not eat eggs for multiple years before this. Upon eating anything new, I'd listen, tuning in to what my body was saying, paying special attention to all the signs and symptoms it would give me in time after trying it: a headache, bloating, feeling nauseated, dizzy, becoming pale in color, or having more severe left-side back and upper abdomen pain. At times, I'd get the hot and cold sweats as well. After a couple of days, I tried one more bite of an egg white. If I got any of the same symptoms again, that indicated that my body wasn't ready to eat that food. I would wait a couple weeks and do the same process with this egg white all over again. In the meantime, I would do the exact same process introducing a different food free from the time of trying any other new food. Some new foods were compatible with my body, so I would slowly increase one bite to two bites after a day. Then three bites and so forth. Yes, this was a LONG and tedious process… but it was also VERY important!

The abdominal and back pain weren't as severe as they'd used to be, but the pain was present and heading back in the direction for the worse. *Why? It's not over yet, is it God? Something isn't right.* Thankfully, I wasn't doubling over from the abdominal and back pain. I wasn't getting as much success reintroducing new foods into my diet as I wanted. Ultimately, I decided to take a break from re-introducing new foods back into my diet. I stayed with eating the same foods we had ate throughout the extended online program. It didn't take long for me to realize that eating just those specific foods weren't making the symptoms or pain decrease. *What is going on?*

60

Expectations

Kelly

As I just said in the last chapter, I wasn't getting as much success reintroducing new foods into my diet as I wanted. Point blank obvious is the reality of this statement, what **I wanted**.

For the normal person at this point in the gut healing program, they should have been feeling much better, having improved their health. I wasn't the normal person in the program, though. I had MUCH more going on inside of me, much more that would be addressed in the near future. But I did think I should be feeling better than I did at that time. Which leads us to the topic of **expectations**!

The truth of the matter is that **expectations**, for myself and others that I've talked with about this subject, we seem to find that when we put SPOKEN or UNSPOKEN expectations on someone, on a circumstance, or on ourselves, in the end we often feel let down when the expectation wasn't met.

In my health struggle for the first many years, I had expectations and high hopes of getting answers to my steadily declining health. Well, thus far on the journey here, I still had no defining answers other than what I researched and believed to be true for myself, I having pancreatic cancer. My expectations continually got me nowhere but down-and-out when I'd work with health professionals, EXPECTING them to tell me what was wrong with me. What happens when that high hope and expectation comes shattering down to the reality of someone telling you, "I have no answers to help you." Faced with the reality of our expectation not being met, we may feel sad, confused, let down, or even depressed.

Is it wrong for us to have hopes and expectations? I've had a lot of experiences that felt like errors in my life because of putting MY expectations on myself and others. What happens when the people or circumstances don't line up with MY expectations? I'm let down. I might even lose faith in myself or an individual because of my expectation(s). Sometimes I get confused and need to refocus to figure out where I went wrong. And every time, I need to let this be an AFGO (another fabulous growth opportunity) moment to see the error of my way. Once I realize my error, and swallow my pride by embracing an AFGO moment, I am then humbled with 20/20 vision to see the error of my way. I begin to live with not letting my expectations take control and block relationships, health realities, daily life realities interacting with other people, or goals and dreams, etc.

"Expectation is the root of all heartache." -William Shakespeare

Have you ever gone into a premeditated discussion that you'd rehearsed over and over in your head for what had felt like hundreds of times? Maybe it was when you were having to have a difficult conversation with your boss, spouse, child, or friend. Maybe it was introducing yourself to someone you wanted to get to know, trying to get the courage in telling yourself what you would say when the time came. There's lots of life scenarios that this could happen in, but the point is, when put in the midst of any premeditated situation did all of our rehearsing actually go as planned? I'm willing to guess NO. And that's exactly the point. Our expectations got in the way of how we thought something should go, what a person would say, or how a scenario would play out.

Why do we have to play out any life scenario in our head a hundred times? Is it wrong to NOT think about this? Yes, I think it's responsible to think things through as to what MAY happen. But I don't think we should get stuck in our thoughts and spoken/unspoken expectations of how, why, when, or what will happen.

What do I mean by the "spoken and unspoken?" You know, the expectations we speak to others and the unspoken ones we don't speak to others but still expect? As children, we grow up with rules, the dos and don'ts. Our parents verbally speak many expectations, but there are other expectations we somehow feel the do/don't but they're not spoken to us. We learn about the

242

spoken and unspoken from a very young age. Right? Following me? Do you think it's at all possible that with these spoken and unspoken expectations and rules, that this plays a role in how we interact, speak, handle conflict, and live our lives? I think so.

I'll just ask a couple more things for each of us to ask ourselves and to think about. Am I living my life with spoken or unspoken expectations? Am I putting MY expectations on myself or on others, and is it affecting them? If I am, is this right for them, and is it right for me? Why do I do this? Do I want or need to change my thinking, analyzing, and views so that I'm more aware of how MY expectations affect others and myself?

We are all human and we all make mistakes. I don't think any person, or any circumstance, will ever meet our expectations. Sorry to burst anyone's bubble! I've had to address "my view of expectations" because, honestly, it was messed up. And you know what? As I continue to sort through that mess, I'm learning that I do better without any expectations. Laying aside MY expectations and going into anything and everything with an open mind, free of expectations, has set me free at a whole new level of living my life. I've found that it not only helped myself, but it helps others too. It seems we all get blessed when that happens!

Wherever life leads us, I hope and pray that instead of letting our expectations take control of any life situation, that we'd each take a step back and let it be an AFGO (another fabulous growth opportunity) moment to live in and get blessed by!

61

Reasons and Seasons

Kelly

It was now the end of September 2015. Mom and I had completed the online gut healing program, having been done with it for over a month. However, we were still eating the same as we did on the program. I hadn't expanded my diet too much. I was still feeling pretty miserable.

The month of September is always garden harvest time! This September was no different than others in the past--Mom and I stood together in the garden, working and talking. We discussed many subjects, including her skin rash which was present and itching, and the left-side abdominal and back pain I continued to have. "The itching flares up only when I'm hot and sweating, like right now!" she chuckled. "Otherwise, it seems to be improving." She smiled.

Slowly, but surely, wins the race, flashed through my mind. "Mom, you look healthy and vibrant! You look younger than you did before starting the program!"

Mom looked up from picking green beans and said, "God love yah, girl!"

"God love yah, girl!" a line from one of our many favorite movies, "The Divine Secrets of the Ya-Ya Sisterhood", a 2002 American comedy-drama film starring Sandra Bullock, who is one of my favorite actresses. We laughed, then Mom followed by saying, "I FEEL a lot better too!"

I, however, continued to battle bloating, dull and achy abdominal and low back pain, nausea and dizziness that were present day and night, and headaches getting worse again, especially when I was tired to the point of exhaustion. I was still constipated too, which aggravated me. I had moments of feeling "okay", but that varied from minute to minute and hour to hour.

JE September 14th, 2015

Not feeling so great... sore throat, itchy eyes, ears, and even (my) face. This is the second time with this strep throat stuff, although it's not as bad this time around. I'm still constipated and living on daily enemas. Yes, it's very old already. Lord, it sure would be nice to have BMs on my own to push this junk out of my system. I'm a mess. Give me patience, Papa.

God was giving me ample opportunity to grow patience. Take for instance, going number two. I may not have been able to have BMs on my own, but I was doing enemas twice a day, which took ample time to do. Fortunately, the enemas were enough to keep up with the detoxification process. The horrid, yucky toxins--in many forms including gallstones, continued to come out during the enemas. The gallstones passed until there were none left. I smiled thinking, *"Well, never ever would I have thought gallstones would, or could, come out of a 20-something year old!"* Ha! My patience was paying off well!

People come into our life for a reason, for a season or for a lifetime. I've found this to be true. Have you? In my health journey thus far, I'd met many professionals that had been helpful to me, to whatever degree it may have been. They came in many different forms: The reflexologist, the acupuncturist, the FMDs (functional medicine doctors), some MDs (medical doctors), the three leaders of the online gut healing program who were a part of our weekly webinars on the program, Dr. Daniel, my NUCCA chiropractor, my mom, Amy, my massage therapist and friend, Hallie, and even more massage therapists (cranial sacral therapies) coming in soon to this unfolding story, and other individuals as well. My point is that these people were each helpful in their specific way. Not one of them was better, or worse, than the next one. *Well, except for the one chiropractor who'd lied on his website about his credentials and stood me up on my appointment date.* All of them were aiding in helping "better" my health, teaching me, guiding me, and walking along side of me with their gifts of various helps.

Some of these same individuals had spoken--prophetically in my view, words as to what was going on with my health, or specifically what was going on inside my body. The Reflexologist had told me my stomach and pancreas were having problems, and then had asked way back in the beginning of telling my story here, "Have you been having any abdominal pain or digestive problems lately?" Also, Hallie, the massage therapist, had said, "It feels like you have a fire burning inside you." And I did. They and others were here for me in this season of my life, for a reason—to help bring me back to ease—wellness of health.

On September 21, 2015, Mom surprised me with a craniosacral massage therapy (CMT) appointment. I'd had CMT done once before, in the year 2012.

Looking back to that time in 2012, I literally had no idea what kind of results I would be getting before going to the appointment. On a phone call before that appointment, I remember the therapist, Cathy, asking me a bunch of questions, and then telling me how to prepare for the appointment. I was slightly confused because I thought I was just getting a regular deep tissue massage. Craniosacral massage therapy had NOT been on my radar back then!

What is craniosacral massage, you may be wondering? It's a gentle, noninvasive form of bodywork that addresses the bones of the head, spinal column, and the sacrum. It allows the cerebral spinal fluid (this is in our spinal column) to be normalized. The goal of craniosacral massage is to release compression in the areas which are blocked, therefore alleviating stress and pain. This type of massage works directly with the myofascial tissue (the thin, strong, fibrous connective tissue that extends throughout our body to provide support and protection to our muscles and bones). Myofascial tissue actually holds EVERYTHING in place in our bodies! If we didn't have myofascial tissue, we literally would fall apart--unable to stay together. Not kidding! It's like glue!

At the first 2012 CMT appointment, I'd laid on the therapy table, then Cathy gave me a couple minutes to relax before she started working. I'd battled sciatica since right after high school. Added in with my gut issues, the sciatica always seemed to linger, sometimes flare up, all depending on how my gut felt. Why? Because my pelvis was tilted, which I came to find out in that very first appointment with Cathy. I'd walked away from that first appointment in jaw-dropping amazement. *She barely even touched me! Yet, I feel AMAZING. And, my sacrum and pelvis feel the best they've ever felt!* Cathy had been able to help relax my pelvic muscles via the sacrum, which aided in the releasing of the sacrum itself so that my pelvis that had been tilted would ultimately shift back to where it was supposed to be. Those were the days when I was over-exercising, running 3-12 miles per day preparing for triathlons. Despite how awesome that first appointment was, I hadn't gone back again to her until 2015, when Mom surprised me with the appointment.

The long-short here is the last few years of 2013-2015 my tilted pelvis had gotten worse again. I, myself, had told Mom about "craniosacral massage therapy" at times throughout the years--during massage schooling, how beneficial it can be. And now, with the second appointment being made for me BY Mom (who actually listens to me when I talk, most often), I was anxious to see if this therapy would, again, be helpful as it was three years prior. *I wonder if correcting the pelvic tilt will aid in better digestion?* I was eager to find out!

This season of illness was bringing people into my life to help me reverse my health. That reason, alone, was enough for me to keep on putting one foot in front of the other, to see what results would come from my time with each of them.

62

Words – Visions – Dreams

Kelly
The craniosacral massage therapy I'd tried in 2012 had helped a lot! And, so it did again now in 2015. A few months later I went back for one more appointment, and after that another appointment 1.5 months later.

Within 1.5 months between my second and third appointments, I can confirm my knowing that my pelvis wouldn't return back to the previously jacked-up wrong position. I had two therapists at these appointments, Cathy and Donna, working on me at the same time. I told them that I was having abdominal and back pain. In the second of three total CMT sessions, Donna had said while her hands were placed on me, "Kelly, this spot here on your left side feels hot. It almost feels like it's on FIRE."

Thinking of my good friend, Hallie, the massage therapist, I said, "Yes. I've been told, 'It's like a slow burning fiery heat, penetrating from inside my left side'."

She replied, "Yes. Well said! Just below that spot, in your intestinal area, it feels cold, damp and um, (cough-cough) squishy." Donna had started coughing while Cathy watched her intently, then Donna said, "It's like this spot is eating you from the inside out."

"What else do you feel or see, Donna?" Cathy inquired.

Let me just say this now. Donna has a unique gift--she's able to feel and see things in peoples' bodies that aren't visible to the human eye. Donna has an intuition, a knowing about things. She was having one of those revealing, knowing moments during the second of three appointments with me, and I'd only just met her on the first appointment here in 2015. She'd not been a part of my VERY first appointment in 2012 with Cathy. Donna knew something, and was about to tell us more about what she saw and felt. She struggled to clear her throat, then proceeded with statements addressing the "squishy" (which were the biofilms that I'd been passing in daily enemas, and continued to pass, that she had not known of. I actually hadn't TOLD either of them of these very personal happenings—biofilm discharges detoxing out of me, up until just after this point).

Donna spoke more, while Cathy and I listened. We had all been honest and open with each other during my appointment. But then, *how much information is too much?* I thought. I was kind of embarrassed to tell them about the biofilms I was passing. I wasn't offended when Donna stated what she did to Cathy and myself. I'd told them I had been doing a "detox" program, having just completed it recently, not telling of the actual biofilms--the "Squishy" Donna had named in my intestines. Then, I got bold and openly shared a bit of what was happening at this time.

Cathy asked, "Did you pass this stuff while you were on your cleansing program?"

"Not that I knew of right away in the program. But through it, yes, I did, and I still am... just not as 'intensely' as during the program while taking detox supplements. But yes, in general I have been detoxing really heavy in the last few months." I stated.

"Are you sure it's not intense right now?" Cathy asked. *Am I sure?* I thought. *These biofilms that Donna is talking about are what Mom and I researched. Oh man. She's speaking prophetically!* I just nodded my head, yes, to Cathy's question. I was in my head having my own thoughts. *No need to cause a stir with too much information.*

Cathy continued asking more questions about the program while they both worked on me. She asked specific questions about my digestion process, my digestive system, and about the abdominal pain I had told them about. Again, I answered all of her questions. My pelvis had been tilted, which was WHY I was there. I was not there for the "Squishy". Together, the two therapists were able to get my pelvis back to its neutral--"normal" position again.

Craniosacral massage pressure isn't very deep. Donna and Cathy weren't palpating or pushing deep into my abdomen. Donna had simply had her hand on my abdomen where she felt and saw what was going on deep inside my body, inside my intestines. Obviously, God was using Donna to show me more of the truth--the biofilms "were eating me alive". And she was right, of course. The biofilms were eating me alive, from the inside outward.

Prophetic words, visions, and dreams. Maybe you've had them yourself. Or, maybe not. Maybe you know someone that has gone out-on-a-limb and spoken one of these to you or someone you know. Whether you believe in prophetic words, visions, and dreams or not, it's your decision—your choice. I'm not here to convince you one way or the other. I am simply sharing what I've found to be true for myself.

A handful of people in my healing journey had spoken prophetic words to me. The reflexologist, then Hallie, and now Donna. I can't speak for them on HOW they knew what they spoke to me, but they KNEW without question and stated what they saw/felt/knew. I don't know if it was easy, uncomfortable, or really awkward for them to share their findings, but they spoke regardless.

Did I openly receive what they each had to say? Yes! I, myself, have uttered prophetic words. I've had dreams and visions of things that have come to pass. I'm in no way, shape, or form bragging. I believe God can use anyone as a messenger to speak to us and to others. I also think that God can use a person at the exact time He deems fit, to impact another person for His reasons that we don't understand at the time, or may never understand, or will come to understand at some point in our life, later. The point in my saying this is; I do believe people come into our lives for a reason. Sometimes people speak a truth into our heart that is helpful, something we need to hear. For me, I'd like to think that's exactly what all three of these individuals did, spoke prophetically into my life. They were preparing me for what was to come, or were confirming what I thought I knew, in the words they'd spoke.

Okay, so here's where it gets tricky. Just because these individuals spoke words that turned out to be prophetic, does that mean when someone says something to you or me, and it gets labeled "prophetic", mean that it WILL happen? No, I don't believe it will happen FOR SURE. Why? Because this is where man's "free will" comes in, just like I talked about in "Everything Happens for a Reason". Free will has the ability to change outcomes of what COULD BE with the choices that we or others all make.

Let me give an example of me knowing God is speaking to me, because truly, the Holy Spirit speaks to us humans all differently—communicating particularly for each one of us to hear His voice. It was a beautiful summer day, back when I had this particular experience. I was outside enjoying the sun's rays on the dock, watching the water, then closing my eyes and just soaking up all the peacefulness and warmth. As I laid there on the dock, a dollar amount was put on my mind, laying solidly on my heart. I hadn't even been thinking about money! In that moment, I got that same familiar feeling I get when God is speaking to me. He definitely spoke to me. And, I was to give a specific individual this specific amount of money--gifting it to the person.

As soon as Papa God had spoken to me, He reassured me and then was quiet. I was now sitting up on the dock looking around, at full attention. No one was around. There was no noise. It was me and the still lake, and the still small voice of Papa God in my head, stirring my heart. I moved myself onto my back and looked up to the sky while starting to audibly talk to my Papa God. My heart was blown wide open as I spoke, asking "*why?*" Quiet, and more quietness was the answer. My heart couldn't shake what I'd been told initially, the dollar amount and who was to get it.

251

When my heart can't shake a feeling, such as this was, I know that the words I'd been told must be done. After those couple days, asking and wondering, *"Do you really want me to do this, Papa?"* I still hadn't shaken that feeling. It took me a couple more days of praying, being sure that I was to give this specific dollar amount to the person.

It was time, I needed to write out a check for this specific dollar amount. So, I did. I also wrote a letter to the recipient and put both the check and the letter in an envelope. More days passed, and then the individual received it.

Okay, before finishing this story, maybe you can see that MY free will could have stopped this from happening. Right? I could have ignored the words to give money to so-and-so. So, I ask you, was this a prophetic telling of what I was to do? Yes, I think it was a prophetic word. How do I know? Well, let's find out! The individual received the envelope who'd received the letter and the check, and after a double take look at the check, spoke of the need for that specific dollar amount (not wanted, but truly NEEDED). I had NO idea the individual even needed money, let alone needed a determined amount for something specifically needed. I was absolutely clueless. But God is NOT CLUELESS! The individual was now able to use the money as needed! Pretty cool, huh?

What if I hadn't listened to my Papa God, and instead let fear consume my thoughts, and my free will respond with a *"NO, I will not give the money"*? The ending might not have turned out how it had, and the money could had come through another source, or not come at all. Who knows for sure but God Himself? On behalf of myself and this individual, we are both thankful we didn't have to find out how it may had turned out otherwise.

The point in my sharing this story is not for an accolade, or to prove to you that God speaks to me. I tell you because I believe God uses words, visions, and dreams to help us on our journeys in life, giving us courage to step out in faith, comforting us in a storm, or giving warning to help guide us to a better or chosen path.

Thus far in my health journey from illness to wellness, the prophetic words spoken to me by the reflexologist and Hallie had come to fruition. Donna's words were now, too, but would be in even more fullness in the days, months, and year to come. Donna knew there was a deeper issue, that the "Squishy" (biofilms) were wreaking havoc inside me, eating me alive. She was right. But as of right now in the telling of my health journey, those biofilms weren't being addressed at the deeper level that they needed to be. *What's next, Papa?*

63

Doctor North

Kelly

Mom and I talked about where I should go from here, having completed the online gut healing program, in regards to my health. We both knew I needed more professional help, because the biofilms were still detoxing out of me. And, because I was still unable to have a bowel movement on my own-- being constipated, multiple daily coffee enemas were still my best friend.

Together, we decided it would be a good idea for me to do a phone consult with Dr. North, who was one of the leaders involved in the online program's live webinars we attended each week. I called his office, he being out of state in the south. Getting a voice recording, I left a message for him.

Dr. North's assistant called me later that same day. We set up a phone consult for me to speak with Dr. North about my various symptoms and the continued abdominal and back pain. I gave the assistant my email address so paperwork could be forwarded to me for me to complete. I'd send it back ASAP.

Paperwork. Again, LOTS of questions to answers about digestion, the food I ate, what my bowel movements were like, the symptoms experienced when eating, food intolerances, sleep pattern or issues... just all sorts of questions I'd been asked so many times before! There were also questions I would have never thought as to WHY they were being asked!

My appointment was scheduled for the next week after I'd made contact with Dr. North's office. However, a few hours later after the initial contact, I was called again, the assistant saying, "Someone just cancelled their appointment for tomorrow afternoon, Kelly. If you want to take the appointment you can."

"Yes! I will take the appointment! Thank you for offering it to me. I really appreciate that." I replied! Then I got busy finishing the paperwork and sent it back along with three test results from when I was working with the FMD only a half-to-one year earlier. Surely Dr. North would want to know that information, I thought!

September 29th, 2015. Dr. North called me for our first consult, which came to be monthly phone consults for the next near two years after. As our conversation started, I told Dr. North a brief history of my last five years of left-side abdominal and back pain, telling him the symptoms I'd experienced and how they'd continually gotten worse until I started the on-line program.

"After I'd started the program, I was able to function through daily life easier. I could be free of pain for a few hours, or up to even a half of a day. Once in a great while I even made it through a whole day of having no pain, which is UNHEARD of! The symptoms all drastically changed for the better during the program." I told him. "I still have abdominal and back pain, along with most of the other symptoms too, again. If anything, they all seem to be coming back in full force."

"Kelly, tell me what your 'current' symptoms are." He inquired.

"I'm constipated. I've been constipated ever since I started the detox part of the online program (which Dr. North is a leader in, along with two other professionals). Prior to the program I had diarrhea anywhere from 5-15 times per day."

"Okay." He said, questioningly for me to proceed.

"I get headaches daily. Most of the time they are enhanced when my body needs to eliminate toxins. I battle nausea and dizziness a handful of times per week. I get bloated, and with that I have more intense abdominal pain due to the pressure. I get tired and fatigue easily. Afternoons are when my energy level is the lowest. I have left-side upper abdominal pain that is deep underneath the ribs. It extends down to just below my belly button. However, it always hurts underneath the ribs. The pain varies in intensity. I have left-side, middle, and low-back pain. The pain goes straight through my body into my back, three dimensionally, that feels like a stabbing knife."

Dr. North listened, asking many very direct questions. I answered his questions honestly. Then he said, "Tell me more about your left-side abdominal and back pain please, Kelly."

"The left-side pain is underneath my ribs. I have to reach under my ribs in order to attempt to grab at the *burning spot*. I've been told it feels like "FIRE" by two different massage therapists. The pain is mostly on the left side, but goes into the right side at times. The left-side abdominal pain started off as a dull, achy pain five-and-a-half years ago. Over the years, it has continually gotten worse. It goes through my body 3-D, like I was saying before, making my back hurt. Along with the left-side abdominal pain, I have left-side back pain. The middle-and-lower back-pain is just to the left side of my spine. The back pain is so deep inside that I can't grab it or touch it."

"What are the symptoms associated with the abdominal and back pain, Kelly?" He inquired.

"Currently I have headaches, low-back pain, nausea, dizziness, hot and cold sweats, and feel REALLY sick. Over the past five-and-a-half years I've gotten more food allergies and intolerances to foods. I've had diarrhea before, like I said, and now am constipated since doing the detox part of the program. Yellow spots have grown in the whites of both of my eyes. The whites of my eyes have a distinguished yellow tint in them (jaundice). I get abdominal cramps, and left-side pain 24/7. I am always fatigued," I said.

From this one initial appointment with Dr. North, we talked each month and started getting somewhere in discovering what my real health issue was. Dr. North has many titles behind his name. His knowledge in "Food as Medicine" is remarkable. He is licensed and practices as a homeopathy doctor, a dietary clinician, a botanist, and has a wealth of knowledge in other areas of health as well. Thank God for Dr. North being part of the online gut healing program. Had I chosen not to do that program, I would not have crossed paths with him. I thank God for making a path of helpers coming into my life, lightening the way for me to reverse my health.

256

64

Let's Talk Frankly

Kelly

On my very first appointment with Dr. North, he asked me VERY specific questions about my left-side pain. He wanted to know when the pain started. Then, asked to what degree the pain was and how it had gotten worse, or better, in the last many years since the onset. He had reviewed the paperwork and test results I'd sent to his office, before our appointment. He was well informed of my health situation.

Dr. North asked, "How long have you been constipated while doing the program?" And then, "Can you tell what is coming out in your daily enemas?"

"I'm getting loose stools with LOTS of biofilms in it." I replied. "The biofilm is always the first part to come out. Then, I may have some biofilms throughout the rest of the enema, but definitely not as much as initially. There's some formed stool but mostly it's sludgy." I informed him. *Remember, you can tell a lot about your health based upon your stool!*

"What does this biofilm look like, Kelly?" he inquired, kindly.

I answered, then elaborated, "I really think the biofilm is what is constipating me." He asked more questions. As Dr. North spoke, he educated me about these specific biofilms I was passing. He suggested I could "do some research" and told me more about it.

I will be the first to say, what grows inside of us and comes out in our poo, when forced to vacate our bodies, can be judged as a disgusting conversation." BUT, if I wanted to get to the ROOT-cause of my illness, I had to be completely honest, transparent, and vulnerable. I call this "Being REAL".

Dr. North's major concern was for my left-side abdominal pain. As for the specific biofilms I was passing? They were a BIG part of that pain. He proceeded to tell me, "I'm going to design a protocol specifically for you. It will give your body exactly what it needs. In the protocol I'm going to send you, there will be a homeopathic remedy for you to take immediately upon receiving it."

"Okay. I will." I replied.

"Don't wait for the other supplements to arrive before taking it." He instructed.

I responded, "I will do that. Thank you." After Dr. North answered and explained other questions I had for him, we set up my next month's phone consult and then ended my appointment.

Since I was at work, and my next client would be walking through the door any minute, I resisted the strong desire to do an internet search about this specific biofilm. There would be time for that later. For the time being, it was back to work for me.

My next client walked through the door at "Helping Hands Therapeutic Massage & Body Work". My focus was now solely on the client and their individual need for healing.

When I got a break in my work schedule later, I googled "biofilm" and did exactly what I liked doing, researching. Dr. North's words kept running through my mind. I found exactly what the good doctor was talking about. He'd told me about the different stages of "Rope Biofilms" (RBs) and how they mature through each phase. It was quite repulsive, thinking of what I was reading about was living inside of me and wreaking havoc in my body, and how these toxic cells have the ability to communicate with each other within the biofilms. Yet, I was so interested, more like so captivated, that I continued reading.

Wow, these things are killing me from the inside out. These RBs didn't come into my body on their own, because they cannot live in oxygenated environments. They started their cellular life inside of me, growing from within my acidic (lack of oxygen), inflamed, body. I was passing all five stages of these RBs in my daily enemas. Yikes! But woohoo! Shaking my head, I did what any research nerd does when she finds something really interesting... calls another research nerd--my mom, who was not at work with me this day to talk.

JE September 29th, 2015
I had my first phone consult with Dr. North today. He is an IMMENSE help! He figured out, well, a LOT! Facing my reality, a hellish nightmare... HELP ME LORD! Thank You for Dr. North, Papa God!

65

Toxicity Confirmation

Kelly

Being out of town, Mom answered her phone promptly knowing I'd had my appointment with Dr. North, immediately asking, "How did your phone consult with Dr. North go?"

I relayed the conversation, telling Mom everything. I told her Dr. North's thoughts and his intuitive knowing of what he sensed was going on in my health. "Mom, I've read more about these biofilms. He suggested I do some research. He was RIGHT! This is the toxic junk coming out of me." I spoke excitedly! "Remember how I'd told you about the craniosacral appointment with Cathy and Donna, specifically what Donna had said, 'she'd felt my abdomen was cold, damp, and squishy'?"

"I do remember you telling me, Kelly." Mom stated. "How could I forget that confirmation?" Mom and I then talked for a good length of time. We ended saying we were BOTH really thankful for Dr. North going deep, starting to address the ROOT issue of my health.

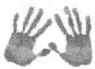

The next day after my first phone consult with Dr. North, and from then on, I paid even closer attention to what was coming out during my enemas.

Enemas were time consuming, but they were much needed for cleansing my intestines and getting the pathogen die-off quickly moving out of me. I was detoxifying AND healing my body, one enema at a time.

Within a few days after the phone consult with the good doctor, later stages of RBs (rope biofilms) were coming out in my enemas, all without additional "helps" in the form of detox supplements. This toxic stuff had certainly been festering in me for a LONG time.

Where do rope biofilms reside?
Rope biofilms (RBs) can reside anywhere in the human body during the first stages--mucous stage, but they prefer the small and large intestines where they have easy access to food. The RBs "feed off" of their host. Since they develop from inside human bodies (created and grown from heavy metal toxins, sugar, and all kinds of toxins such as drugs--prescription medications and recreational drugs, and from chemical exposures including GMOs in food) and then feed off-of the human. They don't have their own DNA... SO NO TEST CAN DETECT THEM. You cannot see these rope biofilms in X-rays. They are pretty much UNDECTABLE. These statements, above, can open up a whole can-of-worms in the field of medical diagnosis of "cancer". However, I'm not going down that road here.

In the intestines, the RBs continue to form and grow up to five stages, and basically suction themselves to the intestinal walls. As they metastasis, they have the ability to block the intestinal tract (hence, aiding in my being constipated). Rope biofilms are most active between one to six o'clock in the morning. They release toxins that suppress and hinder the immune system. They do not require oxygen to develop and grow. They actually will die WHEN exposed TO oxygen. They create cellularly, growing in an acidic environment, morphing from stage one to full grown, at stage five.

In a more recent medical conference in Dec. 2016 in Washington State, Dr. Klinghardt MD, PhD shared some thoughts about rope biofilms. "It is the first time in human evolution that our bodies are taxed with so many environmental toxins that are stored in the body and eventually impact our cells. As increased concentration of heavy metals have been found in rope... rope biofilms are POSSIBLY collectors of some of these toxins, helping us to survive our polluted environment."[8]

---

[8] Dr. Dietrich Klinghardt "Ropeworms – What Are They", Dec. 4, 2016
https://ropeworms.com/ropeworms-biofilms-klinghardt/

Interesting suggestion by Dr. Klinghardt, of "ropes being a 'help' to humans living in this polluted world." So, these RBs were actually helping me, is what he is suggesting? What I saw as my hellish nightmare, he is suggesting was a possible help? *Go figure.*

What symptoms can be produced from rope biofilms?
Also, in the article, Dr. Klinghardt said, "Rope biofilms can alter human attention and reaction. They can cause multiple symptoms including but not limited to: weight gain or loss, food allergies and intolerances, common colds, coughing, back pain, rashes, headaches, indigestion, hair loss, abdominal pain, imbalanced gut flora, nausea and much more. They are suspected of being involved in cancer, heart disease, Attention Deficit, Autism, and Alzheimer's. Science, in the world of naturopathy, is learning even more about biofilms and the disastrous effects they have on people's health, including almost all chronic illnesses."

If you're interested, do an internet search of Dr. Dietrich Klinghardt's article, "Ropeworms are Biofilms" to investigate further--reference found at the bottom of the prior page. And, if you are interested in learning even more about biofilms in general, visit Chris Kresser, "Kresser Institute", at his website on the internet for the article, "Biofilm: What It Is and How to Treat it"[9].

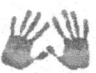

Dr. North's remedy came a week-and-a-half after our first phone consult. I took the remedy immediately. Then a few days later, the rest of the supplements he wanted me to start on arrived, which I started taking as noted in the supplied instruction paperwork.

In the last three years, every time I'd started taking a new supplement, I would get really sick. This time, now, was different though! I didn't get sick immediately upon taking ANY of them! This was a HUGE change! I had times that I felt bad after taking them, but the supplements weren't causing me to be bloated, nauseated, acquiring a pounding headache, or feeling outright lousy. This was a wonderful change!

[9] Chris Kresser "Biofilm. What It Is and How to Treat It" March 6, 2018
https://kresserinstitute.com/biofilm-what-it-is-and-how-to-treat-it/

I'd learned a great deal of helpful information while doing the gut healing program. I needed to continue daily implementing many of those healing methods I'd learned. If I didn't do these strategies regularly, I knew that my healing process would take longer. I was determined. I continued doing daily coffee enemas, of course, and many of the other detoxification methods such as castor oils packs, medicinal teas, detox baths, using essential oils—diffusing and applying on myself, using food is medicine, taking nutritional supplements, and more strategies for improving my health.

This entire healing process was like pulling off layers of an onion, taking time (years) and patience (acquiring patience with every possible situation that arose), and a whole lot of tears in between.

Lord, I trust You. You are in control. Please, show me the way and direct my path. I know You will, thank You.

66

Laughter = Beautiful Music

Kelly

I was learning a LOT during this entire healing process. One thing that I was continually learning, then accepting, and eventually embracing, was that I NEVER knew how I would feel from one minute to the next.

I might feel AWESOME physically at one moment, and the next minute the pain could grab ahold inside of my body stabbing me. Stabs were always a painful surprise. But, as I've said before and I'll say it again, I found joy in the simple things because of this daily challenge. That's the honest truth. Whether I felt good or not, I was always trying to find joy in my circumstances no matter how I may have been feeling.

What are the first thoughts that come to mind when we hear the word "laughter"? Funny? Comical? Contagious? Sore abdomen? Noise? Freedom? When I think of laughter, I think of a lot of those words and more! Did you know that laughter decreases stress hormones and releases endorphins, the natural "feel good" chemicals in your body?

When I was sick, I can look back at a season of life where I had virtually no laughter. Please, DON'T feel sorry for me. Let me explain! Remember when I've said that it hurt my gut to cry (sobbing) and that's when I learned to cry more "beautifully", doing so silently? Well, I also had to learn to not laugh because laughing caused a lot of abdominal pain too. Try as I might, there just wasn't another option for laughing. So, for a few years I barely ever laughed. And when I rarely did laugh it hurt like crazy.

It has been said, "laughter is the best medicine". Sometimes in life, we have to give up things that are important, actually needed and valuable, for a season of time because they just aren't the right fit for that season. You know what I mean? Like when a spouse gets sick, and you, being their spouse or caregiver, discontinue your weekly bowling league, or favorite activities for a season of time until life gets back to a new normal—your loved one back to being well again, able to take care of themself.

Laughing, to me now-a-days, is truthfully music to my ears. I can't tell you how many times other people's laughter moves me. Or my own laughter, or my family's laughter moves me when we are all together. Being sick and living together (as a family of four) with a lot less laughter happening, with my health teetering on the brink of destruction, was pretty heavy for all of us. As a general rule of thumb, if you know our family, we often worked hard and played hard together. Actually, as I'm writing this here, years after the facts of this health challenge, we still do work hard, but we each are pulled in different directions with our jobs, so we have less free-time for our own interests and hobbies, so it's a lot less time together playing now.

Anyways, the dynamics of our family were pretty upbeat with a lot of laughter in all the time we'd spent together while I was growing up! Then, after becoming sick, laughter still happened with other members of our family, but rarely was I joining in. Over time, it seemed they were laughing less, too. It was sad, but that's the truth of the matter. My health had sort of "blanketed" laughter, even for them. But they shared plenty of laughter with others, so they still got their feel-good endorphins released.

To this day, I still remember the first time I laughed while still "detoxing", and it actually didn't hurt me! Our family was sitting together at the kitchen table. Having just finished a meal, spontaneous laughter started. It was contagious. We all laughed, unable to stop. You know that feeling when you're laughing and it's pure, innocent, carefree, and coming from the deepest part of your being? Well, that's what it was! As I laughed, I had a check in my spirit, and took notice to what was happening. I was laughing HARD for the first time in years! And it felt GOOD! It was almost surreal. Our family of four shared OUR first real free-flowing laughter ALL together for the first time again! After that meal, as Mom and I were standing in the kitchen doing dishes, Mom tenderly stated as tears slipped down her face, "Kelly, you were laughing tonight. I couldn't help but just sit and watch you when you were laughing, because it was such beautiful music to my ears."

Tears were flowing down my face now as well. "I know, Mom. When I started laughing, it was almost as if I was pulled out of myself, looking at myself sitting at the counter from outside the house through the window. I was looking in and taking in the whole scene, being able to watch myself sit and laugh." Mom nodded her head. "And when I was laughing, I had turned and looked to you. You then looked me so deeply in the eyes that I knew you were thinking the same thing, 'She's REALLY laughing. This is the first time in YEARS! What beautiful music!'" I'd spoke.

There are so many aspects of life that each of us can so readily take for granted. For me, laughter was certainly one of them. Now days... I laugh freely without pain. I can laugh without thinking twice about any consequences! I can share spontaneous laughter with family, friends, strangers, and even with you here while reading! Laughter. It's a true joy, one that I'm forever grateful for.

As we each go about our day, let's listen to the music of both our own laughter and other people's. Let the music open our eyes, hearts, and ears to the beauty laughter brings into our lives!

67

Glyphosate – Toxic Poisoning

Amy

I recall hearing a number of years ago, a person questioning us, his listening audience from all around the world during a conference online, "Are we 'humans' with a 'genetic expression', or are we a 'genetic expression' having a 'human experience'?" I remember laughing out loud at that, then shortly thereafter NOT laughing and finding myself really thinking about what was said—a very thought-provoking question.

Have you ever thought about WHAT it is that makes you human? Or, have you ever thought as to how your body is intricately designed? Do you know what you, I, and every "living and breathing" thing is made up of? Kelly and I just talked about this again recently, what makes up our body and how each person is so alike, yet we are so different from another human being.

The answer to what makes us human is "cells". Every living thing is made up of cells—our DNA. When a living cell is fed what it specifically needs to function, it thrives and is productive within its environment, working with other cells to become its full potential and expression. When living cells are missing specific nutrients designed for their specific makeup, or are being poisoned by something being put on or into them, then that cell, that living organism, or that human being, will not thrive but instead self-destruct.

Chemicals are used in our food system here in America. There's a well-known chemical produced by a very large and well-known company—who is one of the world's largest chemical companies, and is the most widely used herbicide in the United States. About 100 million pounds of this chemical are applied to U.S. farm fields and American's lawns every year, according to an environmental agency that is supposed to be protecting Americans. Proof of this statistic is not found on an internet search anymore, so you'll have to trust my information is accurate. The facts simply disappeared from the web in recent years while publishing this book. *Go figure.* I don't use actual names here for the sake of our own 'safety", not wanting to disappear as did the information on internet.

Glyphosate is a toxin and an active ingredient in the well-known chemical mentioned in the last paragraph. Glyphosate levels in American farmland soils AND air have soared in recent decades. Did you know glyphosate kills human cells, particularly embryonic, placental and umbilical cord cells? What is being sprayed on food crops within industrialized farming--the practices of using chemicals and seeds designed to grow with use of this chemical, and spread onto lawns to kill weeds but not grass is literally killing us as humans, amphibians, insects, plants, and mammals. Again, this information is not found on an internet search anymore, so you'll have to trust my information as accurate. I use NO SPECIFIC company name or product here. You can probably name the company yourself.

All of us Americans, and many people across other countries around the world, have a pervasive exposure to glyphosate and other chemical toxins on a regular basis. It's unavoidable in the 21st century. We need to eliminate glyphosate from our body before it ruins our immune system, resulting in chronic inflammation and infections, all leading to poor health. I'm hoping this is not new information to anyone, so far. Surely you have heard the arguments about chemical poisons in our industrialized food system. How does growing genetically enhanced, science-based crops that are then used as ingredients in GMO foods cause problems with our health?

When laboratory designed foods made of GMO ingredients come into our digestive system, which cannot recognize the GMO particles AS food, then the immune system sees the particle(s) as the enemy and is ready to fight. These GMO designed foods are only a PART of what is causing so much ill health all around the world. Since our bodies cannot recognize the DNA of these foreign foods, the GMO food ignite a defense pattern in our immune system to hold back the "invader". After years of these patterns taking place, our bodies become inflamed, having inflammation, then illness eventually sets in. The body fights hard until it is overcome by the toxins. The timeframe of this happening is different for each individual. The immune system then can no

268

longer fight any enemy domestically when overcome by toxins. At this point, more GMO particles entering the body become a bigger problem--the person experiencing this battle may take notice to food allergies, headaches, skin rashes, hot flashes, and many other symptoms which lead to developing chronic diseases, and many other illnesses leading directly to an early death. The truth is, this system of making prepackaged food made with foreign agents disguised as "food ingredients" doesn't help us at all. It harms us and should be outlawed. It actually is outlawed in some countries, by the way.

There's more going on here than meets the eye. We were told in the 60's a "new type of genetically modified wheat", containing glyphosate and various kinds of gluten, "produces twelvefold the amount of product compared to older versions of wheat", and that "it would solve the world's hunger problem". This was not the beginning of our food system being poisoned, but it made a bigger impact on soils and humans being poisoned. On the surface, the modified wheat seed may look like it solved the world's hunger problem. But in reality, these foreign agents in food, GMO designer foods, and the chemicals used to grow food crops are all cellularly killing us as a human race from the inside out.

I hope we each do our research and find out for ourselves what is good vs. what really does harm our health concerning GMOs, the processes and chemicals used in growing these types of crops and products made from those.

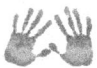

Family is important to me. Is it to you also? I came across a group called "Moms Across America" recently, on the internet. These moms are responsibly informed, helping to educate others, and are making an impact in our world through their various efforts to clean up our food system in America. Check them out online. Do a search on them, momsacrossamerican.com.

I encourage each of us to do our own investigating. By watching any of the documentaries, movies, or videos from the list provided from the "Moms Across America" website, which have a good, reliable information base to start from, having not seen many of their videos, I can tell you that "Food Matters" is an informative documentary to start with, or "Genetic Roulette: The Gamble of Our Lives". Also, "Super-Size Me" is very eye-opening to anyone who thinks "fast food" is nourishment to our bodies.

A statement from the "Moms Across America" website--"The movies and videos everyone should watch to understand what is going on with our food supply and Genetically Engineered crops in the USA and other countries."[10]

Seriously look into this website to get informed, if any of this just shared information on glyphosate is new to you. If you love your family, you'll definitely want to keep them safe from harm as much as one possibly can. Please, do your research and then decide what is best for you and yours concerning feeding your family.

---

[10] Moms Across America, https://www.momsacrossamerica.com/

68

The Perfect Storm

Kelly

In "Glyphosate – Toxic Poisoning", Mom shared valuable information that we should all be aware of. GMOs are also at an all-time high of being designed, manufactured, and dispersed across our country in grocery stores everywhere. Glyphosates are wreaking utter chaos in people's guts, damaging people's health. Glyphosate poisoning of people's bodies is at an all-time high, a BIG cause for so many cancers diagnosis and deaths.

Are biofilms a byproduct of GMOs in processed foods? I believe yes, definitely, it is but not all science experts in the fields of "health" and "nutrition" are in agreement, at least not yet. I think the altered DNA from GMOs in humans (AND in animals/pets) have negatively altered human intestinal cells and bacteria, forming a new life form INSIDE of us—living off of us and is therefore causing cancer. I've come to the conclusion that IF biofilms can develop inside our bodies, igniting a cellular birth of mucous (inflammation) because of the GMO foods we eat, then the toxins contained within these processed foods are surely the fuels that feeds the biofilms to later stages of growth leading to toxic overload—cancers of various kinds.

"Seriously" you ask? Yes! I was eighteen years old when I changed my SAD (standard American diet) to a healthier diet. I'd ate and drank whatever I wanted for all those years before that (mostly under my parent's supervision, of course). I had unknowingly set-up a perfect environmental scenario in my gut for these biofilms to develop and grow; in a cold, damp, acidic environment, and eventually having multiple problems such as allergies, leaky gut, SIBO, and food sensitivities. The inflammation (biofilms, stage 1) was imbedded in me with no means of escape up until the online gut healing program. So, the biofilm organisms grew in stages, up to stage 5 inside of me. When I began to detox, by taking supplements that gathered up pathogens in my gut, and more specifically by doing coffee enemas to carry out these biofilms—pathogens, was how I started to reverse my health. The supplements and specific food I consumed (as medicine) in my diet were aiding in killing the biofilms. The biofilms are very hard to disrupt, but it CAN be done.

Remember in "Toxicity Confirmation", I'd said the rope biofilms (RBs) have a human DNA and they are "undetectable" in testing? I'd also said, "They feed off of the human". In turn, they were stealing nutrients from me, causing MANY problems including malnutrition.

Growing up, I hadn't practiced ANY kind of detoxification. We Americans are lacking in total body detoxifying practices, which should be done at least once annually but better to do semi-annually--spring and fall.

PH (Potential Hydrogen) also plays a role in establishing a "perfect storm" environment for RBs to develop. Our gut PH should be alkaline, which supports a healthy body. I've talked about the importance of PH before in "What am I Drinking?, so I'm just reminding us of the IDEAL alkaline range is between 8-10, but 7's is good too. Anything under 7 is considered acidic. The lower a person's acidity, the more susceptible they are to illness and disease. Testing PH is fast and very easy. There are a few different ways to test for it, including testing saliva or urine, that one can do at home needing only "PH Test Strips" costing anywhere from $7-$13 that are easy to find on-line or at a natural health store or a food coop near you!

Did you know by looking into a person's eyes, seeing the appearance of the eye(s), is another good indicator of our health? The conjunctiva (which is part of the whites around our pupils) can tell a lot about one's state of health: if they are red, inflamed, pale, creamy/blurry, or yellow colored, dull, telling if one is sickly or if they are vibrantly healthy.

Back in 2013, I'd started getting a yellow spot in the conjunctiva of my right eye, although both eyes were yellowish in color (jaundice) before that. I figured it would go away with time. I didn't know for sure that this yellow spot was a helpful indicator of my ill health.

After a few months of having this yellow spot in my eye, the left eye was following suit. I then went to my eye doctor seeking answers. He immediately told me, "You have an inflamed pinguecula in both eyes. The right eye is worse than the left." The doctor then gave me some eye drops in hopes of helping to reduce the inflammation. "If the spots don't disappear within a few days, I will order you something stronger" he'd said.

"I'm leaving for Colorado with my brother in a couple days. I won't be able to get those eye drops if I need them." I'd responded. The doctor proceeded to give me all the information needed if I'd have to pick up stronger eye drops while on our alpine skiing adventure. I did purchase the stronger eye drops while on vacation, and used both bottles of drops with NO improvements.

Once home from Colorado skiing, I hadn't gone back to the eye doctor because deep down in my heart I had a feeling it was correlated with my left-side pain. This was all back in 2013. Mom and I had talked about it and agreed, even though we didn't know HOW it correlated with my left-side pain directly at that time. We saw this as a symptom from a deeper issue going on inside of me. Amazingly, at that time in 2013, the yellow spots began to improve when I had started going to Dr. Ann, the homeopathy doctor. She'd helped me understand the importance of an alkaline PH environment in my body.

Changing my diet was slowly helping to improve my gut health and the yellow spots in my eyes. Illness and disease stem from a weak immune system. The bad pathogens attack the "weakest organs" in our bodies, our "weakest link(s)". This, then, is when pathogens multiply, causing illness to not just lurk in our body, but grow into disease. If we're not feeding and providing our bodies nutrients needed to function and fight off pathogens, then we are feeding illness and disease, which then metastasizes, wreaking havoc inside of us. It's scary to think about, I know, but something we all should be aware of, too.

As Hippocrates says, **"All diseases begin in the gut."** Let's make sure we are taking care of our gut, feeding it good, wholesome non-GMO foods!

69

Essentials

Kelly

"Coffee" enemas were not the only way I eradicated rope biofilms (RBs) from within my gut. Supplements, food as medicine, remedies and other specific helps from Dr. North were all aiding in killing the biofilms. But also, in this process of detoxing, I used essential oils IN the enemas at various times.

Like I've said before, I'm a health research nerd. While researching essential oils one day, I found that lemon juice AND essential oil enemas also worked to get rid of RBs. If you knew me personally, you'd know that I stand behind what I say when recommending something, providing the information I know for myself to be true. Furthermore, if I don't know it to be true for myself, I'll clearly state that fact. I concocted a self-made mixture of purified water, lemon juice, and essential oils for some enemas periodically for a day, specifically: Frankincense, Lemon, and two other combination oil mixes. These helped me to detox. The oils absorb directly into the blood stream, killing any and all bad pathogens and bacteria coming in contact with the oils. "Essential oil enemas" weren't something that my body wanted regularly, so I only did this specific oil blend when I sensed my body needed one, sometimes doing a few back-to-back. I was to the point in the detoxification process that I spent a LOT of time in the bathroom doing enemas, usually two enemas per day, and sometimes three. My body was detoxing HEAVILY. It was essential that I kept up with the die-off process happening daily.

Physically, I was tired from all the time I spent in the bathroom doing enemas. Detoxification is NOT easy! It is hard on a body, even though it is essential to keep up the pace so that the die-off would not stay inside of me making me feel more ill. I had only been doing enemas for just over a couple months at this

274

point. I was physically wanting to be done with enemas. HA! But, deep in my heart I knew, *it's going to be a good length of time before I am done detoxifying my body.*" Despite my desire to be done with enemas, stopping the process was NOT an option. I KNEW that I needed to get rid of all this toxic junk, bad pathogens, inside of me because they had been slowly killing me. Essential oils were going to be another player in the detoxification process!

You might be to the point in reading my story finding yourself thinking, *"What was the one contributor that helped the MOST in reversing your health?"* I've been asked this question a great number of times through the years. Truthfully, there wasn't any single one contributor that was what ultimately "healed" me. It was a great many contributors combined that helped me heal. Some of the biggest were: coffee enemas, using food as medicine, nutritional supplements, Dr. North's remedies and protocols, detox baths, and colonics. There wasn't one contributor that was the miracle worker. It was the combination of everything, including the duration of time in whatever season of healing that I was in, AND my being at peace with my situation that all contributed, being vitally important, in the process to heal.

Essential oils are an amazing aid to healing and improving one's health all-around. Essential oils are proven to aid in healing many ailments, illnesses, and diseases. Essential oils are highly concentrated, so they have a strong aroma, although a person can dilute the oils as well. To fully understand the concentrate of these oils, to make a bottle size of 5ml of Rose essential oil it would take 22 pounds of rose pedals! That's a lot of roses, so it's no wonder Rose oil is one of the most expensive oils to purchase. Only the most powerful healing parts or pieces of a plant are used to make an essential oil.

I first started using essential oils when I was in high school, to help with headaches and seasonal allergies. When I was introduced to these oils, I was skeptical of them actually doing anything. HA! *How can a simple oil help with allergies?* I'd thought to myself way back then. Using a mixture of Lavender and Peppermint oils, equal parts of both, and rubbing a few drops onto my temples helped ease headaches. We used this combination of oils often, having a bottle available within reach at home and on the road.

Back in my mid-teens, Mom had been having allergy and sinus issues while she was visiting at a friend's house. Her friend asked her, "Do you want to try some essential oils to help with your sinus symptoms?" They had a short discussion. Mom did want to try the oils, so together the two of them combined the oils needed and Mom experimented with the concoction. Within five minutes, Mom's headache was breaking up. Her eyes stopped itching, her nasal passages began to open and soon started draining. She was feeling better in just ten minutes!

When Mom left her friend's house, getting back on the road she'd called me saying, "You should try these oils, Kelly! They've brought me immediate relief! I'm sure they will help with your seasonal allergy's symptoms too!"

What the heck. What do I have to lose? I thought to myself. *It's worth a try!* "Okay." I replied hopefully.

When Mom came home, she had a bottle of each of the individual oils. Her eyes danced in anticipation as she grinned at me, holding the oils as if they were gold in her hands. "Are you ready to try them?"

"As ready as I'll ever be!" I laughed. Soon after, my headache started to subside within minutes after using the oils. "Mom! You're RIGHT! The oils DO work!" I'd exclaimed excitedly!

For the next few years, I continued to use essential oils for my allergies. It wasn't a cure all for eradicating allergies, but the oils helped immensely with alleviating allergy "symptoms".

Essential oils are used for many reasons, including: cleaning your home, purifying the air, helping fight cold and flu symptoms, relaxing your body, soothing sore muscles, alleviating pain, balancing hormones, improving digestion, aiding in healing skin conditions such as cellulite and wrinkles, and are also used in homemade personal care products and homemade laundry detergents!

One REALLY neat aspect about essential oils is that they have the ability to cross the blood-brain barrier. Did you know most of the molecules of the substances used in chemotherapy are too large to pass through the blood-brain filter/barrier, which is why scientists and doctors say chemotherapy doesn't work on brain cancer? Some of the smaller molecules of chemo get through, but not the whole combination of the drug that's intended for its use. They don't know for sure, but it seems that in order to cross the blood-brain barrier, only molecules less than 800-1000amu (atomic mass units) in molecular weight can get through, some experts have said. That being said, when it comes to essential oils, certain oils have less than 500amu.

Have you ever heard the phrase "Frankincense is GOLD!" Well, it is! It has less than 50amu. Hence, Frankincense oil has proven itself to play a VITAL role aiding in deteriorating brain tumors, and kicking brain cancer (and other types of cancer as well) in the can! Based upon firsthand experience, frankincense oil aided my health in my healing journey. When I started having abdominal pain in 2010, I slowly started learning more about the different essential oils and experimenting even more with them. Different oils helped with certain ailments, and some helped with multiple ailments! I started researching specific essential oils that could help with my left-side abdominal and back pain. Then, I started using Frankincense oil on my left side regularly. And guess what? When I applied it to my abdomen, where the cancer was deep inside of me, it didn't hurt my skin at all, but felt like it was burning deep INSIDE my body in the firey-hot spot I've spoken of so often.

I eventually implemented essential oils into my business, both in retail sale and using them in some of the massage therapies we offer at "Helping Hands Therapeutic Massage & Body Work" They've made a great impact in improving my health and the lives of others! They are certainly essentials in my life and lifestyle!

70

Healing from the Inside Out

Kelly
JE October 12th, 2015
Thank you for coffee enemas and detoxing all this nasty, toxic stuff, Papa God. Please remove it ALL and let me know when they are all gone Lord! I trust You and THANK YOU for this AMAZING journey these past five-plus years, Papa! It's been rough, but truly amazing!

Another month passed, nearing the end of October, 2015. It was time to speak with Dr. North again! During the monthly consult, I told Dr. North the specifics about the RBs I was passing.

Dr. North listened intently as I talked, and then said, "Fill me in on anything else I should know, Kelly. Tell me, how you have been feeling? What has or hasn't changed?"

I shared, willingly. "The 3-D pain in my left side has improved a lot! When my body is ready to detoxify itself, that is when I mostly get the left-side pain. I usually only have this pain once or twice a day for the most part. I still have days that I don't feel 'well'. The left-side abdominal and back pain has improved versus last month, when it hurt constantly." I paused, thinking, then continued. "The headaches have decreased. Dizziness and nausea only happen a handful of times a week. I'm still constipated... that hasn't changed. Hot and cold sweats still come and go, although there are not as many of them."

"Okay." He said still listening intently.

"I still wake up during the wee hours of the morning, feeling sick. That has decreased though. I still fight fatigue and low energy. When my energy is low, I'm physically tired. Taking an afternoon nap would help." I joked. "I've never been a napping person."

"It's good that these changes are happening, Kelly. We are making progress! I would like to see you making even bigger progress now. I'm going to design a new protocol for you. The protocol that I have you on now has been very helpful. This new protocol I'm going to design will hopefully bring even bigger results." He said warmly.

He continued to talk and asked me questions. Dr. North told me that the new protocol was going to be more direct for the healing of my leaky gut. And, the new supplements would help seal the loose junctions in my intestines. This was where the biofilms had first grown, in my intestines where my junctions were loose from leaking gut, unfortunately inviting BAD pathogens to live and pass through. "The aloe vera juice we are going to have you take is going to help soothe your digestive system, bringing more healing as well." He stated. I would also be taking another homeopathic remedy like I had in my first protocol from him. "Take the remedy upon receiving it. The supplements will, again, arrive a few days after the remedy. This new remedy will take care of your salt craving." he advised me, both of us knowing that my adrenal glands were fatigued. The salt cravings I had were a good indicator of fatigued adrenal glands. They were stressed, fatigued, from being sick for so long with the rigorous detoxification process my body was going through. I needed all the energy and healing I could get, and addressing my adrenals was vital to reduce my stress level.

Dr. North's remedy arrived in the mail shortly thereafter, and I took the remedy upon its arrival, as instructed. Within the next 24 hours of taking the remedy, I no longer had any salt cravings. *AMAZING!* I still enjoyed having the added flavor of sea salt added onto some foods, however I no longer needed large amounts of salt to feel satisfied. Soon after the other supplements arrived, and within a week's time of taking those I noticed that my symptoms were, again, slowly improving. More days passed. The headaches decreased in frequency.

A day quickly came where I only had two headaches per day; 1 headache right away in the morning when doing my coffee enema, ending with the released stool from enema-induced therapy, and another headache towards a day's end when a build-up of RB die-off would pile up inside of me. This was HUGE progress! *This is surreal to go through an entire day without any continuous headaches,* I thought to myself!

The first thing to come out in my daily coffee enemas were always the rope biofilms (RBs). They were plugging me up--stopping me from having a bowel movement on my own. However, with each enema I was eradicating more of the toxic organisms that were living inside of me, living off of me, and I was beginning to really heal from the inside out! Protocols and remedies, along with enemas and other daily helps, were all working together for me to have GOOD results!

71

Steps in the Right Direction

Kelly

JE October 26th, 2015

My body is really and truly exhausted, Papa. Help me to hang in here and get all this toxic junk out! To be FREE and truly begin to heal again, to have energy and feel good. Not to mention, have my own BMs again. I look forward to those days, whenever they may be. My body knows when it needs to detoxify and I'm listening and abiding, Papa God.

During the course of the next month something new was happening! The left-side pain had decreased—was improving! The burning hot firey-hot spot was DROPPING! **BOOM!** The first time I felt the "dropping sensation" deep inside of me was when I was lying in bed on my left side. It felt like something dropped inside my abdomen, going in the direction of my thighs, (dropping over, but if I'd been standing it would have been dropping down). I didn't know what was happening, but I took notice! The same dropping sensation happened again the next night. The thought, *I bet this burning firey-hot spot, the cancer, is beginning to fall apart,* went flying through my mind. The dropping happened yet again before I spoke with Dr. North in November of 2015.

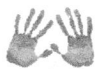

So, what were the days like, and symptoms I had, at this point in time? I still had "really bad days", but they weren't as often or nearly as severe as they'd used to be. If I had to compare the bad days to the years prior to this, they didn't even compare. Bad days now consisted of headaches, severe low-back pain, nausea, dizziness (sometimes), hot sweats, left-side and upper-abdominal pain (hot and achy), bloating (sometimes), constipation (which enemas always helped with), low or sometimes no energy, and an overall bodily weakness.

A "normal day" at this time consisted of some, or all, of these symptoms: low-back pain, always present to some degree like it had been for the last three years although not as severe, a headache or two a day, left-side abdominal and upper-abdomen pain--mostly a dull ache, but could be a dull burning sensation, and being physically tired, fatigued.

Activity, work, and heavy detoxing played a role in being fatigued. The intensity from all of the detoxing my body was doing was exhausting my energy. I would go to bed at night feeling utterly worn out, unable to go to sleep right away because my body was so weary, but unable to "relax" because of the stress it was under. My head COULD pound with tremendous headaches into the night. The left side pain was 3-D, and try as I might I could never access my fingers or the Thera Cane deep enough into my body to reach that firey-hot spot to bring any kind of relief. I'd roll about, a lot, while in bed because of the left-side pain. When awakening in the morning, I'd feel like I had hardly slept at all. Sleep wasn't always like that though. I had nights that I DID sleep well.

I always slept especially well after my monthly massages! I averaged 6-8 hours of sleep a night--which for a young adult is an okay amount, but when a person is sick, that's not ideal, but those few select days that I slept really well I could get 9-10 hours. Those longer sleeps were SO wonderful, to wake up in the morning feeling like I had truly slept deep! I felt rejuvenated, kind of. My body was sore all over from the intensity of detoxing. I had been detoxing heavily since June 2015, and it was now mid-November, being almost five whole months.

Slowly but surely, I was seeing and feeling healing results! Each day was filled with healing. There were a variety of different healing "helps" I'd do. Some of the methods still included: coffee enemas, castor oil packs for liver cleansing, detox baths, light exercise, quiet time, using essential oils, looking at all realms of healing physically, emotionally, mentally, spiritually executing what came to light, eating healing foods, spices, herbs and drinking herbal teas

282

and lots of water, and doing lots of self-care! I didn't have extra time to do anything else but to help myself. I needed to focus on healing, and that took all the time and energy I had while still doing my job of running my own business. It was a process, juggling everything, but I enjoyed it never-the-less. I was finding the right balance in it all, and I had people who had my back when I needed extra help in all areas of life, special thanks to my family. Also, a special thanks to those few select individuals that knew the true state of my health, who were always there for me and praying for me too.

Healing takes time. I WAS healing, from the inside out. I was truly seeing the healing begin, taking BIG steps in the right direction.

72

Slow and Steady Progress

Kelly

November 23rd, 2015. My phone rang. It was Dr. North. "Hello!" I answered.

"Hello, Kelly!" Dr. North said, "Please tell me, what has or hasn't changed in the past month? How are you feeling? What's new or different in reference to symptoms? Give me an update on your overall health progress." His voice was always jolly, full of care and light-heartedness in greeting AND otherwise!

"I continue to make slow and steady progress towards healing. Headaches are fewer, only one or two per day. Nausea and dizziness happened a couple times this month. The left-side abdominal pain is slowly, continually, getting better. Low-back pain is still present but that, too, is continually getting better. My skin, hair, nails and eye health have all been improving the last many months. I'm less fatigued. My energy is improving, somewhat. Prior to this month, I didn't have much extra any energy at all." I stated. "The biofilms continue to come out right away in the enemas. I'm still constipated, but I think that is due to the toxic junk die-off. Overall, progress is being made. Subtle changes, which I know… healing takes time!" I laughed lightly, genuinely.

"Good. I'm glad to hear that we have some changes happening! The supplements and remedy worked well for you then?" Dr. North asked, knowingly. More questions were asked and I answered them. I asked a few of my own questions and he gave me helpful insights.

"I have something new, and weird, that has happened a few times since we last talked. It's never happened before." I stated.

"Okay, tell me about it," he replied openly.

"The firey-hot spot in my left side, underneath my rib cage? Well, I was lying in bed one night and all of a sudden, I felt a dropping sensation. I felt it deep inside the upper left portion of my abdomen. Since then, the dropping has happened a few other times."

"Okay." He said, still listening.

"Also, when I've done my coffee enemas lately, I have this feeling that whatever has been dropping needs to come out of my body, but it won't..." My voice trailed off. "I have another question too. When I was going to a functional medicine doctor, he had me do a 'Comprehensive Stool Analysis Test' (CSAT). The reason that he recommended that test was because he wanted to see if there was anything 'abnormal' going on in my gut. I'm wondering if a CSAT isn't something that might help us find out exactly what is going on inside my abdomen? A lot has changed since the last time I did the test."

"Yes, Kelly, you brought up a very helpful point. It would give us a lot of information based upon the results. I can order you a CSAT that you can do right in your home. Upon completion of it, you will mail it directly to the testing lab. I think this would be a very good test for you to do again." Dr. North replied.

"Okay. Mom and I were talking about it recently, wondering if a new CSAT would be helpful." I added.

"I would like you to do the CSAT." He stated confidently. We then talked about the good progress I was already making. The progress was small but the fact that I was making progress was important! Healing takes time. Time would be a big key. "I'm going to design another protocol for you." He continued to share the new protocol for me to follow. "One of the supplements I'm going to have you take will help with the gut-brain connection: crossing the blood-brain barrier in order to 'wake up' your neurotransmitters. The gut-brain connection will help with reversing, or eliminating, constipation along with many other things. I want you to be able to have a bowel movement on your own, hopefully by your next phone consult. If not, then we are setting up the terrain for the bowel movements to happen in due time." He informed me.

"I'll send out the CSAT to complete at home. The next time we talk I'll go over the CSAT results with you." We soon finished the consult, Dr. North saying, "Until then, bye-bye!" I smiled at his well-known "bye-bye" I'd come to really enjoy hearing.

The Comprehensive Stool Analysis Test kit came in the mail. I did my deposit during a morning enema, packaged everything appropriately and then returned the pre-addressed box of samples to the lab, overnight delivery, to get tested. I'd get the test results back in three weeks or so, and then we would review the results together on the next phone consult with Dr. North.

73

Awestruck Wonder

Kelly

Throughout the next month, I continued to experience the "dropping sensation" in my abdomen. There was never a certain time of day, or any indication when the dropping was going to happen. I'd experienced it when I was on the floor stretching, lying in bed while trying to fall asleep, and even while working on a client doing my job. I never had any warning when it was going to happen! Each time the "dropping sensation" happened, though, my upper abdomen, specifically my left side, felt better!

Hmmm... the "dropping sensation" is always on my left side. It would drop from the firey-hot spot deep within the inner most part of the upper abdomen, falling an inch or two, seemingly. At this stage, the small and large intestinal area was feeling less inflamed, less than it had been just two months ago. *That "dropping sensation" has been the rope biofilms dying,* I thought inwardly. Now that firey-hot spot was firmer too, not squishy. The firey-hot spot in my abdomen had changed considerably in the past 2-3 months. I could touch the area without much pain due to the outside pressure I applied to that spot now. I could even reach down underneath my ribs at times without as much pain!

The "dropping sensation" continued sporadically for the next weeks and months. I felt the drop going lower and lower each time it happened. One time, when the dropping happened, it felt like whatever was dropping had dropped close to my bladder. That same week my bladder couldn't hold as much content as it normally did, until the drop happened once again. And when it did happen again, within that same week I started to notice more interesting stuff coming out in my daily enemas. It may sound weird that I actually enjoyed this. It almost felt as if I was doing my own science project. And this research nerd enjoyed it! I was finding some kind of satisfaction and fun in this... and even some humor to help lighten up the serious atmosphere that illness can bring. Deep in my heart I felt "a knowing" that these new weird black pellets coming out in my enemas were directly correlated with the "dropping sensation". The pellets then continued coming out with each enema. *Is this stuff coming from the firey-hot spot in my abdomen?*

At this same time, I had something else "new" come out in my enemas... more rope biofilms, but they had a bluish-green color to them. These came out a couple more times over the course of the next month--bluish-green colored RBs. *Talk about toxic stuff!* I thought. *Am I getting to the root of my abdominal and back pain?* God seemed to be telling me *"YES"*, in my heart. *I'm in awestruck wonder, Papa!*

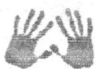

On a whole other subject... One early December day in Minnesota I awoke at 6:40am to my cat, Goofy, who had jumped back up onto the bed next to my head, deciding it was time for me to get up! In the process, she noisily knocked things onto the hardwood floor from my bedside table, meaning it was, "Time to get up Kelly! It's time for an adventure!"

Chuckling, I crawled out of bed feeling worn out from a restless night of sleep. It felt like I hadn't slept at all. I reached out, pulling Goofy into my arms. She purred contently in my embrace. After petting her, I set her back on my bed. She jumped down onto the floor, running out into the living room. She looked out the sliding door in eager anticipation of me opening the door for her. "Be safe, Goofy. Love you." I'd said while letting her out.

After getting my morning coffee brewing, I went outside to feed Mr. Rabbi. I'd returned back in to the house, got my brew ready and did my daily morning enema. Afterwards, though, I still didn't feel well. My patience was lacking from the restless night and feeling ill. I avoided speaking with members of my family that morning due to my mood, moodiness. I completed my work-out before breakfast. At breakfast I spoke to Mom, telling her about my miserable night. Afterwards, I went outside for a walk hoping to clear my head and prepare for my work day. Later, as I got into work at my business in town,

Mom--who is my receptionist, told me, "Your work schedule has changed drastically for today. Two of the three currently scheduled clients have cancelled their appointments."

"Okay. Thanks for letting me know." I replied. Since I now had extra time in my schedule and it was time for Mom's monthly massage, I told her I'd work on her. She agreed, willingly. It was decided that we'd do a "Raindrop Technique" with essential oils and massage incorporated into the session. This would take 1.75 hours.

During Mom's appointment, we talked while I worked. Halfway through the session I had her turn from her back onto her stomach. As I worked her back now, I applied the essential oils. My stomach had been feeling uneasy. Five minutes later, I felt like my stomach couldn't hold whatever was going on any longer. I ran out of the therapy room into the nearby restroom in the second therapy room, and much to my delight I had a bowel movement ALL ON MY OWN! Happy dance! This was the first bowel movement I'd had in a couple months, all on my own! This happening was HUGE! Just then I realized that Mom was still laying on the massage table in the other room, having not said a word to her WHY I was leaving.

When I returned, I apologized saying, "Sorry Mom, I didn't even think to tell you where I was off to before exiting the room!" Then proceeded to tell her the good news!

"Oh Kelly, I'm just GLAD you finally had a bowel movement on your own!" She replied with a muffled voice which is typical of very relaxed clients.

Dr. North had said he was hoping that I'd have a BM on my own during our last phone consult. *Well! It happened!* I thought to myself. I smiled and focused on my work.

JE December 2015
I realized these last few days that I sweat easier. I guess I've noticed that lately, but man, it feels good! I'm healing and getting healthier, Papa!

And so I was, healing and getting healthier. I'm in awestruck wonder!

74

The Truth Revealed

Kelly

It had been a rough couple of days while starting the new protocol of supplements. For instance, after nearly a week of adding just some pure fiber into my diet, I knew that it wasn't working with my body. *Great,* I thought. When I took fiber in the past, I'd bloat and the left-side pain in my abdomen and my back would nag constantly. Same was true this time, it hurt. Headaches were present immediately upon drinking the fiber solution, and my stomach was upset. I'd be gassy but unable to pass it, therefore being bloated. I was sluggish and tired. I stopped taking the fiber after the first seven days in order to see if it would help determine if the fiber really was the issue. I continued to take all the other supplements I was on, though.

Many months back during the gut healing program, we were educated about fiber, slowly adding it into our diets, fibers such as chia seed, or flax. If the fiber didn't work and we were having really uncomfortable symptoms, we could stop taking it for a few days then try it again. That being said, the 8th and 9th mornings I skipped taking the fiber and did my usual morning enemas at this time. I wasn't getting AS much toxic junk out as I had months earlier. I was thankful the rope biofilms seemed to be slowing down! However, there were still more toxins inside my body that needed to come out, and I knew it. Ever so subtly, over the course of the last two months, while working with Dr. North, the abdominal pain HAD improved!

Do you like a hot cup of something warm? Something medicinal? Something that's GOOD for you? Well, if you've heard of "Golden Milk", it's a lovely medicinal AND a taste-full tea. Mom and I have been making our own rendition of it for years... and MAYBE you've even gotten a taste of it while visiting with us! If not, rain check! Anyways, one day while making our version of "Golden Milk" tea, renamed "Wonder Woman Tea" which is made with fresh grated ginger and turmeric root boiled in clean pure water then sieved and the tea mixed with ground black pepper, coconut milk, ground nutmeg, ground cloves and cinnamon, raw honey and pure molasses, Mom unintentionally added some kick to it. The kick? RED PEPPER! *Ha!*

You may be thinking, *how does one unintentionally add red pepper to this recipe?* We have multiple of the same style salt and pepper shakers, some of those having regular black pepper and one of those having red pepper in it, all sitting in different areas of our kitchen. Mom had grabbed the closest black pepper shaker while making the tea, it being red pepper, not black pepper!

I'd sipped about a quarter of a cup of my tea before going outside for a walk. While I was walking outside, my abdomen felt warm, and soon my abdomen and stomach began to feel very uncomfortable. It wasn't until I got back inside the house 30-40 minutes later, that Mom and I were talking and figured out the *mistake*. Well, that *mistake* was actually a pretty nice one for me because once again I ended up having a BM on my own shortly after ingesting the tea with added KICK! This medicinal tea with the added spices was doing its thing, and I was pretty happy to say the least!

Later that same day I had a second BM again, all on my own! I let out an excited, "WAHOO! Two BMs in one day!" I was ecstatic! Having only those two BMs on my own, I was back to the two daily enemas in a matter of 24 hours. However, some exotic, weird colored biofilms came out once again. This hellish nightmare--in my eyes still, was exactly as described: hellish, a real nightmare. But it was one nightmare that I needed to go through in order to get well. In my heart I not only knew that detoxing these was key, but also felt deeply as having a responsibility to do so in respect for myself, for my body.

I received an email from Dr. North's receptionist. In the email were the results of my stool analysis test I'd completed three-and-a-half weeks earlier. I eagerly opened the email for my results! Reading them carefully, the information confirmed the deepest knowing in my heart about what was going on deep inside my body--pancreatic cancer. I was truly detoxing the cancer, the evidence showing in the samples of stools I'd sent in. For real--I WAS DETOXING THE CANCER!

December 21st, 2015 the phone rang. "Hello." I answered.

"Hello, Kelly. How are you doing?" Dr. North questioned, warmly.

"I'm continually doing better. I've had a few more interesting incidents happen since we last spoke."

"Okay. Fill me in on this news." He invited, warmly.

"I've had two bowel movements all on my own, in one day! Since then, I continually have the urge to have a bowel movement but it just won't happen on its own. The biofilms are slowly decreasing. However, they are still coming out in daily enemas. I truly believe I'll know when they will be done, as I feel that my body will tell me. I'd still like to know if there is a certain amount of time that it takes to get rid of these toxins?" I inquired.

"First, that is GOOD NEWS regarding the two BMs on your own! Excellent! Secondly, about the biofilms... You are right, Kelly. You WILL know when they are done. I can't tell you a specific amount of time that it takes to get rid of them. Actually, I find it very interesting that your body is still detoxing them, because I haven't sent you any specific supplements to target and extract them. Your body is eradicating them all by itself."

I was flabbergasted! *My body is detoxing the RBs all by itself with no help from the supplements? WOW!* I thought to myself. *The body never ceases to amaze me!* Shaking my head in mock astonishment, I muttered, "Wow". I was speechless and amazed.

"Tell me, what else has been happening regarding the left-side pain." He invited.

I quickly regained my thoughts, answering his question, "It's been improving. Slowly and subtly the pain is diminishing. The left-side abdominal

292

and back pain were worse when I was taking the fiber you sent me. I quit taking the fiber for a few days and my symptoms did improve. I tried taking the fiber again a few days later and the symptoms came back. I haven't taken the fiber since." I told him.

"Okay." He commented, still listening for more feedback.

"Headaches are minimal. I still had a handful of them this last month." I continued, "I rarely get bloated unless I feel sick in my abdomen area. When that happens, which isn't as often, it's usually due to my body having so many toxins built up that need to come out. Doing an enema takes away the severity of the symptoms. In turn, I have more energy and can sleep through the night without waking up in pain."

"All right." He stated.

I voiced other thoughts and ended with, "Overall with the changes, I do feel better." *Slow and steady...* flew through my head in private thoughts.

"I'm so glad that improvements are happening!" Dr. North announced. "Now, let's go over your 'Comprehensive Stool Analysis Test' results. Kelly, these results have a LOT of helpful information regarding your state of health."

"Indeed." I agreed. I held the printed copy of the test results in my hand. I looked at the results while he spoke. The truth about my health was FINALLY being revealed in my test results, the culprit being seen in my stools for many months now.

"You have a bacteria overgrowth, Kelly. This kind of overgrowth is VERY rare. You aren't taking a supplement that is associated with this imbalance. There is an overgrowth of bacteria in your pancreas, Kelly, causing a big disruption in your body." He continued, "This overgrowth causes tumors and cancer."

My deep knowing was finally being confirmed by Dr. North, who wisely informed me, "You have a lot going on inside of you right now..."

75

Reacting to the Truth

Kelly

My consult with Dr. North continued, he confirming the deepest knowing in my heart--*I had a tumor in my pancreas and it was cancerous.* My body didn't react, as if seeming to understand that it didn't need to. My body and mind had known I had pancreatic cancer for a good long time, and so I AND my body were doing everything we knew to fight my way back to health. Our bodies KNOW what they need. We just need to listen, agree, and do all we can to bring health back into ourselves.

Dr. North and I talked about the supplements I'd now be taking, and using specific foods as medicine to eradicate the present toxins from my still overly-toxic body. "A new protocol is needed for you. One that is designed for exactly what you need at this point in the healing process. Your pancreas needs all the support that it can get." Dr. North said, knowingly.

"That would be good!" I said while smiling really big. "I'm going to be honest with you Dr. North. In the past five-and-a-half years, I've done extensive research about this 3-D abdominal pain that extends from the abdomen into my back. I've also looked closely at pancreatic cancer symptoms. I've had every symptom over these years, except for blood in my stool." I informed him.

"Okay." Dr. North said, listening to what I was saying.

"Cancer is a fancy word that the Western medical field uses. You and I both know that cancer is made up of bad pathogens and toxins. I want to thank you for all your help and continued help that you've been. I've tried a lot of ways of natural healing in those first five-and-a-half years, and went to many other naturopathic professionals for help." I paused, then continued, "Dr. North, you have been the person that has truly ADDRESSED and gotten to the root cause of this left-side pain. I am SO very grateful. Thank you!" I spoke.

"Kelly, you are so very welcome." He replied warmly. Dr. North was TRULY addressing the left-side pain I was having. We continued our consult, at the end of it scheduling then next consult in a month's time. He ended the call saying, "Happy Holidays! May this new year, 2016, be one full of continued healing for you, Kelly."

"Thank you. It will be. 'Happy New Year' to you!"

We disconnected and I took a deep breath. Dr. North had gone deep in discussing my CSAT results. He had made it known that we had A LOT of work to do in this next year, but that I was headed in the right direction. I was grateful, and greatly encouraged! I had HAPPY tears while sharing a big hug with Mom. I whispered into her ear, "We finally have evidence to our own heart's knowing, a confirmation. I don't feel any different, other than thankful we are finally going to address the ROOT cause." I was truly humbled and thankful.

Many people can read this and think, *you had to of been devastated with the test results despite, your somehow, knowing what you knew in your heart to be true.* Or, *you have pancreatic cancer*--which in Western medicine is quite often thought of as a death sentence--*and you act like it's no big deal?* And you could be thinking a lot of other things, too… and if so, then please just hear me out.

First: No, I wasn't devastated, nor even surprised by my test results finally indicating what was going on in regards to my health. Remember all those toxic rope biofilms and exotic, weird colored RBs that had been coming out of me during enemas? Well, this was literally some of the cancer coming out of my body.

Second: You're right, I didn't act like it was a big deal. I already knew in my heart of hearts what I knew to be true--I had pancreatic cancer. Having the confirmation from the CSAT was honestly reassuring.

Although we now knew for sure, having proof, what I was dealing with, did I TELL other people besides "my tribe" of a select few individuals? Actually, no--for the exact reasons I've stated before. I wasn't ready for other people's opinions, sympathy, or anything that would deter me from focusing on what I NEEDED to be focused on in regards to my individual healing process. This being said, Mom and I did tell "our tribe" of people that knew more of my health situation. They had my back. I was comfortable with these people knowing because I knew they would SUPPORT my choice. Their support was a critical part to my healing, too, in so many aspects.

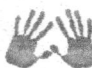

I'm going to re-state what I've said before, but needs to be said again. Had I gone the traditional Western AMA route for help with my left-side pain, I know I wouldn't be here today alive, full of life and good health. I wasn't willing to go the traditional medical route. Their way of treatment to killing cancer wasn't right FOR ME. My parents respected that decision I made for myself and fully supported me. They listened to my heart, and I honored my "knowing heart" in abiding to that which it was telling me to "go the road less traveled", using alternative, all-natural, complimentary, health options for healing.

Mom also believes that I wouldn't be here today had I taken the road MOST OFTEN traveled. The prescribed medicines—chemo and radiation drugs, would have killed me, she said. My grandma, who knew my health situation all along the way, also had said after the worst was over, "If Kelly would have gone the 'medical route' she wouldn't be here today. I'm so glad that she chose the route she did." Thanks Grandma. I love you, and love that you honored my choice, too.

Everyone gets to make their own choices in life. I made my choices, and I'm here today BECAUSE of those choices, and am choosing to share my choices for healing with you for so many reasons. I have NO regrets. You are free to think whatever you want about the choices I've made. You are entitled to your own opinion. I do respect that, because, it's your life and it's your choice, just like it's my life and my choice!

76

Cancer
Can East and West Meet?

Kelly

The pancreas sits across the abdomen, behind the stomach, in front of the spine just below the lower ribs. The pancreas is about six inches long. There are two main functions of the pancreas, including: An exocrine function that helps in digestion, and an endocrine function that regulates blood sugar.

Pancreatic cancer is one of the more deadly types of cancer. By the time it is detected, a person usually has only a small number of weeks or months to live, rarely ever living beyond a year's length. Why? Because the tumor is hard to detect. It can rarely be palpable with the human hand, nor is it easily detected via imaging tests. Some signs and symptoms of pancreatic cancer include, but aren't limited to: dizziness, nausea, abdominal pain, 3-D pain that extends through the abdomen into the back and low back, headaches, malabsorption of food, inability to be comfortable in any position--especially sitting, an inability to digest foods, fats, and nutrients, having weight loss, appetite loss, diarrhea, digestive issues, being bloated and uncomfortable after eating, jaundice (yellowing of eyes and skin), unable to sleep restfully, and overall feeling fatigue. Most often, the signs and symptoms are mislabeled, drugs being prescribed, all of which further delay detection.

I was misdiagnosed by the Western medical community, being labeled IBS (irritable bowel syndrome) in the summer of 2010. As time went on, years, the severe pain I had was partly due to the tumor sitting directly on my pancreas. Since the pancreas was unable to do its functions properly, I could not digest my food, and other organs were stressed while trying to compensate for the pancreas.

As I started a deep-detoxification process in 2015, specifically utilizing coffee enemas, I was killing the rope biofilms, the layers of the tumor. Some of the other healing methods I utilized included: using food as medicine, healing mentally, emotionally, physically, and spiritually, soaking in detox baths, doing castor oils packs, using essential oils, doing hot water bottle compresses and various massage modalities, chiropractic care, acupuncture, stretching, lots of self-care, doing some series of colonics, exercising lightly, doing ear candling and nasal douches, having quiet time, taking various supplements and herbal remedies, getting sunshine (vitamin D), addressing nutritional deficiencies, doing lemon juice and essential oil enemas, getting needed amounts of sleep, drinking healing teas and lots of pure water, and getting fresh air every day. All of these methods of healing were important to my continued healing. One single healing method wasn't going to be a cure all. Instead, in order to regain my health, I needed to use a vast variety of healing modalities. Keeping track of my progress in journals, having support from family and friends, and taking each day as it came were all important too.

Our Western medical community tells us the only way to treat and cure cancer is with chemotherapy and radiation treatments. Doctors prescribing chemotherapy, and health teams who are part of their patient's radiation treatments, are required to wear hazmat suits, face shields, and gloves. They wear these because these therapies are made up of powerful toxic substances the healthcare providers themselves don't want to touch. These toxic substances that are being used to fight cancer are, and is proven, cancer CAUSING substances in and of themselves! Does this seem backwards to you? It does to me—and harmful to say the very least.

Chemotherapy was first discovered in the 1940s in Italy, when nitrogen mustard gas had been dropped on post-mortem autopsy bodies. The number of lymphocytes in the post-mortem bodies declined then. In turn, a select group of doctors determined that they should use mustard gas as an antidote for people that had leukemia, lymphoma, or an over-production of lymphocytes. This same "mustard gas" was used to KILL soldiers in world wars. Some of the same chemicals being used today in medicine today contain this powerful toxin, "mustard gas", including chemotherapy. The powerful toxins in chemotherapy used to kill cancer cells, not only do they kill SOME of the cancer cells, but they also kill all healthy cells as well. Furthermore, damage is done to a person's organs, making it VERY hard for the body to get the toxins out of their bodies and to then become well again.

Did you know there are two kinds of cancer cells? **They are "mother" cells and "daughter" cells**. Chemotherapy can kill the "daughter" cells. However, it DOESN'T kill the "mother" cells. This means a person treated with chemo can be generating new cancer cells stemming from the "mother" cells that will not be detectable for many years. In time, the new and now stronger growing "daughter" cells metastasize more deeply than before, often leading the patient to an unhappy end. This makes me so sad, and very mad.

Radiation, like chemotherapy, is detrimental especially for women's breast health. In what way, you wonder? Radiation exposure is a procedure also used in mammograms. When the breast is examined via mammogram at yearly check-ups, healthy breast tissue is at great risk. Radiation throws toxic rays into the breast tissue. Each year of radiation exposure to the breasts continually degrades healthy tissue and exposes the body to radioactive toxins which actually aid in the growth of cancerous tumors in breast tissue.

For more information about the real dangers of chemotherapy and radiation therapy, consult "The Truth About Cancer, A Global Quest", documentary by Ty Bollinger[11]. You can find this online, on the internet as well. On the "Truth About Cancer" website, one can find a ton of information from interviews Ty has had with hundreds of professionals in both Eastern and Western medicine realms of healthcare around the world, discussing specific therapies that work for specific cancers, and also exposing therapies that cause more human damage and death. Also, they give information on nutrition and a whole lot more!

As a cancer patient sits and receives critical news regarding their health, the patient likely thinks that their doctor knows what is best for them. Unfortunately, the doctor will recommend only what they were taught in Western, AMA (the American Medical Association) funded medical

---

[11] Ty Bollinger, "The Truth About Cancer, A Global Quest" series and transcripts, January 2015, "Cancer: Step Outside the Box" July 2016. website support.thetruthaboutcancer.com

school's training programs at universities all across the United States. Despite all of the medical school training, it is sad that nutrition barely gets talked about. Doctors training through the AMA are not taught "food as medicine" in medical school.

Medical students are taught to be law abiding, following the rules set in place by the AMA. Medical doctors can, and will, suffer adverse consequences when they don't abide by the regulations of the AMA and the governing law. So, if a doctor DOESN'T prescribe chemotherapy or radiation therapy to patients with diagnosed cancer, they have a REAL potential to LOSE their license to practice medicine. It saddens me greatly that our American government and the AMA aren't willing to intertwine BOTH Eastern and Western therapies to address not only cancer, but so many other ailments, diseases, and chronic diseases and illnesses.

Eastern modalities can often be looked at as "voodoo". But WHY, then, have the Eastern practices been around since the beginning of time and have so often been proven therapies, and the Western practices having only virtually evolved in the last 200 years? WHY can't we utilize both practices and therapies rather than just one Western way? Why can't the AMA doctors refer patients and clients to other professional practicing Eastern modalities, and visa-versa, for testing, diagnostics, and prescribing? And why don't health insurance policies cover Eastern practices? Good questions.

Doctors are people we go to for answers. If our doctor isn't knowledgeable in one area, one is sent to a "specialist". But, is it WRONG that we aren't getting other options of help than only Western medicine? Which leads me to my question... CAN East and West meet to collaborate, work together, to help a person get to the ROOT of their health issue? I do believe it can be done, but in the highly controlled society that we live in today in the USA, for the most part it's not going to happen. There's too much to lose, money that is, for those in control pulling the strings.

I respect professionals in BOTH branches of medicine and healthcare, East and West. Without one, we would be incomplete. I believe what I just stated. I would LOVE if East and West could come together.

I highly encourage anyone, everyone, to do their own research and find out what's right for them concerning treatment for cancer; Eastern medicine, verses Western medicine. Just because what's right for us in one season of life doesn't mean it will be right for us in another season. I hope we can each allow East and West to meet in our lives, so as to better help and heal from the inside out!

77

Selfcare – Self-help – Selflove

Kelly

When I've spoken to people in real life about aspects of what it looks like to care for one's self, using phrases such as "**selfcare**", "**self-help**", or "**selflove**", I've found it interesting how some people react, appearing to not want to hear examples or, opinions, recommendations, or advice on the subjects. I wonder why? I also wonder if the phrase "**selflove**" is misinterpreted as meaning conceited, if one is not familiar with the use of the phrase "**selflove**".

If any single one of us has a problem or issue with an aspect of our life, and we ourselves ask for advice, why do some of us appear to not want to hear another's answer? Is it because it isn't what we want to hear? Is it because we don't like to feel like we are being told what to do? Is it because we might be intimidated that someone knows something we don't? Or, maybe if we get responses to our asking of advice, could it be we don't actually want to have to put forth an effort to ultimately reap a result out of "fear of the unknown" and actually doing life differently?

I'm going to get even more personal in asking questions. Since cancer is at an all-time high, epidemic proportions, do we want to ask questions, do research, to find ways to help ourselves; finding self-helps and doing self-care, which are both a product of self-love, to diminish the likelihood of a cancer diagnosis happening to us? Wait, do we even want to face this reality of the possibility? If we don't, then I guess it's safe to say you should stop reading this chapter. Sorry, but that's the truth. But, in the case that you want to help yourself, your children, your significant other, your grand kids and friends, etc., then read on!

There are a lot of all-natural methods to cure cancer naturally, without toxic medicines--which deplete our immune systems. I can say this because I did it. I'm SHARING my story and healthful information because I'm passionate about getting the truth out. Some of the non-invasive lifestyle changes and treatments include, but are not limited to, the following: eating an organic--clean diet, eating specific cancer-killing food, drinking cancer-killing teas, juicing, doing a thermography session, taking homeopathic remedies, practicing cleansing organs in the body yearly or using the "Gerson Therapy" to detox, doing colon hydrotherapy, addressing vitamin and mineral deficiencies, using essential oils, cooking with herbs and spices, practicing traditional Chinese medicine (TCM), embracing homeopathy, getting regular massage therapy, take in a series of acupuncture sessions, getting exercise in daily to sweat out toxins through the skin, drinking pure clean water, eating oxygenating foods, doing self-care tasks daily--taking care of yourself physically, mentally, emotionally, and spiritually, doing chiropractic care regularly, taking natural remedies, decreasing stress in life, using photodynamic therapy and hyperbaric oxygen chamber therapy, doing far-infrared and near-infrared saunas, doing pulse electromagnetic frequencies, aiding diet with additional supplementation, eating (organic) apricot seeds, absorbing natural sunlight, eliminating amalgam fillings in teeth, and balancing energy. All of these are practices of true preventions for illness and disease. Do some research on any or all of these therapies to gather more information for yourself and loved ones if you're interested in helping yourself to become even more healthy, daily.

Okay, so that was a long list. How many of the things on the list have you done in your life already? Most all of these just listed treatments cost money out of our pockets, since health insurance companies most often do not cover these costs. How about doing one practice on this list in the next week of time? Or, how about you pick a few that you'd like to implement into your lifestyle daily if you don't already, like exercise or nutritional supplementation? Speaking for myself, there's a few treatments on the list that I haven't done that I DO want to try... specifically the oxygen chamber therapy and pulse electromagnetic frequencies prick my interest!

What we feed our bodies each day impacts our health. Below is a list of some foods, herbs, and spices that can aid in diminishing cancer cells. Please keep in mind, everything on the list should be certified ORGANIC! And make sure to always wash your produce before eating, to remove insects or their eggs!

Herbs and spices include but aren't limited to: *Turmeric, ginger--PROVEN to be STRONGER than chemotherapy to kill cancer cells, garlic, black pepper, rosemary, curcumin--found in turmeric, oregano, parsley, cilantro, dill, coriander, basil, thyme, and cayenne pepper.

Leafy green vegetables are the foundation of any healthy diet, since they are exceptionally rich in minerals, vitamins, antioxidants and enzymes. Leafy greens are rich in antioxidants known to combat cancer, including beta-carotene--a type of vitamin A, and vitamin C. *Spinach, kale, collards, mustard greens, arugula, swiss chard, leaf lettuces, beet greens, and dandelions are some common greens found in supermarkets, or that you can grow yourself!

Cruciferous vegetables are powerful cancer killers, and, are some of the best vitamin C foods available. *Broccoli, cauliflower, brussel sprouts, cabbage, onions, garlic, and mushrooms.

Berries are high in antioxidants. *Blueberries, cherries, raspberries, strawberries, goji berries, aronia berries, and blackberries.

Carbohydrates or orange-colored foods, which are high in carotenoids. One of the carotenoids, called beta-carotene, is an essential nutrient for immune functioning, which is a detoxifier for liver health. Also, they fight cancers of the skin, eyes, and organs. *Sweet potatoes, squash, carrots, golden beets, and pumpkin.

Nuts and seeds *Chia seeds, flax seeds, sesame seeds, pumpkin seeds, hemp seeds, sunflower seeds, walnuts, almonds, and brazil nuts.

Healthy unrefined oils Did you know that your brain functions BECAUSE of GOOD QUALITY FATS? That's why we NEED to eat GOOD fats daily! *Coconut oil, flax oil, cod liver oil, cold pressed extra virgin olive oil, grapeseed oil, ghee, all nut oils, and clean animal fats.

Food IS medicine, and fueling our bodies with nutrient-dense food IS vitally important for good health!

What goes into our bodies is critical. This is yet another important topic to discuss--a product that goes into our body, for women; **tampons**. Guys, if you love your gals, PLEASE do not only read this information, but share it with them if they menstruate! And women, please read for your own benefit and share it with other women in your life.

Each month women have their menses--menstrual cycle, AKA what we women most often call a "period". The products that many women use, tampons, sitting readily available on store shelves to buy, are filled with chemical toxins. Whether they are fragrance-free or not, they're toxic because they're made of toxic full ingredients--bleached and pesticide filled rayon, cotton, viscose and wood shavings, all aid in causing "Toxic Shock Syndrome", which also leads to cervical cancer and uterine cancer that are both prevalent. If these toxins are next to the most vulnerable tissue of women, the uterus, should this be a concern? It doesn't matter if you're a man or women, I would think it should be a concern. If we are utilizing products that are filled with toxins, putting them right into our body, we are putting our most precious tissue for reproduction at risk for disease, illness, and very possibly women becoming unable to conceive children--infertility.

So, what can we do to put a stop to this issue? Could it be so simple as to buy organic chemically free, toxin free tampons and pads? YES! A couple of popular and SAFE brands for women's menses are "NatraCare" and "Seventh Generation", but there are a number of clean brands out there.

Ladies, do you think your body gets tired of using the same tampons products, or do these products cause you discomfort? Do you dislike using sanitary pads? It might be time to try using a "menstrual cup"! This product is easy to purchase online and is a SAFE alternative. It's also VERY cost effective.

Our bodies aren't something to be continually put at risk for disease and illness. What we put into our bodies IS important. Today, and from here on out, we each have a number of "**self-helps**" that we can choose to implement into our daily lives. "**Self-help**" is "**selfcare**". "**Self-care**" is showing "**self-love**".

78

Unlocking Vulnerability

Kelly
It was the end of December 2015 when the remedy, and then a new protocol of supplements from Dr. North arrived in the mail. I started on those immediately as they arrived.

Like most often times, once I took the supplements, I started getting sick. However, I knew the difference between a "good sick" and "bad sick". This WAS a "good sick" I was experiencing. The new supplements were specifically designed to kill the toxins and eradicate them from inside my body. Headaches became more prevalent again, and dizziness was happening at times. I wanted to sleep more but my body, or my mind, wouldn't let me. I had restless sleep. My energy level was pretty low. The yellow spots in my eyes continued to get better though, so that was an improvement! My body was a lot less sore than it had been for the last few years, and in turn it was continuing to unlock. YIPPEE! I'll get more into that in a bit here.

I continued to do my daily routine of numerous forms of healing. At this time, it mostly included coffee and lemon juice enemas, alternating between a detox bath or castor oil pack—placed over my liver, using essential oils, doing light exercise to get me sweating, daily self-care, taking my supplements, drinking LOTS of water, eating a totally organic diet which consisted of 60-70% vegetables, 30% meats, and 10% nuts and fruits, and drinking Essiac Tea[12].

---

[12] The Original ESSIAC® Tea – Rene Caisse's Original Formula
https://www.essiacproducts.com

Essiac tea dates back to the 1920's, formulated originally by Rene Caisse Notice that Essiac spells Caisse back-wards—Rene's last name! Essiac tea is a proven remedy to cure cancer. Each morning and night I'd drink this tea on an empty stomach. I felt it working deep inside my abdomen a short while after drinking it. It was definitely helping in the detoxifying process!

Each day I continued eliminating the rope biofilms via my enemas, and then my low-back and abdominal pain would be immediately relieved. Sometimes the RBs where green-blue in color. I often found myself thinking, *the detoxification process is like peeling away layers of an onion.* The epicenter, which each layer surrounded, was yet to be eradicated. The epicenter was being addressed by removing the layer upon layer protecting it. This unpeeling was significant in my healing process.

Each day was different, bringing new subtle joys here and there. I took notice to those "joyful" moments. Detoxing and healing weren't easy, though. My whole entire being was exhausted from this long process. On hard days I focused on getting through the day, and that kept me moving forward. I set small goals to help me make it through the day. Papa God and Mom were the two constants in my life, day in and day out.

How much longer? I asked Papa God. It'd already been six months of detoxing. I was slowly and subtly progressing in positive ways in my healing journey. In turn, my body was beginning to unlock via helps of massage therapy, exercise, and stretching. Massage therapy helped specifically to loosen my abdominal, my hip flexors, and muscles in my back, especially the left side. The tight muscles were trying to protect the 3-dimensional area of pain deep inside. Each day I'd massage my abdomen with my hands, 2-5 times throughout the day. I'd make sure that I massaged it first thing in the morning upon waking, and before I went to bed at night. This would help my abdominal muscles to relax while sleeping, I hoped! If there was time for doing more self-abdominal massage in the day, I'd do so as well! Hallie, my massage therapist and friend, was always able to help me during my monthly massages too. She'd penetrate deeper into the muscles then I could, to reduce the tightness. And another great part of seeing her was that my own hands got a break!

I continued stretching and using my "Thera Cane" every night before bed too. When I had first started using this self-help tool, a "Thera Cane", doing specific stretches for my very tight hip flexor muscles, it painfully hurt. However, I knew that the hurt was a good and helpful pain. The process of working these muscles took time; specifically, years to unlock them! These muscles kept me in a fetal position during some of my roughest years of illness. They seemed to want to stay in their locked position. Consistently working them, though, along with other helps, were key in getting them to loosen and to ultimately, at some point in the future, STAY unlocked. As the unlocking of my hip flexors started, my right hip would pop upon moving it in a certain position. And when it popped, it helped lessen the low-back pain! The popping would diminish when my pelvis muscles loosened-up enough, when the pelvis--sacrum were in alignment. Then, I'd be able to dig my "Thera Cane" deep into my hips AND be able to self-massage my abdomen deeper.

I had times throughout the many years of illness that my pelvis would release when I least expected it. It would happen without any indication or forewarning. An example of this was one time I was doing some light stretching exercises on the floor. I audibly heard, and felt, my sacrum--pelvis, un-lock. As it did, I felt warmth penetrate outward from the back of my pelvis towards my hips. Immediately, I had more feeling in my upper legs. The entire pelvis area would be looser than it had been in years prior! I could skeletally move easier and more freely.

In order for my body to be unlocked at a deeper level to promote FULL healing, I had to examine all aspects of my life. As the unlocking happened, I first had to realize an important aspect of letting go of stuff; AKA practicing **vulnerability**.

To be vulnerable is to be at ease, to be open and to be transparent. Vulnerability is something that is greatly misinterpreted. To be vulnerable is not a bad thing UNLESS a person is doing so for the wrong reason(s), such as an abusive situation.

I'd started with my heart being vulnerable on December 29th, 2011 when I came to know peace in my heart, told in the chapter titled "A New Heart". The walls built up around my heart had to be broken down, promoting forgiveness to everyone for everything, and to live in truth. Being vulnerable wasn't easy. I had hard, deep conversations with God, and with individuals, mostly members of my immediate family, while learning to be fully real, transparent, and vulnerable. As my heart started to heal within, in relationships with my family and with other people, I began to heal emotionally, mentally, and even some areas physically in the years since 2011. I had become more vulnerable, and it was good! I started to love people unconditionally. I was open and honest with them, being vulnerable. Some people just don't understand WHY I am this way, seemingly getting a notion that if I am nice to them for no reason, I must want something.

As my heart learned the beautiful power of vulnerability and the freedom which comes in practicing it, my mind learned it too. I had no idea that vulnerability was going to help unlock my locked-up, tight body as I was learning this practice.

At this point in my journey, December 2015, being vulnerable greatly aided in unlocking my body. On this journey towards WHOLE healing, from the very beginning I'd began to use other methods to help me understand what vulnerability encompassed even more. By being vulnerable to trying new things, like applying food as medicine, it changed my life for the better. My mind was able to think clearer because the foods weren't causing me to have "brain fog". My bodily organs were beginning to work together better as a whole, as a complete functioning system. Dr. North's remedies and protocols were also a big impact in being able to function better.

Bottom line: In becoming even more ill physically to become well, I had to learn to be more vulnerable--learning to ask for HELP, to speak kinder, to be REAL and to share life with people even when I didn't feel good. It wasn't easy to change.

Some really cool thing happened too. I'd meet complete strangers who would start sharing their life story with me, which was pretty amazing. The person sharing, most often times, didn't even know me. Yet, they were willing to be REAL with me, sharing their heart. This made a big impact in my life. It helped me to realize that vulnerability not only affects ourselves, but others in our lives. People can sense other's openness, or sense them being closed-off too.

Vulnerability is really an asset in everyday life. We shouldn't have to build or put-up walls around our hearts, or minds, to protect ourselves from being hurt or from learning something new. We shouldn't live in fear of being hurt with words, actions, judgements, and feelings of shame. We are human. Life happens and we make mistakes. Forgiveness is key. We live life and learn from our mistakes, making amends and moving forward. Vulnerability can be a beautiful thing, IF we are willing to allow ourselves to be so.

As I began to heal my body, organs, mind, heart, and being, I was learning the beautiful power of vulnerability and living in the fruit of it!

79

Reaching the Unreachable

Kelly

On a cold Minnesota Saturday in early January of 2016, while Mom and I had been running errands in the metropolitan area., that I had my scheduled monthly massage appointment with Hallie. I looked forward to every monthly massage!

"How have you been feeling, Kelly?" Hallie asked.

"Honestly, it varies from minute to minute. One minute I feel fine and the next minute I feel like I'm going to throw up." I replied. "I have times of feeling well, but lately it's been pretty rough. The supplements I'm taking are killing this toxic stuff in my body. It's been hard. My body is so tired of detoxing. BUT, as hard as it is, it IS good! I need to get this junk out so I can be well in health and truly begin to live life!"

"You are doing such a good job! Oh Kelly, I'm so glad you are here!" Hallie smiled, hugging me.

"Thank you, Hallie. I'm glad I'm here too." I smiled. Hallie left the room while I prepared myself for the massage.

When she returned, she started working on my back and spent extra time on the left side. Like always, she knew exactly what areas needed extra work. As she worked, I felt her touch the spot in the left side of my back that always hurt. She stopped on top of the spot. I took a deep breath and let it out. "Pressure okay Kelly?" she asked.

311

"Yes. You can even go deeper. That's the spot that's always painful to various degrees. I can never reach deep enough in to access that spot." I sighed.

"It is SO tight." She told me, continuing to work. Soon she had me turn over onto my back, "I'm going to work your abdomen now, Kelly."

"Sounds good." I replied.

"I'm sorry, my hands are a bit chilly." Hallie smiled. We shared a chuckle as we both had cold hands. *Our poor clients!* I thought.

"Actually, they really don't feel that cold." I said, as she continued her work.

"That's probably because your abdomen is so warm." She spoke. I paid close attention to how my abdomen was feeling as she worked. It was really tight. The left side, just under my ribs at the pancreas, was tense and hard. This spot seared with throbbing heat, which included 3-D pain extending straight through my abdomen into my back. "Deep breath in, Kelly." I was instructed, filling my abdomen with air. I slowly let my breath out as she gently used her thumbs to reach deep into my upper abdomen, just under my ribs. I finished letting breathe out as Hallie gently finished working the two points she was pressing. "Another deep breath in." she whispered softly. I drew a deep breath in, and as I exhaled Hallie again reached deep into my upper abdomen, underneath my ribs. This time she had accessed the firey-hot, searing, 3-D spot. I knew as she accessed that spot something good was happening. As she was right on the spot there was no pain, it was as if she was suffocating the burning fire!

FINALLY! After five-and-a-half years of trying to reach that burning spot someone was able to reach the unreachable! It felt surreal. In that moment, I experienced true thankfulness and SUCH RELIEF. I couldn't utter a word. I was speechless. I didn't want the moment to end. Taking another large breath of air, Hallie reached deep into my abdomen again, pressing other points around the firey-hot spot. I continued to take more breaths correlating them with her work. As she finished working the area around the spot, she decided to go back to the firey-hot spot. "You found it, Hallie. That's the spot that the pain extends through my abdomen into my back, burning in a 3-D effect." I whispered softly.

312

"It's so tight in here, Kelly. It's hard, as if it is protecting something." Hallie stated gently. She reached into my abdomen working just above the hot, searing, firey-hot spot. It felt so good! Again, there was no pain as she pressed into it! Hallie continued working, listening with her intuitive hands and entire being as she always did with me, and other clients too, I'm sure.

Time flew by and my appointment came to an end. We each took a deep breath, then exhaled together. We shared a smile and she left the room. *Wow! Did this really just happen? Hallie reached the unreachable! This feels surreal!* With joyful tears swelled in my eyes before slowly getting up and dressing, I stretched by back and neck, both cracking from the stretch. A few tears dropped, in appreciation.

"How are you feeling Kelly?" Hallie asked, as I walked out of the therapy room towards the front office to meet her.

"OH MY! Really good! I feel SO much better! Thank you, Hallie!"

"That hot spot, Kelly? It's like a rock--HARD. I got a visual of a 'cement scraper'. It's as if that spot doesn't want to break up. It's got a firm foundation, and a strong fence built around it."

"You're exactly right, Hallie." The muscles in my abdomen and back were staying tight trying to protect that area. Hallie and I gazed into each other's eyes and shared a deep knowing smile.

That day we had shared a special moment that I will never, ever, forget.

The next day after seeing Hallie, I started to CONSISTENTLY have lengths of a few hours at a time without any left-side abdominal pain or back pain. There was only one exception though, the deep firey-hot spot INSIDE my abdomen, the epicenter. Something had changed though. It no longer burned with an angry vengeance, but instead had a dull ache, and a very small burning feel. At times, it would itch. Feeble attempts were made to reach the itch.

If you aren't aware, an itching sensation while an injury is in process towards healing IS a sign of actual healing happening! GOOD NEWS!

The days I didn't feel well, at this point, were not as severe, nor painful as in the past months and years. The abdominal and left-side pain were reducing drastically. I was beginning to experience bits of what "feeling well" felt like for someone with optimal health. This was surreal!

80

My Little Dude

Kelly

January 11th, 2016. "Good morning, Mr. Rabbi! How's my Little Dude?" I called out as I started outside the door to approach his heated outdoor rabbit hutch. Normally, Mr. Rabbi would see me coming as I walked to his hutch, then he'd happily hoppity-hop-on-down from the top floor of the hutch to the bottom floor to meet me at his enter-and-exit door. Today though, he barely lifted his head when looking at me from the top floor of his hutch.

Oh, no! I thought to myself with immediate concern. Opening his ceiling door on the top floor, I peered in. Mr. Rabbi sat hunkered down, shivering. *His heat lamp is penetrating enough heat to keep him warm. He shouldn't be shivering. What is going on with my Little Dude?* I thought. I reached in, petting him. He leaned into my hand not attempting to move away. His food from the night before sat untouched. *Oh, no!* I thought again. Mr. Rabbi ALWAYS ate his fresh produce. This was NOT normal.

I put his new, fresh food in place of the old and waited for him to move towards it. He didn't. He continued to lean into my gentle touch, with his soft white fur nestled into my hand and forearm. "What's going on Mr. Rabbi?" I asked. At times like this it would be nice if animals could talk human.

After going back to the house and telling my parents about Mr. Rabbi, Dad and I went out to check on him. He was still sitting in the same spot, shivering. However, he had eaten a nice portion of the fresh food that I had just gave him. *GOOD!* I thought, and reached in, petting him again. He again leaned into my hand, a warm embrace. Dad and I decided to take Mr. Rabbi into our heated garage so we could monitor him more closely. Picking him up

315

gently, holding him close, he nestled into my neck. He seemed to welcome the closeness and warmth. Once inside the garage, we put a blanket inside a cardboard box for our mini-lop furry friend to sit in. I gently lowered him into the box. He sniffed his new surroundings, looking around curiously. He had been in the heated garage a few times before when it was really cold outside, so this wasn't totally a new environment for him.

Bun-Bun, my other cat who is very furry, black in color and lives in the house with Goofy, came into the garage walking close to Mr. Rabbi. They looked at each other, and then Bun-Bun walked away. Mr. Rabbi nestled into his box, unaffected by the friendly look-see! Giving Mr. Rabbi some more dark, leafy greens and a container of water, he ate and drank.

It was around noon time when I'd come into the garage after a brisk walk. I looked down at Mr. Rabbi, noticing a couple scratches on his skin where the fur was a bit separated. My stomach dropped as I crouched down to my knees examining the scratches closely. I got up, ran to the door into the house yelling, "Mom! Come here!"

Mom, hearing the urgency in my voice, came running. "Look at these scratches! I bet these have to do with the reason why Mr. Rabbi isn't feeling well?"

The scratches were already scabbed over. It looked as if they had been there for a couple days. I hadn't seen any blood on his white coat. *When could this have happened?* I thought. After making a few phone calls to veterinarians, Mom found one who was willing to look at my Little Dude.

I, myself, was feeling pretty sick that day too, so Mom took Mr. Rabbi to the veterinary clinic. The vet examined him, then had his assistant clean the injured area of scratches. He told Mom, "Mr. Rabbi has pneumonia. It could be due to the scratches." He also said he thought Mr. Rabbi was dehydrated, so he injected some water underneath his skin to rehydrate him. In addition, the vet gave him an oral medication to help with his high fever.

When Mom and Mr. Rabbi arrived back home, I greeted them inquisitively. Immediately I went over to see my Little Dude. He was lethargic and weak. I got down on the floor and leaned in close, drawing him near to me, all

316

the while petting him. I softly and lovingly talked to him, despite him being lethargic and medicated. He ever so slightly leaned into my embrace.

"Hang in here, Mr. Rabbi. I love you, Little Dude." I softly whispered to him. I got up from where I had been laying by him, looking over my shoulder as I walked out of the garage. That's the last time I saw my Little Dude alive. I'd walked downstairs to continue writing my health journey on my computer. Little did I know that those would be my last words to Mr. Rabbi. Within the hour, he passed away.

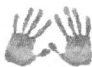

The day before Mr. Rabbi's death, my brother, Troy, had brought Mr. Rabbi to the outside of a sliding door on our house where I was working intently on this writing project. Upon seeing the pair, I scrambled up from the floor to open the door. Troy was petting Mr. Rabbi and I reached out to pet him too. I decided to bring Mr. Rabbi inside the house to help me work on my computer for a little while. He wasn't supposed to come in the house, but this day I'd made an exception to the rule.

Mr. Rabbi sat next to me on a blanket I had sprawled out on the floor. He snuggled in close to me. Within a few minutes he was curiously looking around. Bun-Bun had peered at Mr. Rabbi curiously. The mini-lop wanted to go see Bun-Bun, but wouldn't because he seemed to not want to step off of the blanket we were laying on. I smiled at my two furry amigos. Mr. Rabbi then turned toward me, standing up on his hind feet. He put his two front paws onto my low back. I turned at my torso, watching him, lovingly. Mr. Rabbi watched me closely too. We held our gaze with one another. Soon, he dropped back onto all four paws and hopped up right next to me. He crawled underneath my arm, nestling into my side. We'd shared a special moment together. Resuming my writing, he lowered his head wanting to be pet more, so I stopped to pet him. He laid his head down on the blanket, thoroughly enjoying the attention. I chuckled, stopped petting him, and he laid with his head down momentarily and then he put it back up. He then sat there watching me type on the computer keypads while snuggling close, as I continued typing away on my keyboard. This was one fine memory to have with Mr. Rabbi before he left this world. He was a great friend and pet!

Mr. Rabbi taught me a lot about life. With his help, he aided in bringing healing to my life with my feeling love and having compassion toward him, like with all animals in my life I've cared for. He gave me joy on days when I didn't have much. He was part of my joy in the simple things every day. Throughout the year-and-a-half I had cared for him, he helped bring healing to me in a way that no human was able to. I am forever grateful for the time that my Little Dude and I had together. I'm also thankful for the joy and love he brought to our entire family, including my two cats, Bun-Bun and Goofy--who was Mr. Rabbi's favorite amigo to go on adventures with!

JE January 11th, 2016
Mr. Rabbi passed away tonight. I sure am going to miss my Little Dude. He came to our family's home when I was at one of my sickest points. Today, as he lay there, not breathing and still, I could only think about if it would have been me lying there instead of him. This only caused me to bawl all the more. Thank you, Lord, for the precious time Mr. Rabbi and I had together. He was a big part of the reason I got up every morning when I was in so much pain.

81

Eating Our Emotions

Kelly

Throughout the month of January 2016, I had started taking new supplements, and again I got really sick. I was nauseated, having hot and cold sweats, feeling like I could vomit most of the time. I had headaches. I knew the supplements were killing the bad pathogens in my body, and in turn they were setting up a terrain for healing in my gut. I continued to take the supplements, knowing I was benefiting and healing with their help. I wasn't going to stop taking the supplements just because they made me feel worse.

During this time, I started to eat more organic foods that aided in promoting continued healing and functioning of my pancreas specifically, including: baby microgreen sprouts of kale, broccoli, and brussel sprout, and also strawberries, asparagus, blueberries, broccoli (full grown), cauliflower, cherries, sweet potato, dark leafy greens (especially spinach), and taking also taking probiotics in capsule form.

My diet at this time also consisted of lots of steamed, dark, leafy greens (Swiss chard, beet greens, kale, collards, and dandelions), steamed or roasted vegetables (broccoli, asparagus, turnips, rutabaga, squash, carrots, sweet potato, beets), grass-fed meats (antibiotic free and nitrate free bacon, turkey, chicken, and very little beef), fish (wild caught, not farm raised mahi-mahi, tuna, cod, and salmon) and fruit (strawberries, blueberries, raspberries, and avocados. Yes, avocados are a large seeded fruit that grow on trees). I also continued eating good fats and utilized a variety of healing herbs and spices into our cooked food. These were all organic, whole, foods. My diet was becoming more diversified than what it had once been! I also drank a LOT of water, 1.5-2 gallons per day, to aid in the detoxification process. In addition, I'd drink kombucha (a ferment), green tea and bone broth daily, liquid chlorophyll, ginger detox tea, lemon water, coconut water, and aloe vera juice.

Taking my supplements, using food as medicine, working with Dr. North, and researching more specific ways to help speed up my healing process, I was slowly and subtly progressing in healing. Massage therapy, exercise, and stretching daily all aided in detoxing too.

Food IS medicine. What we put into our bodies is OUR choice. But it doesn't just lie on the fork, spoon, or fingers in which medicinal food enter into us. It lies deeper—in our psychology. Food can be a really touchy subject with people. I'm willing to guess we all know people (and maybe we are this way ourselves) that love to eat, OR have a love-hate relationship with food, can eat and not gain a pound, can look at food and gain weight, who gravitate toward unconscious snacking when watching TV, or just in general enjoy eating comfort foods. Wait, what are comfort foods?

"Comfort foods are foods that provides consolation or a feeling of well-being, typically anything with a high sugar or other carbohydrate content and is associated with childhood or home cooking" is the general definition. Sounds pretty "comforting", huh? What comfort foods come to mind when you hear the phrase "comfort food"? Apple Pie? Warm bread with lots of butter? A mound of melt-in-your-mouth pancakes with melted butter and warm syrup? Fried chicken? Steak and potatoes? A warm, chocolate brownie with a side of ice cream? A thick-crust pizza with extra cheese? Or, how about spaghetti with a thick, rich sauce and chucks of hamburger in it, topped with parmesan cheese and a side of garlic bread? Anyone's mouth salivating yet? Thought so!

Okay, now that we've salivated and swallowed a few times, let's take a look at WHAT foods we choose, or gravitate toward. I'll be honest and share mine with you. I love "snack lunches", multiple foods that can be seen as "snacks". Growing up, that is what Mom called our lunches filled with a variety of foods! Most often they were fresh raw veggies; broccoli, carrots, snow peas, cauliflower, and celery. Then some summer sausage and marble cheese sometimes layered between crackers, a portion of fruit (apple, blueberries, or any seasonal berry, half an orange or clementine), and probably a cookie or three for dessert. There was ALWAYS dessert—store bought or homemade cookies or bars. Snack lunch was so fun to eat. I just loved those!

This being shared, now it's time to think of what foods you gravitate towards. Then, to ask the question of WHY we gravitate toward these specific comfort foods? What's the connection to the food? Once again, I'll use myself as an example with snack lunches. When I was growing up, I did NOT like to eat big meals. Truth be told, I still don't! Anyway, my brother would be gone to school and I was still at home, a preschooler, so it was my mom and me at home. If Mom asked me what I wanted for lunch, guess what my answer was? Yes, you're correct; "SNACK LUNCH!" It consisted of whatever snack-type foods were in the fridge, and cupboard.

Through the years as I grew up, when asked the same question, "What would you like for lunch or supper", can you imagine what my reply was? Yes, it was still "snack lunch!" And, today it is STILL the same, but it's changed in a couple ways. I've identified the WHY I want to eat snack lunches. I didn't like big meals, heavy, feeling-full meals. And, it's no longer about the emotional connection of eating these same desired comfort foods. Yes, I have fond memories of eating snack lunches with my mom, but that's not why I eat them now days. I don't eat all the same snacky-type foods I once did, the junky stuff anyway. I no longer eat any grains, but instead eat wild rice (a grass), and I don't eat any dairy products, so my snack lunches look different than they once were, AKA no dip or cheese. Truth be told, I think I've always been a "snack" kind of eater. Never liking big, heavy meals, snacking was my route! I'm actually a LOT like one of my grandmas in that way. Maybe it was a genetic thing. One of my grandpas had once told my mom when I was still young in grade school, "Kelly needs to quit snacking. She needs to learn to eat regular meals." Mom tried encouraging that often enough. Despite her encouragement, it just didn't work.

We ALL have emotional connections to comfort foods. WHY do we eat what we eat? What is the connection? WHY a specific food? What memory comes back when we think of that food, or eat that food? Why do we grab that same bag of chips or snack mix when turning on the TV? Again, what is the connection? What emotion comes with this food? What thoughts? What memories?

Emotional eating is something that is actually VERY prevalent in our society. We should be aware of this. Maybe, for some people, it's time to stop eating our emotions and start working through them instead? For others, perhaps they really don't see a need to, or don't have interest in asking, "Why do I eat what I eat?" Maybe you were never aware of something called "emotional eating". Maybe you've wondered why you just can't pass up a warm chocolate chip cookie straight out of the oven, sided with a glass of ice-cold milk. Maybe it's because there's an emotional connection that could be addressed so that you don't have to have those chocolate chip cookies every single time you smell them, or crave them.

I don't know your "whys". I don't have all the answers for you. I just seem to ask the questions and present an avenue for us to research for ourselves. I know for myself why I eat what I eat... and I'm glad I ask myself these and so many more emotional eating questions.

It's everyone's life and everyone's choice. You eat what you eat for specific reasons. I eat what I eat for many reasons. Can we change our eating patterns that are not serving us well, to choose foods that are beneficial for our lives and health?

As Hippocrates says, **"Let food be thy medicine and medicine be thy food!"**

82

Subtle Encouraging Shifts

Kelly

Near the end of January 2016, I started to feel a little better, sporadically. I had a few days in which I could go a few hours without pain earlier in the month due to the massage therapy with Hallie. But now with added helps from Dr. North that I'd been taking since shortly after our last consult in December of 2015, the end of this new month of January I was having less severe left-side abdominal pain, and the back pain was getting better subtly. I was mostly not having headaches, nausea, or hot sweats. This was surreal, a few hours of relief. I felt that my body was closing in on getting all the bad pathogens out.

I needed to keep doing all of what I had been doing in order to kick this disease out of my body. Those few hours of "feeling REALLY WELL" encouraged me to keep being determined and focused on getting through the rough times, even though there were fewer of those both days and nights. Truthfully, my body was exhausted from detoxing so heavily for the last seven months. However, I couldn't stop detoxing now! I was reaping the rewards of my efforts! Each day I'd put one foot in front of the other, pressing onward. *"God, help me!"* was my go-to prayer.

Often, during those trying times, Mom would give me a hug and wouldn't even have to say a single word to me. Her loving presence helped soothe me. It wasn't always easy when I had moments of frustration. Most of the time, I choose to not dwell on my pain or the frustration(s) when they arose. Instead, I'd stay focused on healing and moving forward as best I could. I was doing better overall, but I had a way to go in the healing process. I'd smile thinking that with each day I was one day closer to optimal health.

I whispered my prayerful thoughts one night before I drifted off into a restless slumber. *"Lord, help me to be patient. I trust You and Your perfect timing, Papa. You continually give me the strength, encouragement, and discipline to stay focused... and I'm so very grateful. Help me, Papa. I'm so tired. I love You and couldn't do any of this without You. My thankful heart is my best offering."*

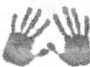

January 27th, 2016. My phone rings. I answer, "Greetings, Dr. North!"

"Hello, Kelly. How have you been doing? Fill me in with how you have been feeling in the last month. Inform me about any changes or anything new that has happened." He invited warmly.

"I continue to get better slowly, subtly. I've had one bowel movement on my own since the last time we have talked! However, I'm still doing daily coffee enemas so that I can have a daily elimination." I stated. "The left-side pain is still present, varying in degree of pain from minute-to-minute. I've been able to go a few hours in a day where I have no left-side pain a few times! THAT has been a wonderful shift!" I spoke cheerfully.

"This is great!" He shared my enthusiasm.

"The left-side pain in my abdomen and back gets worse when I'm not feeling well. Headaches arise when this happens, along with some bloating and gas." I informed him.

"Okay." Dr. North said.

"I'm still expelling the rope biofilms during enemas but they're not as prominent. On that note, I feel like I finally have the desire to have a bowel movement on my own, but I'm still unable to do that. I continue to see the pellets in my daily enemas too." I stated.

"Kelly, you are making such good progress!" Dr. North exclaimed. "I know that this healing process has taken a long time, but we ARE making good progress! At this point in time, we are TRULY getting to the root of the issue and eradicating it from your body. As we continue this process of purging the bad pathogens out, we are supplementing good nutrients and bacteria back into your body. We are doing a 'two-in-one', purging the bad out and implementing the good in with KEY healers." He clarified.

"Yes." I agreed. And I truly did agree, knowing strongly in my heart that I was on a "best" path for myself to get the help I needed to become well again.

"Kelly, I want to talk a little more about your Comprehensive Stool Analysis Test (CSAT) results from last month. I want to restate that your results offered a great deal of information. I'm glad to see that the inflammation that is present isn't too high, considering what is going on inside of you." He paused. "I have a few things that I want you to start implementing into your regimen each day." Dr. North explained further, then I willingly agreed to his plan for me. "Great. In addition, keep eating these foods..." Dr. North listed a few specific foods that would help my body to heal from the inside out. "What you have going on in your body takes time to heal. For the next year, Kelly, you will continue to heal and detox. Although in the course of the next month I want your healing to take a drastic change eradicating the rest of the bad pathogens, then you won't have as much pain, and the healing process will happen more quickly. Your body will begin to heal itself, with some help, and will start to work as it was designed to. You have made so much progress, Kelly. Let's continue to aid in moving forward in the process of your healing to wellness!" Dr. North stated warmly.

"That sounds REALLY good! My body is so tired of detoxing, Dr. North. I know the toxic junk needs to come out, but I'm exhausted from detoxing so heavily for such a long time. Don't get me wrong, it is a GOOD thing! Pushing the toxins out is rough!" I chuckled.

"Kelly, you are doing such a good job. Keep up all of your great work." Dr. North encouraged me.

We spoke more about the last CSAT results. As the phone call came to an end, we agreed on a date and time to talk again in one month.

Sleep was a continuous battle for me. I'd wake up feeling sick in the early hours of the morning. I'd be able to go back to sleep, although my abdomen

325

always seemed to ache. I continued to sleep on my left side, as this created less pressure on my abdomen. I'd average 6-9 hours of sleep a night on a good night. Mostly, it was 6-7 hours of sleep/night, not the recommended amount for an ill body to heal. Interrupted sleep because of pain while my digestive system was doing its job, the organs detoxifying through the night, made deep rest a challenge. However, I was having subtle, encouraging shifts happen during the days.

83

The Spot Is...

Kelly

I started taking actual fiber one-half-hour after I woke each morning, after my January consult with Dr. North. The first five days were difficult because I became bloated, feeling sick. After those five days, my body reacted less severely to the fiber. Then, I took the "remedy" Dr. North had sent me to improve my gut and brain connection so that I could have a bowel movement on my own. I also starting taking the other supplements, daily, from the new protocol. The remedy would always come in the mail first, after our monthly phone consults, then the supplements would arrive shortly thereafter. That was the routine.

At this time, the rope biofilms (RBs) were getting to be nearly nonexistent, and so were the pellets! I'd get some of each, every couple of days, but that was it! I was still doing daily coffee enemas, although I had a physical desire to have a bowel movement on my own. Still, though, I was unable to go number two on my own. My abdomen didn't hurt as much after eating. I wasn't getting nearly as many headaches during the night. The hot and cold sweats came only when I was feeling really ill, then I'd have fevers, which was "normal" for me, based upon the last few years.

I continued to wake up between 12:45-3am due to the abdominal pain, when my liver was working to digest and repair, trying to push out the toxic build up from within my body, getting extra help from the supplements. I averaged 1-2 nights/month that I could sleep between 8-10 hours, one of those nights being a day when I'd got a massage from Hallie!

JE February 6th, 2016

Had a massage from Hallie today. As I got off the table, the thought went through my head, "I wonder if this is what it feels like to feel 'normal'... besides my deep dull achy pain spot in my left side?" I look forward to the day that I can feel healthy and well, without pain and symptoms. Thank you for this journey, Papa God, I know You are constantly making good out of ALL of it. I trust You. Let the healing happen in Your time as You see fit. Set me free, Papa.

My digestive system had started to make some new subtle shifts near the end of January into the beginning of February now. The deep burning spot in the left side on my abdomen was much smaller in total area. It no longer extended the length of my pancreas, but now burned in one small area just to the left of the middle of my body under the ribs, straight thru into my back. In the back, it was located just to the left of my spine, about a 1-2" spot that burned, itching deeply inside my core. The spot was diminishing as I continued to detoxify my body!

As you've read thus far, coffee enemas (CE) were a huge part of the detoxification process for me, my daily best friend. So, I'd just like to share a little bit more about CE's history without boring you!

Coffee enemas have been around since the early 1900s. Max Gerson first started using coffee enemas for his patients suffering from tuberculosis. Later he used them for his cancer patients. Coffee enema therapy is often referred to as "The Gerson Therapy"[13]. Dr. Gerson addressed two of the biggest and most influential factors in illness: nutritional deficiency and toxicity. He used raw fresh juices to address the nutritional deficiencies, and coffee enemas were used to force toxins out of the patient's tissues. In turn, this helped to cleanse and support the liver so that it could eliminate toxins properly. Dr. Gerson understood that when the liver gets overloaded, then toxins are continually getting released INTO the body. Coffee enemas were the proper support that the liver (and gallbladder) needed for the detoxification process to start to get the toxins OUT OF the body. Years later Dr. William Kelley learned the importance of coffee enemas from Dr. Gerson. Dr. Kelley started using coffee

---

[13] Dr. Max Gerson, M.D. "How It All Started" https://gerson.org/how-it-works/

enemas for himself when he found out he had pancreatic cancer in 1969. He, too, saw the importance of coffee enemas and continued to use them for his cancer patients.[14]

I'd done a few hundred, or quite possibly more, coffee enemas since Mom and I'd started the online gut healing program as well. Coffee enemas LITERALLY saved my life. It didn't matter how many enemas it was going to take until I got all the toxic junk out of my body, because with the help of coffee enemas I was alive.

A real laugh-out-loud moment. The smell of coffee is Mom's favorite aroma, although she doesn't drink it. Nor do I drink coffee, but I cannot say it's on my list of "favorite aromas", to be sure! Mom and I don't think the same anymore of "morning coffee" as most people refer to their morning coffee. We don't drink it, but we sure can shove it up our WAZOO!

I had a deep knowing—in my heart, for a length of months now, that the day would come when I would know without a doubt in my mind that I would no longer need to do coffee enemas. I'd told Mom, more than once, that my body would know when to discontinue CEs. My body would one day be free from the toxins and RBs, and then I'd be able to have bowel movements on my own. My organs would be able to keep up with the detoxification process and my body would begin to function as it was meant to. I patiently awaited that day, doing everything I could, doing my part in this healing process. I felt a deep knowing in my heart that things were changing for the better, and that it wasn't going to be too much longer before I was out of the woods.

---

[14] Dr. William Donald Kelly, D.D.S., M.S., online book "The Original Metabolic Medicine's Cancer Cure Do It Yourself Book One Answer to Cancer, Reviewed after 32 years 1967-1999". http://www.drkelley.com/CANLIVER55.html

84

Not Out of the Woods, Yet

Amy

Kelly just ended the last chapter saying, "I felt a deep knowing in my heart that things were changing for the better and that it wasn't going to be too much longer before I was out of the woods." The being "out of the woods" time was approaching quickly. She was correct. Healing was happening, but she wasn't out of the woods, yet. The best results were soon coming.

During the season of January 2016 going forward, while Kelly was still detoxing, we were also preparing for a family trip to Hawaii. Kelly had **set a goal** during the summer of 2015 when we booked our family trip to Hawaii. The goal was **to be well** by February 2016's end, right before we would leave for Hawaii. It looked as if this goal was on course for her, with the subtle changes in her daily health. This was so encouraging!

With only the few people that knew exactly what she was dealing with, pancreatic cancer, we now felt as though it was okay to let others know what specifically was happening with Kelly those last years, up to this time of February 2016.

Kelly had been diligent, staying focused on her health and solving her illness through the all-natural routes that often times are unacceptable to the masses, especially to health insurance companies who do not cover the costs of these therapies. Thankfully, she had not had to deal with opposition--people questioning her about her choices of healing, and possibly leaving her having a divided mind about what she was choosing to do to rid herself of the toxins. That, in and of itself, was a huge blessing, not having to second guess herself if anyone had suggested her choice was not the right one (for

330

her). Kelly knew what she wanted for healthcare shortly after the start of her stomach pain, the summer of 2010. She was now seeing the fruits of her labors, five-and-a-half years later. *Kudos, kiddo!*

Knowing that our family trip was coming up in only a month's time, there was an "expectation". That expectation, spoken out loud by Kelly, of her "being well by the time we leave for Hawaii", because of the goal she'd set for herself, was pressing in now to fruition. Would she be WELL by the departure time for our family trip, or be at least on the other side of this illness? Shortly, time would tell. My hopes were high, but I was also open for whatever would be, whether she had this illness in the bag or soon after the trip.

What I can tell you for sure is that our girl trusted in God and His sufficiency for her well-being during this whole long health ordeal. That faith, wild and untamed, was a faith that I recognized; trusting in her Papa God with whatever the end results of healing would be. A faith so strong in a heart so young is rarely seen, at least in my view of this world of human beings. She knew what she knew, and she would not be swayed even by her own family's questioning of her choices. Now, that does not mean that every choice she has made "in faith" is always going to be, or always has been, what she believes it will be, because she is not "all-knowing" as God Himself is. What I'm saying is, I admired the faith she demonstrated throughout her illness.

Speaking of an all-knowing God, do you have faith to carry you through bad days or seasons of grey and unknowns? What keeps you, or me, from fully trusting Him in whatever comes our way, or fully trusting that "we will know", "our situation will turn around", or "His will be done" WILL be done?

I was raised going to church, being told about God in religion classes, and hearing the scriptures on Sundays and holy days. I've always BELIEVED in God. I'd cried out to Him on a number of occasions in my early years of growing into an adult, and in my young adult years. But, I never "knew" Him, I just knew OF Him. Knowing of, or knowing things about God, doesn't make faith real.

Where does faith to believe in this all-knowing God come from? The peace that comes instantly from grabbing onto Jesus' hand in our human experience, during one of our hard, or worst-of-worst situations, is often when faith will become REAL to a person. Ask someone who has an uncommonly unwavering faith where it came from. Really, ask them. Ten-to-one, they will tell you they were at the bottom of the barrel, ready to give up. It was there that I, too, came to faith in God grabbing hold or Jesus' outstretched hand, in my worst-of-worst times--at the end of the barrel. At the end of our barrels, drowning in our sorrows, we can take hold of Jesus' outstretched hand and start a new way of living our human experience, seeing ourselves as we truly are-- humans in a fallen world, who are loved and forgiven by this all-knowing triune God—Father, Son, Holy Spirit.

Kelly's faith sustained her from believing any lie (an evil force) that would condemn her concerning her healthcare choices to address her illness. She trusted God's will to be done, not knowing the outcome of living a longer life with good health or living a half-life for any amount of time. How do I know this? Because we talk about faith and real things that happen in life that are very disturbing, painful, amazing, and wondrous. We have deep talks. A lot.

Why did God give, allow, or afford Kelly ultimately to heal? I don't know the answer. I know she put great effort into what she believed would heal her, convictions of what was a "right way" FOR HERSELF. But do I think that is WHY she was healed? There is something to be said about "obedience in following our convictions or 'knowing' in faith". I believe her determination and her obedience helped herself immensely, knowing she was doing the very best she knew to do for herself.

When crying out in prayer for the people I love & cherish, I'll always end prayers to God with, "…but Thy will be done, not my will, not so anyone else's will, but Thy, God's will, be done." And with that, I will leave the outcome for Him, knowing there is a spiritual battle of forces, "angels of light" verses "angels of darkness", that war in an unseen realm here on earth over the daily lives of every human being. God hears our prayers that impact our own and any person's daily life. Which brings me to my next point.

I believe I have a responsibility "to act out in faith" when moved in spirit to do some act of kindness or carry out some conviction of heart--a prompting, if there is an action needed. Although, it IS a choice, called "free will", to follow those promptings of the spirit of God within me, or not to follow through. Our free will impacts other's lives, for the better or worse. Now, if my choice to

332

follow through with an act of faith in kindness towards another is not received by the person the act was bestowed upon, I trust that God (who sees all and knows all things) is going to ultimately direct the final outcome regardless of my doing any act out of faith, because the outcome may or may not have to do with anything I acted on—being said or done, or perhaps anything which I may have self-orchestrated all on my own.

I personally loved hearing Kelly tell of her day on the dock sunning herself, in "Words - Visions – Dreams" --she hearing God's voice telling her to give so-and-so an exact amount of money. Little did she know that the recipient really needed the money, the exact amount she was prompted to give. In obedience to her conviction of needing to do this act of kindness, she ultimately did give the gift to the person, who was first astonished, and then grateful to receive it. She was blessed ten-fold, in my opinion, because of the act of gracious giving and obedience in following through with the kindness in an act of faith. *God love ya, girl.*

Maybe you've wondered how God hears the needs of so many individuals to the ends of the earth? That I cannot answer. I do trust that He hears and will respond through all of life, using nature, humans and giftings of materials and work, animals, knowledge and information, weather, and water, etc. to speak and respond to us. What is spoken to me by Him is not audible to my ears, but heard in my heart. How do I know it's Him? The Holy Spirit promptings have to go through a "funneling" of sorts for me to trust it was Him. It's usually quite easy to tell.

While Kelly was in her early years of illness, there were people I asked to pray for her, women that I knew who would do so. I trusted that each person asked to pray would do so as they were led to. There were no questions in my mind of their doing so, when they would, or how often they would. Every so often they would hear from us, usually myself, and were asked to keep praying for Kelly's health situation. Doing a group email was the easiest way for these requests to be made, but every so often a phone call was needed, just to hear a caring voice on the other end.

Kelly was not out of the woods, yet, during this part of her telling of her health journey, but she was definitely heading in the right direction. Family is a great place to practice one's faith. As a family, we have daily opportunities to seek

God's face for our own and for other's needs to be met. As a larger family, including friends and relatives, we can share our hearts, our needs, our hopes and dreams with these people. What a beautiful testimony of faith, to access the triune God of this universe, and see how He will orchestrate our lives and answer our prayers in His perfect time, in His perfect way, for His glory.

If you trust in this faith, a triune God, the Father, the Son, and the Holy Spirit, there is power in that faith; power to move mountains, to heal the sick, and to give sight to the blind. He is always available to talk to, 24/7. Or if you question God's existence, and are curious, just call out to Him. A simple "Help" will do. Watch for how He answers. It just may surprise you.

85

Happy Dance!

Kelly

On February 10th, 2016 I awoke in the fetal position feeling sick. I had barely slept sound the last few nights. My abdomen was hurting all over, and the deep, small, burning spot was on fire. I felt like vomiting and had a headache. I got out of bed feeling terrible.

As I dressed, my stomach felt worse as I struggled getting into my clothes. I hobbled down the hallway into the bathroom and much to my surprise I had a bowel movement all on my own! Thoughts of *Oh! My! Happy dance* went flying through my head! Afterwards, I limped upstairs, still battling pain. As I reached the top step, my low back had increased pain--a harsher degree. I started my morning coffee brew on the stovetop. I felt like I was going to have another bowel movement. I again hobbled to the bathroom, making it just in the nick of time. *Oh! My! Happy dance* again!

In the next 45 minutes, I had a total of five bowel movements! I still ended up doing an enema to extract the rest of what needed to come out, which included some of the "pellets" I've mentioned before that'd become a part of each elimination, and even more RBs, but as of late the RBs were less often.

Finished in the bathroom, I laid down in the guest bedroom across the hallway from the main floor bathroom. Shivering, I covered my head with my sweatshirt and resumed the fetal position on my left side. I was cold, had a headache and had a fever, which was normal when I got sick like this. A few minutes later Mom came in the bedroom. I told her about my eventful morning. *Oh, happy dance!* Even though I felt terrible, I knew that I needed to eat something in order to take my morning supplements. Mom made some breakfast while I laid on the bed resting. By the time the food was ready, I was already feeling much better. The rest of the day I had quite a bit of pain coming and then going, but the pain wouldn't last for very long.

Fast forward: Two days later I had another bowel movement all on my own! I knew (and felt) my body was TRULY healing from the inside out. My body was trying to resume simple functions, like having a bowel movement! The gut-brain connection had reconnected. The two were beginning to communicate with each other, and my body was able to know and trust what was going on inside of it! This meant my body was beginning to operate and function as it was designed to on its own. My vital organs were starting to function and do their individualized jobs! *God, is it truly time?* I thought.

I continued to have bowel movements all on my own throughout the rest of the month. However, I was still doing coffee enemas as the pain was too intense if everything didn't detoxify itself out via normal bowel movements.

Then, right before our family left on vacation for Hawaii that month, the bowel movements I was having on my own just stopped completely. *It's not over yet,* I thought to myself. The rope biofilms and pellets were nearly none existent, and I'd had many bowel movements on my own that month. It was beginning to happen, my body doing what it was designed to do, to function on its own, although more time and healing was needed. *"Trust me, Kelly. Be patient."* God seemed to be telling my heart.

"Okay, Papa. You know exactly what I need. I do trust You. Continue to direct me, heal me, strengthen me and light the path. I place my life in Your loving hands." I prayed out loud.

I had eliminated a large number of the toxins out of me... but it wasn't over, yet. And despite that "YET", it was time to leave for Hawaii! Whether I'd met my goal to be healthy and well, or not, like Mom had talked about in "Plans and Goals", it was time for our Hawaiian adventure. So, physically at my optimal wellness or not, I, my family and my aunt and uncle were to soon fly out on a grand adventure together, one that for me, personally was more than just a vacation or "get-away".

336

86

Dreams Become
Reality in Hawaii

Kelly

Our family trip to Hawaii was to be more than just a vacation or get-away for me. Let me explain.

I'm a woman who does not have a bucket list, even from when I was a little girl. Maybe it's because I don't believe that a person should wait to do something they love, or something they want to do until they retire, or have to have to wait for that "perfect" occasion. I guess I'm more of the mindset, "If the opportunity arises and the timing is right" type, that it may happen, but even than if it doesn't work out, I don't expect that it has to happen. This being said, there have been two things that I've wanted to do since I was a little girl, but for me they were never "bucket list" material. I hoped that they would happen in my lifetime, but I wasn't SET on them happening.

So, what were these two things I'd wanted to do? The first was to go to Hawaii. The second was to learn how to surf. The little girl that dreamed, hoped, that one day these opportunities would happen had no idea if and when it would ever happen, but I was for some reason drawn to these two things.

These two dreams actually happened TOGETHER, just like something else once did in my high school years. Back then, I'd wanted to shoot both a "banded duck" and also a "triple-curly tail (male) Mallard duck". As it turned out, I shot one bird with both assets! It was a crazy "woot-woot, hoorah" experience that knocked the socks off me!

337

Back to my dreams of going to Hawaii, and learning to surf. Let's jump back to about nine or so months, during June-July 2015, when Mom and I were talking one day. Mom was asking me about how many credits I had to do for "Continuing Education" (CE), for my line of work in being a Massage Therapist, and also asked when I had to have my CE credits completed by. I told her, and she asked me what I was thinking about taking for the class. I had an idea, desiring to learn Ashiatsu massage, but wasn't set in my mind on doing this class. As we'd talked, the subject of my desire to go someplace warm got brought into the conversation (if you remember at this point in time, I was ALWAYS cold). "Yes, that'd be good, to go someplace warm," Mom stated.

Long story short, I jumped online to find what states in the USA had an Ashiatsu class being offered, and when. There were five states that offered "National Certification" for this particular class, two of which were warmer states, and one of those states being Hawaii! My mind reeled when I saw "Hawaii" on my laptop screen! Memories of being a little girl desiring to go to Hawaii flooded my mind and warmed soul. *Is this really possible? Is this even realistic? Could I really take my CE class in Hawaii and actually have BOTH dreams I've always desired to do happen? Would I even be able to surf?* Remember, the year before this during the summer 2015 my health was teetering on the edge of destruction. We didn't know if I was going to be alive much longer, especially if something didn't change for the better anytime soon, then. This may sound morbid, but it was my reality. Knowing the current state of my health the summer of 2015, going to Hawaii didn't seem very realistic, but I'd told Mom about my internet search findings nonetheless.

"Kelly, I think you should get in touch with the instructor and see if you can take the training this winter. If you can, sign up for it! We could take a family vacation to Hawaii!" Shocked, in disbelief, as to what I was hearing doesn't begin to describe the expressions that were revealed on my face. Mom chuckled as I digested what she'd just said, and then stated, "Well, this isn't written in stone. All of us need to talk about it. If it works for us to do, we'll need to figure out a good time to go". And then we'd decided that very day for me to pursue gathering information and we'd then have further communications amongst us four—my family.

A week or so later, the four of us, in addition to my aunt Lori and uncle Brad, made arrangements to take this vacation after I'd heard back a confirmation that I could take my CE class in Hawaii. And that is how this vacation to Hawaii came to be a reality!

It still felt unrealistic to me, given my state of health back during the summer of 2015, for me to go to Hawaii AND learn how to surf. Mom and I had talked about the reality of the situation. Hawaii was fulfilling my only two desires I had. Well, besides the desire to BE WELL IN HEALTH. That being said, if I was alive, I was going on that trip. And if it killed me to go, learning to surf, etc., okay, because I already accepted the fact that I MAY die anyhow. Furthermore, in going on this trip, I would do the two things that I'd wanted to do my entire life thus far. This trip was honestly more than JUST a vacation. It could possibly be our first AND last family vacation together. IF I wasn't going to make it, when we were making the plans those six-plus months ago, I wanted my family to still go on the adventure without me.

I had BIG plans, goals, and dreams to be healthy and well by the time we were to leave for Hawaii, but only months of time, at the time of scheduling it all, would tell if that would come to fruition. Again, I faced reality, whatever God's will would be, I would be okay with.

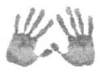

So back to the current time in my health journey, the end of February 2016. It's time to go to Hawaii! Fortunately, the time was here and so was I. Unfortunately, I still could NOT sit without being in pain, and I was back doing enemas daily. The flight to Hawaii is long--really long, over eight hours, not including sitting in airports and driving to and from those. "It was ROUGH" is putting it lightly for my personal traveling experience. To make matters worse, our flight, before heading oversea, had to make an extra stop to refuel before leaving the mainland because of strong headwinds. I battled physically, mentally, emotionally, and even spiritually, during the entire flight. But, despite it all, I was in pursuit of LIVING out my two dreams I wanted to do since childhood and I was healthy enough to do those! I was eternally grateful to be still living and breathing.

As our unit of six people arrived in the tropical state, my mind reeled. *It's really happening. We're here. I'm here. I made to Hawaii!* It was surreal for me. After finally getting to our vacation rental home and unpacking, showering, and so forth, I'd went downstairs after everyone but Mom had gone to bed. I'd been very stressed with travel on this extra-extended day, with pressures and great discomforts. She cradled my face saying, "We are here, Baby! You're here!" We sat on the living room sofa, and I started crying. Even as I write this now, years later, it still brings tears to my eyes because it was one of those really special moments.

Mom spoke memories of making the plans for the trip, some of which I just shared with you, and the unknown of my being alive having been completely up in the air at that time. Mom finished speaking, and a gentle smile pulled at my lips despite my still not feeling well and I being way past the point of exhausted. I was emotional.

"Mom, do you also remember how once we'd made plans for this trip that I'd told you... 'I don't want this to sound morbid, but please hear me out. We both know my health isn't good, actually at all right now. If something doesn't change with my health, I may or may not be alive to go on this trip. If I am, I'll be fulfilling the two dreams I've always desired to do, and I'll be healthy enough to make the trip. That is what I'm planning on! But, if I'm not alive, Mom, I want you all to still go on the trip. Do it for me. Please? If I'm not here to join you all, I'm asking you, please, don't cancel the trip, but go there and do it in remembrance of me to fulfill my only two desires.' Do you remember that?"

Tears had flowed freely down our faces, but Mom knew I'd meant every word when I'd spoken that to her just the past summer of 2015. Mom nodded "yes," she remembered. I continued, "And then you'd said, 'Okay. But you ARE going. I'm not giving up on you and you're not giving up on me, right?'"

"And in agreement, I'd responded back, 'Without a doubt I'm NOT giving up!'" in 110% agreement." With that memory shared, we embraced one another on our first night in Hawaii and wiped our tears... and I responded before making my way to bed, "Yes Mama, we're here. I'm here. I made it. Thank you for helping me to make it here. And thank you for helping make coming to Hawaii a reality." She then said I should get to bed for some really needed rest.

As I lay on the bed in Hawaii that first night, the memory of our past summer's conversation faded as rest entered into me.

87

Hawaiian Adventures

Kelly

My health wasn't where I'd wanted it to be when we departed for Hawaii. It was better than it had been months before, but I had a way to go before I was fully healthy and well. My health situation wasn't going to stop me from doing what I came here to do, if I had a choice in the matter.

A summary of our trip is in store because, honestly, this trip was a milestone marker for me in my current health situation, and it was actually our first time flying to somewhere as a family for a "family vacation", our immediate family of four.

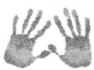

Sunshine. Warmth. Shorts. Tank tops. Flip-flops. Sunglasses. And let's not forget, easy-dry water-wear for some of our daily-dos! These were all "must haves" for Hawaii! We went on many walks daily, looked at touristy "must see" places, checked out a botanical garden, rented bikes for the entire length of days we were there to bike to from place to place, soaked up the sun's rays, and sat on the lanai for most of our meals, to play cards, and to watch and listen to the ocean waves hitting the shoreline. But that wasn't it... there was more, lots more. All day, every day, I was happy to be in warm weather, to not be cold. The sun felt good on my skin. And each day, I continued doing my daily coffee enema regimen to keep up with the detoxification process. So be it. It was what it was.

On day two after arriving to the island, we explored the reality of surfing! Since it was so windy, the places where a person could rent surf and boogie boards required anyone wanting to rent boards to take lessons from their licensed instructors in a designated area of water, a bay, where it was a tad calmer. And so, we, Troy, Uncle Brad, Mom--who'd had NO intention what-so-ever of even getting into the water before the trip, and I, all took the surfing lessons on land and then IN the ocean!

Surfing went well with the help of two instructors. They made catching the waves EASY! It was a fabulous experience! It didn't take much and I was tuckered out, but that didn't stop me from quitting. As I stood on the surfboard, no one could wipe the smile off of my face as I was living out my second dream that I'd come here to fulfill!

Mom, who in her regular "swimming in any body of water thoughts" was deathly afraid of a shark attack, had not even one thought of such a thing while in the ocean water learning to surf! Not once did she think of sharks attacking. *What?* It turns out, a friend back in Minnesota--who KNEW the morning of this happening that mom would be going IN the ocean water, who'd also KNEW Mom's "fear of sharks and whatever was under the water", was praying for her ocean water experience, specifically. Mom was told this once back home on the mainland. *Prayers answered, ya think?*

The entire time we were in Hawaii it was SUPER windy, so much so that a very rare event called "The Eddie Aikau" pro-surfer event took place while we were there. The wave swells have to be over 40 feet high, at the least, for 24-plus hours during the event. Before the event was confirmed as a GO, the waves were definitely that big, so everyone interested in partaking in the event at any level of watching to actually surfing in it, people from all around the world, they'd be on-hold to know if the event would even take place just days before the event WAS "a go". 40-foot-high waves are BIG, BIG swells! Confirmed, the event was a hands-down BIG event! Thousands of people swarmed Oahu in a very short time-span of 24-48 hours.

We, our group of six, all decided to watch some of the surfing event. We rode our bikes to the location where it took place, one-and-a-half miles from our beachfront rental house. A MASSIVE number of fans, natives and otherwise, came with cameras and binoculars in hand, embarking a coved area beach and overtook the land on a beach--standing room for thousands of spectators. The mountainous landscape across the highway from the beach was also a place for observers to watch with binoculars and spotting scopes.

"The Eddie Aikau" was a memorable experience to see pro-surfers catch HUGE, MASSIVE waves that they maneuvered through with such skill and grace, that is made surfing look easy! The competitors were amazing to see riding such huge waves! This was a sight of a lifetime for us, to be upfront viewing the event. At times, the waves came up INTO the crowd standing on low land areas on the beach. My brother lost one of his sandals to the monstrous waves, and my aunt lost her beach towel to the water too! Some people's cell phones and camera equipment were ruined by the water coming in so fast and far onto land, their equipment being on the ground was swept away. It was just kind of bizarre how much water was moving about from the massive swells the wind produced! The wind over ocean waters was so loud, it produced a low HUMMMMM, with us during the entire trip, always in the background of conversations, times of thought, or during rest.

Another highlight on the trip was the CE Ashiatsu massage class I took. It was a marvelous experience! Can you imagine taking an outdoor class on somebody's lanai, a porch to us mid-westerners, just 50-feet from the ocean? The view was breathtaking! And to hear the sound of and see the ocean waves crashing on the shoreline meant there was NO additional calming massage music needed! I was over and above blessed while taking the class!

Speaking of blessed. I was here with the people I loved the most--family. That was joyful in and of itself. And, I was living out my two dreams in one trip.

I'm a coconut fan. Are you? I don't care what form it comes in: coconut oil, coconut milk, coconut water, fresh coconut meat, or dried and shaved coconut meat. In Hawaii, some of us enjoyed our first-ever fresh coconut and coconut water. Canned coconut water does not compare to fresh coconut juice inside the coconut! It was there that I learned how to crack open a coconut, by watching one of the salesmen at a fruit stand in Oahu we'd stopped at. Tropical fruit! YUM! We also tried fresh mango, star fruit, dragon fruit, passion fruit, and pineapple. It was fresh, tasty, and enjoyed by all!

One of our last adventures was snorkeling in Hanama Bay. All I can say is, WOW! WOW! WOW! Never in my life had I snorkeled before, but I'd been talking to a client before the vacation and the client had said, "If there's ONE thing I recommend, it's snorkeling in Hanama Bay." Well, that client was right. Since our family had never snorkeled before, we were in for one of the best experiences of our lifetime! Hanama Bay is one of the top places to snorkel in the entire world! Not kidding, it's true. The water clarity was literally PERFECT. And the variety of beautifully-colored fish we saw just left me utterly speechless. We even got to see rainbow fish too! To top it all off, we watched whales off in the distance, outside of the bay, surfacing and putting on quite the show, splashing their tails. The day we did this adventure was our last full day in Hawaii. We all agreed that we left off on a perfect note.

Hawaii was really a wonderful get-away. Like I've said, to me the trip was a monumental milestone of being alive, breathing in all the beauty in life, and headed in the right direction in my health journey. I may not have met MY personal goal to be "fully well" by the time we were to leave for this trip, but I was surely in the right direction. I was able to take the trip I'd dreamed of taking! To me, it was a once-in-a-lifetime trip for a very special reason, a trip I never thought should happen, but perhaps one day would happen. More important was that I was alive celebrating LIFE with the people I loved most.

The special adventurous time and memories made in Hawaii will be forever cherished by myself and my family too. To go to this beautiful place helped contribute to another turning point in my health situation, by bringing me much joy!

88

Revealing The Root

Kelly

While in Hawaii I'd continued to detox, doing my daily morning enema routine and eating healthful homemade meals. I'd had a couple days of feeling genuinely well while on vacation. The warm weather REALLY helped me, as I didn't have to use extra energy fighting to stay warm in the healing process.

When we got back to Minnesota all my body wanted to do was heal through deep sleep for the first time in years. I was able to sleep deeper, for the most part. Lots of healing was happening while I was sleeping. I'd sleep anywhere from 10-13 hours a night once we were back home! *Awesomeness!*

Another wonderful benefit that happened a few days after returning home from Hawaii was that I'd eradicated two big, full, tumorous masses of rope biofilms via my morning enema! They were bluish-green in color, mixed with blood in them. *Gross. I know.* Cancer is NOT pretty. Sorry, but it was so amazing to see! Immediately after passing these, I felt even better physically and was mentally relieved. The RBs coming out of me before this time were all surrounding and protecting the root of these latest pieces of tumor. Now we were getting to the actual ROOT of the tumor, killing and eliminating the mass. I was LITERALLY expelling the cancerous tumor right out of me.

In the days to come after passing those two nasty tumorous masses, I took HUGE strides for the better. The pain was nearly non-existent in my left side! I had considerably less symptoms. My attitude and moodiness also improved. I could smile, laugh, cry joyful tears, and love life easily and it all just felt so GOOD!

345

JE March 5th, 2016
I've slept twelve hours the last two nights and thirteen hours last night. I'm still so very tired though. My body is finally healing inwardly and welcomes sleep. Oh, to sleep. What a blessing!

On March 9th, 2016, I had another phone consult with Dr. North. I shared the wonderful improvements that had happened within the last month, and the latest elimination of mass RBs. "The headaches are nearly gone. The left-side 3-dimensional pain is nearly non-existent. Hot sweats are very rare. I wake up less during the night, and when I do wake up, I don't feel 3D pain. I've had more bowel movements on my own, although they've stopped again. I have more energy, but there is still room for improvement. I laugh and smile more easily. I can go through my days with little or sometimes NO pain! Truly, I feel the best that I've ever felt in my life, and I know that this is just going to continue to improve." I told him.

"These changes are EXACTLY what I wanted to happen for you! This is really good news, Kelly! You are taking great strides in your healing process." Dr. North stated warmly.

As we continued to talk, he asked me specific questions and I answered them. As we wrapped up our conversation, he said, "Kelly, we are looking at one more month of these 'hard core' supplements. In one month of time, when we talk next, we will be focusing on using mostly 'food as medicine' in order to continue in your healing and rebuilding your body's strength with nutrients. We'll be feeding it exactly what it needs via specific foods, using less supplements, although there will be a few. Meanwhile, I want you to focus on eating and drinking better bacteria to help improve and balance your gut health. Keep drinking kombucha. In addition, start drinking (coconut-water-based) kefir and eating sauerkraut. I'll send you a specific bottle of probiotics that I want you to take, and the amounts of these products so you won't react harshly. Also, start with only a couple strands of sauerkraut with a meal. Over time, you can slowly increase to a few more strands, then a spoonful and so forth." He stated wisely.

"I will do that." I agreed.

"Kelly, you are now on the threshold, so-to-speak. One more month and you will be through the threshold! Keep doing the things that we talked about and we will talk again in a month. May you continue to heal and be well!" Dr. North spoke kindly.

"Thank you, I appreciate it! Thank you for all the help you've been and continue to be" I said. *Hmm, "one more month". Smiling!*

Dr. North was right, I needed to slowly keep implementing a good variety of bacteria into my diet to further speed up my healing process. Symptoms arose from implementing the new fermented foods. I had to work through that sick feeling from the ferment's entrance into my body, because I NEEDED these good bacteria in my body! They were vital bacteria I was lacking to digest food (better) and to have a healthy gut. Each day, though, I grew stronger. As I grew stronger, I had less pain and symptoms. In addition, I started to have a few bowel movements on my own again. *Happy, happy, happy dance!* These were awesome shifts in my health!

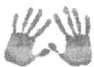

I went to Hallie for my monthly massage in the month of March, too. This day was one of the first times I went to see her that I actually felt well and wasn't in pain. We did our normal sharing of "how you been doing?"

After the massage Hallie told me, "Kelly, I didn't feel the penetrating hot spot that you used to have." We looked deep into each other's eyes and shared a knowing peaceful smile. Healing was happening!

Also in March, on the 20th, 2016 was my 24th birthday. This day was very special for my loved ones and myself. I started sharing, other than with the few individuals that already knew, what I had been going through for the last five-and-a-half-plus years of my life on a social media post. Prior to this time, I wasn't ready to let people know the truth about what I had been and still was going through. The majority of people who commented on the post or contacted me otherwise had had no idea I had been ill. Or, they knew I was ill but not as ill as I had been. I hadn't wanted them to know, again because even though some people would support my decision of alternative healing, others would not, as I wrote about in "Not Out of the Woods, Yet". I didn't want to deal with extra stress when I was sick, stress coming from other's possible voiced opinions being very different than my own concerning my health choices. I knew what I wanted to do with my health situation and didn't need any opposition. My family and I had decided to keep my health situation out of public opinion. I'm still very thankful we'd decided that. But now it was time to be out in the open, and I was mentally ready.

After having shared publicly my health battle that appeared to be being won, some individuals voiced their opinions telling me that "You are going to die if you don't utilize chemotherapy and radiation." Others told me stories of how they knew of friends or acquaintances that had tried alternative therapy but had died. I was respectful to these individuals, trying to explain some important details of my journey to them, but most often they didn't seem to really hear me, or maybe just didn't understand… and that was okay. I knew I was doing what I needed to do. Deep in my heart, I was given insights which I'd acted on from the start of my illness, and answers to what I needed to do, along with helpful people along the way, and I followed through with the flow of it all. God was in complete control. I didn't need to explain myself, or expect other people to understand when I did explain. I knew in my heart of hearts I had been doing exactly what I needed to for myself and for my healing journey. THAT was what mattered.

Papa, thank You. I love You and know You have me on this journey and in this place for a reason. I trust You. You are in complete control. My life is in Your hands.

89

New Shifts Happening

Kelly

Since the day we'd gotten back from Hawaii, as I've said, shifts were happening in regards to my health.

On March 24th, 2016 another new shift happened. While turning my torso at my spine, in order to move my spine audibly popped without my forcing or trying to manipulate a "pop". It was very normal that my back, my spine, would pop. However, this particular spot was exactly where it always had had pain--right next to my spine on the left side in the middle to lower part of the back. This was the location that I always wanted to grab something and stick it into my back for pain relief. As it popped on this day, it no longer ached at ALL like it had the last few years. Someone may see this as a minor deal, but it wasn't. This was actually a major happening for a body that was virtually "locked" from so much trauma happening to it. And then another new shift happened!

The following day, while doing massage therapy on a client, I was standing completely still in a lunge position. Without any of my "self-helps", my pelvis shifted into place on its own. My client was oblivious to my personal happenings, the shift, even though this was audible to the ears. Shortly after the shift, I took notice that I NO LONGER LIMPED! I'd been limping for a few years to protect my left side--my body automatically compensating. In addition, with my pelvis in place, I no longer unconsciously threw my right hip out of alignment, so-to-speak, in an effort to make it more comfortable for my hurting left side. My body didn't have to accommodate for the left side anymore! So, as I drove home that night after work, I realized within minutes of driving that I no longer could sit comfortably in the position I had slouched to--my right side, it being unconsciously thrown out just like my hip while standing had been. Instead, I sat upright, straight, my hip in place for the first time in years while driving! Again, this was HUGE! I could now stand AND sit upright without pain! I was SO excited about this new shift!

JE March 25th, 2016
My pelvis released today. It is continually unlocking, as is the rest of my body, too. I can now stand straight with equal weight on both feet. I can sit upright in a car comfortably and not throw my right hip out to make standing more comfortable for my left side. I'm standing upright and feeling GOOD! It has been such a joy, these "little" but BIG shifts that are and have been happening.

On April 6th I spoke with Dr. North for my monthly appointment, telling him about the latest new shifts and improvements. "I continually improve. The symptoms come less often, as do the sick days. I have increased my fiber and probiotics slowly like you recommended and it's working well. I've only had a couple bowel movements on my own, although I have the urge to go, but can't. I feel like my body is ready to move forward more-so than ever, and that I am really healing now. I find that I still want to sleep a lot. I'm also very sore, my muscles, and fatigued. My energy level has room for improvement but it's better than it's been in the last few months." I chuckled softly.

"Sounds like more good progress is happening!" Dr. North stated.

We talked for a length of time and at the end of the phone consult Dr. North said, "I'm going to send you a supplement that is going to help improve your gut-brain connection. It will help your body to understand you can have a bowel movement on your own without the help of enemas. You've taken these once before and I'm going to give you higher dosages this time. Kelly, keep up the good work. Let this next month be another month of healing and headway in your health!" He encouraged me.

"Thank you. I appreciate your help." I replied kindly.

I was continually learning about patience on this healing journey, respecting it at an entirely new level. Healing takes both time and patience. They go hand in hand. If I wanted to heal, I needed to continue being patient and keep trusting and relying on God. He was the One that was in control. Not me.

"I trust You Lord. Give me patience. Show me what to do and what not to do, Lord. I feel like the time toward optimal health is getting closer, but it's not over yet. Help Lord, give me patience and strength. Use me as I know You are, Lord, for Your glory and Your honor. Your will be done." I said to my heavenly Father, feeling at total peace.

One more new shift! One morning, in April, I woke up feeling lighter and freer. I had a knowing that it wasn't going to be long and this grueling cancer elimination and healing process would be truly over. Then, life would be easier, health-wise anyway--being at ease.

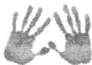

Each day in April was different, bring with it new, healing shifts. Even though progress seemed slow, progress was PROGRESS! Looking back to a year ago, I would go to bed wondering if I would wake up to see another day. I had come a LONG way in one year! It took my body years to become sick, and it would take a length of time to get it back to being healthy. I was making steady steps each and every day toward that.

The beauty of these new shifts happening always took me by surprise. I never knew when they were going to happen, day or night. Yet, they happened... and left me feeling healthier and more whole, healing me at yet a deeper level. I was very thankful.

90

It's Not Over Yet

Kelly

I was making progress in healing. I was slowly but steadily able to expand my diet while eating more probiotic foods. I had increased energy. I stayed active and was starting to LIVE my life; being able to feel comfortable enough to go and visit with friends even though the visits were brief. I smiled and laughed more easily, and boy did it FEEL good! It was like a breath of fresh air for my whole being! To be able to travel in a vehicle without laying down during longer journeys into the city was truly HUGE progress. I was able to comfortably sit, without much or any pain, for longer periods of time too. The days were getting easier and my whole demeanor was becoming more open. Laughing, rejoicing, sharing life, enjoying life, loving and being real with others is so much easier when you don't have physical pain. It was absolutely refreshing and invigorating to be feeling well! And I loved it!

The month of April went by. Within it, I had almost a dozen days of having bowel movements on my own. This was GOOD! I even had a few days that I skipped doing coffee enemas because I wanted to see if my body could get through 24-hours of going number two all on my own. There were two days that it worked. The other days that didn't work were rough, because symptoms would come back then. Those nights, I wouldn't sleep much because it was hard to get comfortable. As bowel movements stopped, back to the bathroom with my coffee I'd go, doing daily coffee enemas again. And guess what? I got more rope biofilms out. I STILL had work to do. It wasn't over YET.

Each day was different. As a whole, I continued to heal from the inside out. I no longer felt fatigued nor had full-body aches that'd felt like a train had run me over and then backed up on me again,

On May 4th, 2016 I had another phone consult with Dr. North. I told him the good news about having some bowel movements on my own, and then how they all-of-a-sudden stopped. He was glad I'd had them, but concerned as to WHY they stopped all of a sudden. "As I started doing the coffee enemas each morning, I started seeing some rope biofilms again." I stated.

"Okay. Apparently, the bad pathogen(s) aren't completely gone if they are still coming out. We need to address this and get rid of them completely." He informed me.

"Yes, I agree whole heartily. Let's get rid of these!" I then asked Dr. North some questions and he willingly answered them.

I've said this before but I'll say it again…as I embarked on this journey of healing, I had a deep knowing that I'd know when it was going to be over. Meaning, I'd wake up and something would feel different--body would be able to function and then I'd be able to have regular bowel movements on my own again. I'd told Mom SO many times, and that I'd KNOW when to stop doing coffee enemas for good. She trusted me to KNOW that, too. For whatever reason, it was helpful to know that someone believed in what I thought I'd know when the time would come TO know!

I trusted that God would make everything known to me about when it was all over. I'd know without a doubt in my mind that it was really and truly over with. I felt at peace and didn't doubt it. Timing is everything. I would be patient.

JE May 6th, 2016
I still don't feel "right" in my left side, 3-D into my back and my entire abdomen… I had bloating, pain, and hot sweats today. Some days it's

frustrating, truly. I'm sick and tired of being sick and tired, Lord. Please help me!

Dr. North's protocol for May was a diversity of supplements that I had taken before. The only new change was to take a rectal suppository.

"Some days, I swear I've done it all." I told Mom, referring to the rectal suppositories. Life was always interesting! Never a dull moment! I researched on the internet the impact of suppositories and learned that the suppository works its way up into the digestive system organs to grab hold of any toxins. Then, it pulls the toxins out of my body via bowel movements. I figured, *"It won't be that bad."* I did my first rectal suppository one evening, not being fully aware of what to expect. Dr. North had told me, "It will be a gentle detoxifier."

As I did the suppository, it began to do its job working its way up into my organs rather quickly, surprisingly. It didn't feel good at all! It was like something was grabbing my insides and I had absolutely no control over it. It had begun to work within three minutes and I was already feeling really sick. My gut and low back hurt. Within another ten minutes I was ready to vomit. I went to say good night to Mom. "How are you?" She asked.

I told her, dryly, with an irritation in my voice, due to the serious discomfort going on inside of me, "Crappy. Exactly what I need to do, too."

"Hmmm, sounds to me like you know what it means when someone tells someone to 'stick it where the sun doesn't shine'!" She retorted. I burst out into laughter at the thought.

"Well stated! That couldn't be truer!" I agreed. "Life is never dull." We shared a smile, and I left going downstairs for a restless night of sleep.

JE May 12th, 2016
I've been tired, sore, and blah feeling near the end of the day a lot lately. Feeling pretty yucky tonight from the suppository. I pray I sleep decently tonight, Papa. Please, please heal me and let me make BIG strides in the next days, weeks, and months. I'm begging You to help me, heal me, and let BIG things happen for the better, Lord. Please, I know and trust You are

working in and through me. Help me to be patient as I wait...and heal. I know You are working wonders in me, Papa. I trust You.

91

Coming Full Circle

Kelly

In the middle of May 2016, Mom drove three hours to attend a funeral of a relative. Before the funeral started, Mom sat quietly looking around. The sanctuary was filling with people.

While scanning the population there, she met a man's kind eyes. She sensed his integrity but had no idea who this man was. She said they ever so briefly held their gaze, then in another moment the man's wife turned and spotted Mom. THEIR gazes then locked, Mom and the man's wife, and the woman's eyebrows shot upward in surprise! The woman pointed a finger towards Mom while mouthing, "YOU!"

The funeral service was to start in five minutes, but that didn't matter as the woman jumped up from her seat and frolicked over to Mom, who was sitting in the "family section". Don't be alarmed, mom knew her, and she knew Mom! Mom and the woman quickly greeted each other enthusiastically! The two of them had been high school friends and hadn't seen one another since right after their graduation. The interaction was very brief, as the funeral was to start. The high school friend, Tiffany, walked--politely this time, back over to sit by her husband for the service. Mom retold this story many times, being asked, "Who was that woman?", during the visiting time after the service! The two talked again briefly before Tiffany had to leave. The friend was currently living out of state, but was back in MN visiting her family. She was actually supposed to have gone back home a few days before the funeral, but she decided to stay for the funeral of their family friend—Mom's relative.

What a gift that was for the two of them connecting after 30-plus years! Nothing is by coincidence!

"Coincidence is God's way of remaining anonymous."
-Charlotte Clemensen Taylor

Sometime early that summer, Tiffany came to our home while driving back to Minnesota from her home state, for a day and overnight to visit with Mom and to meet our family. While visiting us, I remember walking up the stairs and the woman greeting me, engulfing me in a giant hug. As we hugged, I had this sense of, *I've known you my entire life,* wash over me. The weird thing was, I'd never even met this woman before. I only recently knew of her through her communications with Mom at and since the funeral.

Tiffany's stay with us was a quick 24-hour visit, but during this time the two old friends shared many high school memories with my brother and me into the night. We laughed at their funny stories. It was beautiful to see them interact, sharing their past lives with us freely with no holds back, and seeing how they both matured since their high school days. Our bellies hurt from all the laughter shared together.

"Beauty begins the moment you decide to be yourself."
-Coco Chanel

Relationships are full of surprises. If your experience with relationships is anything like mine, you've found out that people come into our lives for seasons of time… some seasons short, others a lifetime, and some sporadically on and off. Old friends we may have lost touch with for a length of time, can come back for another season. As life goes on, we meet new people and they are in our lives for a season, or maybe forever. We meet people when we least expect it, having no idea why they are in our lives at the time they are. Maybe you, too, have experienced this firsthand?

Relationships are intricately complex, seemingly having caused more questions than answers in regard to them. But isn't that what builds our relationship with another person? You know, communicating, spending time together, asking questions, learning about the other person, working through stuff together, and becoming a better individual because we each want to? A lot goes into relationships, not just friend relationships, but especially marriage relationships. ALL relationships take time, energy, love, communication, respect, integrity, and commitment. Whether it's a marriage, friendship, dating relationship, business relationship, etc. Each relationship is a little different, but the foundational pillars for having them are much the same, needing human interactions and great care.

As Mom and Tiffany caught up on all the years they'd not saw or heard from one another, they enjoyed hearing highlights of the moments that went into those years for the other. Just because they hadn't talked for 30-plus years didn't mean that they didn't still care for the other. Their lives had just gone in different directions, and now their paths had crossed again!

Mom had shared with Tiffany about the reality of my health situation the last many years. Because of Mom's sharing, Tiffany randomly shared a recipe she called "GOOP" with us. The ingredients included; ground ginger, ground turmeric, cayenne pepper, lemon juice, apple cider vinegar, and water. As we stood in the kitchen, she told us about it, her eyes dancing with anticipation of the gnarly concoction and us maybe trying it for slashing inflammation!

Mom and I made "GOOP" after Tiffany had left our home, onto her next destination. As I started to drink it, the concoction burned as I swallowed it. Once it worked its way on downwards, I felt the concoction start to heat-up my body! The end result of my taking GOOP, was the next morning in my coffee enema, long, nasty biofilms appeared again in the elimination. I was now doing two enemas per day; one in the morning and one at night. My body was again detoxing RB toxins so quickly that I was having a difficult time keeping up with the process. The great thing about it, though, was that the "GOOP" was causing more die-off and eradicating the rope biofilms/toxins/bad pathogens that had been STOPPING me from having bowel movements on my own! So, our friend sharing her GOOP recipe helped to speed up the healing process and continue to work on the ROOT of my issue!

Isn't it interesting how people come into our lives and the blessings that come out of it? Interesting AND amazing! Timing is everything. Surely God had this reunion of high school friends timed perfect!

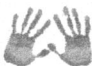

My mom taught me something important about relationships. She said, "Let relationships be like this..." as she held her arm out, her hand stretched out and turned up, fully opened. "Don't cling tightly to people, clenching them in your fist all to yourself. Share your friends with others. Don't hoard them. That way, not only you and your friend get blessed from the relationship, but other people will too."

Great advice and what a blessing it IS to share friends with others! Our friend Tiffany had not only indirectly helped in eradicating the deeply bunkered in RB toxins out of my body via the GOOP recipe shared with us, she'd also said something to me which stuck in the back of my mind for the next two years. But, in order to know what she said, we have to go back to where the discussion had taken place--in our garden on a warm, sunny day in late May during her first visit with us.

Much discussion had erupted the solitude of the garden as the three of us, Mom, Tiffany, and I walked the rows of produce growing around us. I'd just leaned down to pull a few weeds when Tiffany asked me, "Kel, have you thought about sharing your health story?"

I stood up, weeds in hand, as a gentle, curious, smile formed on my face. I responded saying, "Actually yes. I have this 'knowing' that I'm to share my story. I've even written a lot of it already but... I haven't done anything more than write and edit it. I'd like to share it in book style, but I just don't know..."

Tiffany smiled while listening to me and then said, "Have you ever thought about sharing it a blog?" Okay! If anyone knows me, especially the old version of me, technology and I are NOT on the same page. We're not in the same book. Ha! We are not in the same section of a library! I had (and maybe still have a little bit of) a real love-hate relationship with technology. My response in my head to her question was immediately, *"No way"*. Truth be told, I'd heard of blogging but didn't even know what it really was.

I told her I didn't really know what a "blog" was, hence she explained it to me. Our discussion went on, and in conclusion I told her, "Thank you for sharing. I really appreciate it. I will think and pray about this." I genuinely meant what I'd said. We shared a smile and then off we three went for a walk down an epic scenic lake lane--a graveled dead-end road surrounded by woods on both sides, running alongside the lake we live on.

Sharing my story via book style, at that time, was a process that devoted so much time, energy, and money that I had no real interest in partaking of. But blogging? This sounds like a good fit! I grabbed my computer and began researching about blogs not long after the discussion. Around that same time of my research on blogging, our mutual friend told my mom that her son had started a blog and had committed to writing every day for a full year. She encouraged Mom to check it out in an inviting way. Mom did check it out his blog and shared it with me as well. Truth be told, after sitting down and reading a good number of his blog posts, in my heart I knew this was the last little nudge that I needed to confirm sharing my story via blog was the right fit for me.

Two years later I found our friend's words STILL running in my head. I knew without a doubt in my mind that Papa God was telling me I needed to share my health journey with others to read in story form. Blogging was my next step then. And I did, with the help of another mutual friend of Mom's and mine, who'd helped me set it up online. She also helped me to build a website for my business, where my blog is now located.

Today, I want to take this opportunity to personally thank both our friend Tiffany, and her son, for encouraging me to share my story, each in their own way, directly or indirectly encouraging me. Sharing what you each have shared has stuck with me, whether you knew it or not. Thank you for your friendships, both of you!

As for a book version? Well, here it is! With Mom's help to transferring and editing my first 100-plus blogs onto her computer and sharing sections of it at a time with others to review, giving input, we now have the book version. And now I've come full circle in putting my story into a book! Wow! Didn't see that one coming!

92

Plan A, B, and...

Kelly

On June 6th, 2016 I picked up my cell phone. Dr. North was on the other end, calling me for our monthly appointment. As we talked about what's new, what's changed, etc., I told him about our friend's "GOOP" recipe and the effects it had on me.

"I'm detoxing these rope biofilms again with a vengeance, Dr. North! Due to this, I've had to increase to two enemas a day in order to keep up with the detoxification process. I know if I don't keep up with eradicating the toxins, I'll end up re-absorbing them and get even more ill." Reabsorbing toxins means the toxins go directly into the bloodstream, in turn, flowing throughout my body.

"I've never worked with anyone that has had this many rope biofilms coming out after this amount of time." Dr. North stated. "I've been working with you for eight months and they are still coming out, although they had stopped for a short while."

"I know that these RBs NEED to come out, but my question is the same as yours. 'How long are these ropes going to come out?' Obviously, there are still toxins in me." I GREATLY respected that Dr. North was always honest and open with me. At times, he challenged me and I'd learn, growing from that challenge. We talked more in depth and he asked direct questions about my current symptoms: bowel movements--which weren't happening without the help of a daily enema or two again, fatigue, sleep, hot sweats, and he asked about my overall energy and state of mind. I answered his questions truthfully and he put together a protocol that would hopefully help in the next months' time.

"If this protocol doesn't work as well as I hope it does, Kelly, I have a 'Plan B' in mind for next month." He informed me. "The protocol I'm going to have you do this month is a lot like one we've done before. However, it's my hope that we can get the same or even better results this time!"

"Sounds like a plan! Thank you." We discussed more of the protocol, then we scheduled the next month's appointment and said our good-byes.

JE June 9th, 2016

I bawled at breakfast this morning with Mom, due to utter frustration of feeling like this has all gone on forever. Mom said very little, which was a good thing. Guess I just needed a good cry! Tonight, as I write this, I still feel like I need to cry. I worked today and was glad that I only had a handful of clients. I felt really ill this afternoon. It was rough. Freezing cold, back and gut pain, and felt like I had to go to the bathroom (diarrhea) a number of times but was unable to. Felt like puking. Was weak and awoke only to see I was back to having a big limp when walking due to the pain. Did an enema when I got home and got MANY biofilms out. That helped, but still have back and gut pain after eating supper tonight. Very tired and sore in abdomen, back, hamstrings and upper neck and shoulders.

I continued taking the "GOOP" two times daily. The "GOOP" recipe from Tiffany was speeding up my healing process by eradicating the RBs, for which I was very thankful.

On June 17th, 2016, dark blue, translucent ropes and blobs of slime came out in my enema. This had happened a couple days prior, too. This day though, it was a deeper, darker blue! I felt MUCH better after that stuff got out of my body. I knew that the "GOOP" was what was working the toxic junk out, because I hadn't started Dr. North's new protocol since it hadn't arrived in the mail, but would soon. I continued to struggle keeping up with the fast detoxification process that left me tired and exhausted from the eliminations. I didn't know it at the time, but this was one of the final layers I needed to work through to get the nasty rope biofilms--bad pathogenic tumor, out of my body. Thank God for Tiffany, sharing the GOOP recipe with us!

JE June 17th, 2016

Dark clear blue rope biofilms with slime today. NASTY ones that I don't regularly get. It's almost done. Home stretch, Lord! YES! Lots of itchiness in abdomen and pancreas today. The itchiness is a healing itchiness. Thank You, Papa!

Only a few days after the dark blue tumorous RBs came out, I again had my first healthy, normal, BM in this latest new season! It only happened once, but I was grateful for it! It seemed that when I started to wonder, *Am I ever going to be done with this process and be able to go on my own?* that God answered my question in His own way, helping me to be encouraged and to keep me on the right track! Thanks be to God, and for our friend's GOOP recipe!

JE June 25th, 2016

Got a couple rope biofilms out that had a distinct red color to them. Epicenter? Are we getting there, Papa? Hope so! These RBs were NASTY! They were full and healthy-looking, toxic cancer, the tumor itself. Honestly, they did look to be the epicenter.

One thing I've not said, and you may have wondered about how I so clearly could see what I was eliminating in my enemas, is that when doing an enema and eliminating in the toilet bowl, we had a colander for only this specific use…to catch the elimination. Dr. Ann had taught Mom to do this back in the day when Mom was detoxing, in order to actually SEE what she was illuminating in her stools. I did the same, using the "special" colander—setting it inside the toilet bowl, to catch every elimination and actually see these nasty RB parasites. As bad as that may sound, I needed to see for myself WHAT was coming out of me. And as you've read, I did see what was coming out of me, clearly!

The RBs described just before were part of the cancerous pancreatic tumor. I was seeing these with my own eyes. To see what had been festered inside of me, growing and metastasizing, and then dying off so that I could pass it all out of me, was truly jaw-dropping. As gross as it sounds, all I could do was look at the specimens in serious wonder, and then find SOMETHING about this whole ordeal to be thankful about.

Plans. When I think of the word "plan", I look back on what I used to think when I heard that word, and then think about where I am today when I hear it. What do you think of the word's "plan" and "goal setting"? Do you get stressed-out in making plans, or doing everything it takes to meet a set plan? Do you experience a series of fails and successes in setting goals? Or, maybe you just forget having a plan and fly by the seat of your pants?

I used to be a BIG "follow a plan" type of person, and I'd made sure I'd stick to the plan no matter what, while growing up. I liked my routine and didn't want anything to come between me and my plans. I had a pretty narrow-minded view. If "plan A" didn't work, I'd go to "plan B". Rarely did I end up having to go to a "plan C".

These days I have plans, ideas, and goals. But I'm not EXPECTING plan A, B, C, or so forth to work itself out. I'm to the point in my life "it is what it is". I may have a general outlined plan, but I tend to overlook the idea of the "ideal plan that I HAVE to follow my outline". I mean, a great example is how Tiffany came into our lives and enhanced a speeding up of my health journey for the better! What if I didn't allow her "GOOP" recipe into my life? I don't have the answer to that question. The point is, it is really nice when our plans work out, like my plan to heal did. But I must admit, I've found that life can be even more wonderful when our plans are God's plans. God has got the best plans for us, and there are certainly times when we have no idea our plans will be altered for the better by others coming into (or going out of) our lives.

Dr. North had a "plan A" for me. But the thing was, "plan A" might not work how he or I had wanted it to. And guess what? "Plan A" ended up NOT working how we'd both wanted it to. Here's the thing though, Dr. North had a "plan B" in store for me. He'd said that on our phone consult. I, however, didn't know what "plan B" consisted of... and that was okay. Would I be willing to not get stuck in the fact that "plan A" didn't work out when it didn't? Would I be able to embrace "plan B', a change? Would I welcome going to "plan B"? Only time would tell.

Plans can be great. But plans can also be problematic when we become so captivated and set on them, expecting results coming from of our plans and goals. Can we lay aside our plans, allowing time to talk with other people we are rubbing shoulders with? Can we take the scenic route on the drive home instead of the same route we always take? Can we make time to respond to someone who is calling or texting us, or who'd taken time to write an email to us, or who dropped in--all so kindly taking time out of their day to contact us? These things aren't in our daily plans, but they are things that are important to do... bonding relationships, enhancing our journeys and paths in life, and rounding us to become better individuals.

I hope not to get set in my plans and miss learning to embrace whatever is in store for me, whether it be in a "plan C", a combination of "plan A" and "plan B", or using a general outline in daily life. I think I'd rather let the roller coaster of life fill in all the rest! Or better yet, let God have the drivers' seat and I'll enjoy the ride!

93

Fighting the Battles

Kelly

Time for a monthly phone consult with Dr. North! It was July 6th, 2016. Prior to our phone consult I had a feeling that our time working together was coming to an end.

As Dr. North and I talked, I told him how the month had gone--virtually no symptom changes within the last month, but I was still heavily detoxing. I was doing two enemas a day in order to keep up with the RB die-off. Symptoms included left-side abdominal pain, low-back pain, headaches, nausea and hot sweats at times. I was constipated; having the urge to have a BMs but unable to on my own. I was unable to pass gas for hours even though I felt the need, therefore being bloated. The die-off effects would only go away upon doing an enema to extract the toxins from my body. I was frustrated and thought that maybe it was time to say good-bye to Dr. North. *But who else is going to be able to help me?* I thought.

"One more month" went flying through my head. I smiled at the thought of Mom asking me to keep working with Dr. Ann not that long ago, saying, "Please Kelly, just one more month?", despite my frustration.

Dr. North was not pleased about how things had progressed within the past month. Nor was I. "Kelly, I think you need to start easing off the enemas. I know you probably don't want to hear this since that is your ONE form of relief. But the RBs shouldn't be coming out after this extended length of time. You are probably passing intestinal lining that looks like biofilm, but aren't actually rope biofilms." I was stunned at what he said. It felt like a slap in the face, although Dr. North would never mean it that way. My heart sank and I was ready to cry. My thought was, *does he think I don't know what I'm passing in my enemas?* I knew I was passing BOTH rope biofilms and some intestinal lining. The two are similar, but of noticeable difference. "Kelly, I really think you need to ease off the enemas. It's not going to be easy because your body is so used to them. It will be hard, so you will have to start slowly." He was trying to reassure and encourage me. My head was spinning... but I was listening. *If I eased up on the enemas but kept taking the "GOOP", that would give me a good indication of where my body was at?* I thought to myself.

"Okay. I will try easing off the enemas and see how my body functions on its own." I responded wearily. The phone consult continued and after he finished speaking, I asked him some questions. After helping me understand my questions more deeply, Dr. North was going to write up a new protocol for me to follow for the next month.

Dr. North then restated, "Kelly, hang in here. You are doing such a good job. You've made so much progress already!"

"Thank you, Dr. North."

After the consult, I went from doing two enemas a day, down to one the very next day and the following days after that. By mid-afternoon on the first day, my left side and back hurt. As days continued, I'd have a constant headache, sinus congestion, an extra tight abdomen, low back, and hip muscles too. After supper, the symptoms would heighten. I'd go to bed restless and uncomfortable, waking up in the wee hours of the morning sweating and with left-side pain. Sometimes it would burn deep inside, making it impossible to get comfortable. After 1-2 hours of being awake, I'd finally fade into a fitful sleep, only to wake in the morning feeling exhausted. Then, I'd do an enema, feeling much better until after breakfast, when the supplements and "GOOP" kicked in. Together those two protocols were killing bad pathogens, creating die-off effects.

I continued to struggle in the weeks that followed, making it up to a day and a half between enemas. The symptoms got worse as the time between enemas expanded. My throat was very sore and red in the back of my mouth. I started sneezing too. And again, I was awakened in the wee hours in the morning with

367

the FULL left-side burning pain that made sleep impossible until it would finally reduce—having smaller degrees of pain. Each time, this made me just want to go into the bathroom and do an enema to get relief. I knew this pain and the symptoms were due to more RBs dying-off. I just wanted a good night of sleep. Was that too much to ask for? *Trust me.* I was reminded.

"Okay Papa, I'm sorry. Help me. Give me strength, peace, and patience. You and I both know I can't do this alone. I need Your help, Papa God." I whispered weakly.

94

Prophetic Dreams

Kelly

In "Words – Visions – Dreams", I talked about prophetic words and visions I'd had, but nothing about dreams. This chapter, "Prophetic Dreams", coincides with "Words – Visions – Dreams". I'm not trying to prove anything, convince anyone to believe my experience or to believe what I believe. I'm just sharing what I believe to be true, things that happen in a wondrous way that I've personally experienced.

One night of rest in July 2016, during the first week of easing off doing enemas via Dr. North's instruction, I had a dream. I was specifically told in the dream to "STOP doing enemas". In the dream itself, I listened to what I was told and stopped doing enemas. All the symptoms came back with a roaring vengeance, which stemmed from the rope biofilm die-off effect. I became constipated due to not getting the toxic junk out of my system. I also started having sinus congestion, sneezing, and my throat was red and achy feeling. Headaches became a constant nuisance, along with low-back pain that was so intense it locked up my pelvis and abdominal region. I was unable to crack my back, which always brought relief to the low-back pain when I could crack it. The left side in my abdomen varied in degrees of pain and then the firey-hot burning sensation started. All of these symptoms were experienced in the dream. Woe.

When I vaguely woke, sweating, nauseated, and dizzy, I lay there going over the dream while feeling like puking or having to have a BM--neither of which were successful. *This dream... did it mean something?* My mind was a whirlwind of thoughts. Having fully awakened from the dream, I knew in my heart of hearts it held significant meaning. This dream was a depiction of what was currently happening, in real time. I was currently easing off the enemas and it was not going so well. Not well at all, actually. I knew my body needed to continue with multiple daily enemas because it had more RBs to eradicate. I wouldn't be well again UNTIL I eradicated them... ALL of them. Only then would my body properly be able to function by itself having BMs completely on my own.

In real time, Dr. North had told me to start easing OFF the enemas, and I did agree to it. Was he wrong in challenging me to ease off the enemas? No. It WAS actually a good thing he did, because I did need to see where my body was at in regard to being able to have my own BM functions, going normally on my own. Obviously, the timing wasn't right YET.

When is this going to be over, Papa? I murmured, crying out to my Papa God in the darkness of the night after the dream and these thoughts just shared. As I've said before, and I will say again, I knew in my heart that I would KNOW when I would be done with enemas. This inner knowing still held true, and now this dream re-affirmed it to me. After an all-out lengthy conversation with my Papa God, I drifted back into a restless sleep...

As I slept, I had another dream. I was in the process of doing an enema. I finished the enema, and glanced down looking what had come out of me. As I looked into the excretion, there was a very long rope biofilm. It was nearly 3-toxic-feet-long! As I looked at it in the dream, I knew right then and there this particular RB elimination process was truly over with, it would only be a very short time after that excretion that my body would be able to function on its own again. Then, after the eradication of the 3-foot-long RB, I'd have bowel movements on my own without assistance from an enema. Dreams can be prophetic at times, and I believed God was speaking to me through these dreams.

I awoke up from the second dream. Again, I lay in bed, my mind a whirlwind of thoughts. *Papa, are You showing me this as in meaning of what is to come?* And then a deep peace came to my heart about it. "THANK YOU! I trust You" I spoke into the darkness of the quiet night.

Would these two dreams play out to be exactly what was needed for the final elimination of cancer in my body? I didn't know for sure at the time, but what

I did know is that Papa God was in complete control. He was using not only these dreams, but other ones too, to prepare me for the future. When those happenings would come to fruition, to be exact, were details that didn't matter. Papa was preparing me and telling me, *Trust me, Kelly. Be patient. It's happening. Soon, Kelly. Soon.*

If you're wondering, will this 3-foot-long RB elimination come to fruition? Well, time will tell… but in the meantime, Papa God had me exactly where He wanted me. And let me say, He had really gotten my attention! My Papa God was doing a great cleansing work in and through me. I continued to do my part and trust Papa God with my life. My life was in His hands and He was blessing me in more ways than I could begin to imagine, or dream.

95

Listening, Being In-Tune

Kelly

I was on a healing journey to get rid of toxic junk inside of me. So, it should be of no surprise I had the last of my amalgam dental fillings removed in July 2016. When the process of replacing the fillings was done, my mouth felt smooth, clean, and more whole. It was healing, something I could feel inside happening.

While having the last three of my amalgam fillings removed, my atlas and axis went out of alignment in my neck at the cervical axis. I knew exactly when it happened and why it happened. My jaw had been clamped open for an hour-and-a-half. At the hour mark, my jaw all of a sudden got a sharp cramp. I was unable to move so I couldn't talk. However, the cramp only lasted a short, few seconds, so I didn't have to get their attention! Immediately upon the cramp, a shift was felt the right side of my neck, causing my atlas to move out of alignment. As always, when I'd go out of alignment, I acquired a headache going straight into my right eye from the backside of my head. And I thought, *Mental note. To-do list: Go to NUCCA chiropractor!*

I got in to see my chiropractor ASAP. When getting realigned, I get immediate relief. No more headaches or neck pain! Dr. Daniel to the rescue!

JE July 24th, 2016
I slept ALL night last night! Didn't even wake up once due to pain, feeling sick, or even just to go to the bathroom! Feels SO good! Thank you, Papa! Praying for continued gut healing, Lord. I TRUST You and Your perfect timing!

Listening and being in-tune with our bodies. I'm guessing the majority of us have heard people say throughout the years, "I don't feel any pain from that." Or, "I don't have any issues with food intolerance that I know of." And the highly acclaimed, "Oh, it's just old age. That's all." I'm not saying that I disagree with these statements, but I do have a question in regard to those and other remarks, said as quick responses that entail no reflection upon. And my question is: Are we each really listening and becoming more in-tune with ourselves physically, emotionally, mentally, and spiritually, or do we gravitate toward ignoring, having quick responses like these comments just stated because we aren't looking deeper into the WHY we are the way we are, asking ourselves why are we feeling this way? Or, asking ourselves what's the common connection to when I eat this specific food that I feel, think, or develop symptoms or specific emotions? Good questions for EACH of us to reflect on IF we are willing to, and want to become more in-tune with ourselves and our bodies.

Truthfully, this subject of listening and becoming more in-tune with ourselves, our bodies, is a BIG subject. I'm not going to take this subject in every direction, but just hit it at the core--the root. Why do we do the things we do? Why do we act and react in the ways that we do? Why do we eat the foods we eat? Why do we get stuck in the same emotional patterns? Why to do gravitate toward the same type of unhealthy relationships? Why do we eat foods that make us feel "good" for a quick high, but ultimately leave us grasping for more because the high lasts for only a short while? WHAT are the ROOT issues that can answer these questions? Are we willing to face into these questions, issues, our realities? The answers are something only we, each on our own, can answer for ourselves.

Listening, and being more in-tune with our bodies doesn't happen overnight. It's something we have to want, have to work at being diligent in asking ourselves questions, and becoming more aware of and actually thinking and asking ourselves, "WHY do I...?" and then WANT to change.

I described a time when I was at the dentist and literally felt my neck go out of alignment. Becoming in-tune with myself wasn't something that I just woke up with one day. It was a process. My entire healing journey was a process of listening to what my body was telling me. Being willing to face into ourselves and learn about ourselves, what works or doesn't work with us, what triggers and responses we have to those triggers, such as why I walk the way I do—my gate, etc., are all subtle or big things that help us in becoming more in-tune with ourselves when we pay attention, listen, and stay calm. We all have to start somewhere. Starting small is usually best.

If anyone knows me personally, you know that I'm big into "growing into a better version of myself". Reflecting on ourselves and looking into the WHY's of our choices and behaviors are important things to do IF we want to become a better version of ourselves, learning to understand ourselves better. In turn, when we learn to listen to what our body has to say, becoming more in-tune with ourselves, the benefits can be amazingly humbling. And the journey? Well, it may be interesting, full of more laughter, or maybe even tears at times. But is it worth it? You bet'cha!

I would imagine some of you reading here are already on the path to learning to listen and being more in-tune with yourself. And others may have not started, yet. There's no better time to start this process of listening to our body-talk, that I must say is life transforming. You are worthy, you are loved, and I believe that you can become an even better YOU.

96

Forerunner

Kelly
Our warm Minnesota summer was going by quickly. Summer was and still is my favorite time of the year! I love the warmth in the air, the intense sun's rays, seeing the lake, watching the water make waves from the wind and hearing those crash against the shoreline. I love to watch the beautiful wildlife that surrounds us, the magnificent sunsets, and doing a variety of outdoor activities, including vegetable gardening.

At this time on my healing journey, the summer of 2016 would be on its way out in a month, but for only being the beginning of August it was hot and humid. It would soon be time for another phone consult with Dr. North, too. I hadn't made the significant progress that he nor I had wanted, as talked about in "Plan A, B, and...", so I wasn't looking forward to the consult. I'd been back spending nearly two hours in the bathroom doing enemas every single day. *I just want to move on with my life,* I thought to myself. Again, I was reminded immediately, *"Patience, Kelly. Patience. Keep trusting Me. I'm making a way for you."*

"I know Papa. I'm sorry. I DO trust You. Give me the strength to endure this continuous battle, Papa. I can't do this without You. I'm ready to move forward in this healing process, but obviously it isn't time yet. Your timing is PERFECT and I know that." I prayed aloud, while tears trickled down my face. I was exhausted.

JE July 30th, 2016
Talking with Mom after supper tonight, she'd said, "You know, Kelly, you're

the forerunner of these rope biofilms." I had never REALLY thought of it that way, Papa. I now truly understand WHY I'm here dealing with this...and WHY it isn't over yet, Lord. It's because You are using and teaching me so that I will be able to be used by YOU to help other people. **Thank You, Papa, for these rope biofilms.** *I trust You, and all of what You have in store for me, my life, and my future. I am thankful!*

Up until the moments of Mom suggesting my being "a forerunner in this RB elimination", I WAS truly thankful to be detoxing these toxic biofilms, but I WASN'T TRULY thankful FOR having them. I was thankful for the journey and the process. But now, once she spoke this to me, I was truly thankful for something that, in most people's view, I had every reason to be ungrateful for. My now authentic "thankfulness for these RBs" helped me to appreciate something that I could have easily hated and held on to, holding bitterness and resentment about. I choose to embrace the seemingly horrific situation at this time, what I once thought was horrific, now understanding even further why I may be experiencing this. Ultimately, was yet another big step in the right direction, and more steps were coming in the next weeks!

97

What's in Store?

Kelly

August 3rd, 2016. My phone rang. Answering, I said, "Hi Dr. North."

"Hello Kelly. How have you been feeling this month? Tell me about any progress, changes, symptoms, or anything else I may need to know," he invited warmly.

"This month hasn't brought any new changes. I'd quit doing the COFFEE enemas as you suggested. Instead of coffee, however, I'm doing lemon juice enemas. I continue to expel rope biofilms...", and elaborated more on this with him. I'd been detoxing RBs for more than ten months at this point. I was so ready to be done with doing the enemas and expelling the RBs. *Why were they still coming out?* I voiced my thoughts. "I don't really understand how these biofilms can still be coming out. Don't get me wrong Dr. North, I've been sick for a very long time. But REALLY? These have been coming out for a good ten months now." I was ready to cry, but I really just wanted answers, direction, and reasons.

"Kelly, we need to be looking at you individually, versus by the other individuals I've worked with who've had these biofilms. We HAVE been working with you individually, but it is even more critical right now, as this is a 'special' case." He said warmly. "I still think it's the enemas that are causing the 'biofilm' issue. And, I also think these biofilms that you are seeing are actually intestinal lining, which is being sluffed-off via the enemas. I think you need to slowly ease off the enemas and start having the bowel movements on your own. I need to ask you, again, if you are you willing to try going off the enemas? I know that enemas are your one form of relief. It's not going to be easy. We'll have you do it subtly." Dr. North instructed wisely.

Deep in my heart I didn't agree with him. I knew that it was RBs that were causing my constipation. How did I know? They were the very first thing to come out in my enemas. These ropes were what was continually plugging me up. However, I so very much wanted to be done with the daily enemas too. I'd quit the "coffee" enemas already. I COULD do this. I was fighting within-- my mind, my heart, my whole being. *"God, help me."* I prayed inwardly. Taking a big breath, I said, "Okay, I'm willing to try this again, Dr. North."

We continued talking and soon the consult would come to a close. We scheduled my next month's consult and he wished me "...all the best, Kelly. Slow and steady easing off all enemas, like I've already told you. It won't be easy, but give your body time and it will happen."

"Okay. Thanks, Dr. North." I replied.

I was in turmoil, wanting to cry, being so angry I wanted to scream, or express a real impassioned emotion! I walked back into the house fighting the vast mix of emotions that wanted to surface. I had great respect for Dr. North, that he ASKED me if I "would be willing to go off the enemas." He challenged me and made me think outside the box. Dr. North and I were in this healing process together. We both knew that. He needed to make sure that I was willing to go off the enemas, otherwise we were both wasting our time and energy.

The thought of still having more RBs inside of me made me squirm, literally. I was not, and am not, the kind of person that wasn't going to finish something I started, nor was I going to do a job halfway. I hadn't quit so far in my "journey of healing", and I wasn't about to take the easy way out either. I was fully committed to complete healing.

"God, help me make sense of all of this. I don't know what to do. Should I ease off the enemas like Dr. North said, or should I wait until that day comes when the nearly 3-foot-long rope biofilm I'd seen in the dream comes out? I don't know what to do. Make it known to me, Papa. I trust You. Give me peace, strength, and patience." I talked to my Papa God like He was walking right with me. Because, in my reality, He was. He was always with me, through it all.

JE August 4th, 2016

I slept ALL night for the first time in many nights! I didn't wake up during my rest. Not once... not even to go to the bathroom! When I woke this morning, I just wanted to go back to sleep and do it all over again. I was still so exhausted; tired and sore upon awakening. Healing is happening! Help me Lord, please.

I did a lot of thinking the next few days as I continued doing two enemas a day. What would I end up doing? Knowing what to expect--being "plugged-up," is not anything I was looking forward to. Ugh!

On August 15th, 2016, I had an appointment with both of the craniosacral massage therapists, Cathy and Donna. I gave them the latest news of my gut healing process while I lay on the massage table while they worked. They asked questions, and listened to my responses. Cathy reached down and lightly held my right foot with one hand, and my right hip with her other hand. Soon, she was at my feet, holding one foot in each hand. She touched a specific area in my right foot. "How does that spot feel, Kelly?"

"It hurts!" I laughed.

Cathy smiled, saying, "This spot is your right shoulder in 'reflexology' terms, Kelly." I had a 2-hour appointment. It took the full two hours for the two of them to get my body to unlock from the continued trauma it had endured. The muscles had been compensating so much while being sick that it was a continuous process to unlock them at deeper levels. Both therapists were able to reposition my sacrum back to where it was supposed to be sitting. They were also able to unlock my right shoulder, getting my range of motion back. I could feel the healing effects of their work as muscles loosened and bones gently shifted back to where they were supposed to be.

As the two worked, my gut constantly made noise. It hadn't done that for a long time. *Hmm,* I thought to myself, but didn't dwell on it. (Later, though, I

379

reflected back on the appointment, realizing that as my sacrum was put back in alignment, my organs could have also been adjusting to the shift.)

Near the end of the 2-hour session, both Cathy and Donna did some deep stretches with my body that completely unlocked my pelvis and right shoulder. It was then that I'd gotten total relief. *Amen!* "The fascia ALL over your body was flaming hot, Kelly. The fascia was heated due to the impact of trauma, causing the lock-up, tension, tightening of the muscles, and shifting of the bones." Cathy said.

"I can understand how that would happen," I replied, knowingly. I got up from the table, slowly letting my feet dangle before they touched the floor. *Wow, that was exactly what I needed*, I thought to myself while taking a few more moments before standing. I then got up and walked out into the office to pay for the appointment.

As I walked out of the building, I could stand straight and elongated again, without feeling the need to lean on my right hip to stand comfortably due to the left-side pain that would cause the leaning. I didn't limp at all. Nor did I have the desire to protect my abdomen! It'd been a while since I could stand straight without any pain. The low-back pain was nearly gone now, except for a very faint achiness. My right shoulder and hip were both very sore from the craniosacral massage therapy, but it was a healing kind of soreness. In a couple days, my body would be feeling well, having gotten everything worked out, and I would feel amazing again. Little did I know there was more "amazing" results in store for me!

The day following my craniosacral massage appointment I had a BM all on my own! What a pleasant surprise!

JE August 16th, 2016
While working on my first client at work today, I started to feel very ill. I felt awful, to put it mildly. I got hot and cold sweats, a headache and gut ache, feeling like my stomach was going to burst, as if I was going to have an explosive BM, and over-all just feeling terrible. After I checked my client out, she left my office and I got myself to the bathroom. Diarrhea came out. YES! I

380

had IMMEDIATE relief and virtually ALL symptoms disappeared! I was then feeling good until the late afternoon, when I felt the need to have a BM again but was unable to. I'd gone into the bathroom, tried pushing, when all of a sudden, my abdomen hurt (like a cramp) but it was deep inside and taking my breath away. I couldn't breathe. The cramp wouldn't let go. I grabbed my abdomen in an attempt to make it stop. I switched my posture. Neither attempt worked. The bathroom was getting a little darker in my vision and I still couldn't breathe. My vision started to fade so I tried standing up. The thought had already raced through my mind, "Where's your phone, Kelly?"

My phone was on my office desk, in an entirely different room. There was no way of getting help. I grabbed the vanity counter, and leaning I crouched into it, doubled-over at this point. The room was very dark. And then, when it seemed as though I was going to fade, the grabbing sensation in my gut slowly eased off. Mom wasn't in the office, so literally no one was here if I would have passed out... uffda. Since then, my abdomen has been VERY tight. Lord, was this the nearly 3-foot-long RB detaching itself? Or, maybe it is the prelude to the big one detaching itself? The enema I did tonight once I got home brought relief, but I feel something is happening. A shift. I feel it, Papa. We are so close. We're closing in Papa God. Homestretch!

98

Prophetic Knowing
Becomes Reality

Kelly

JE August 17th, 2016

I had two bowel movements on my own today! Thank You for these bowel movements, Lord. I am so thankful!

I'd had a significant change since I had gotten the craniosacral massage; the enemas were easier on my body, not having to work as hard to detoxify. I was so very thankful for the bowel movements I had on my own in just two days. I had high hopes they would continue. Bowel movements came more easily, as if on their own again. Unfortunately, though, that didn't last.

JE August 21st, 2016

Tonight's enema brought out very "healthy-looking" rope biofilms. They were dark red with white edges on them and in them. They actually looked like lines on agate rocks, although these were in biofilm form. After they came out, I still felt like I needed to go more. I sat back down and out came a big blob that had a dark red spot in it. Am I now to the epicenter, Papa? I FEEL closer to "the end" of it, Papa. Is this it? Soon?

As I wrote in the journal entry that night, August 21st, my Papa God literally and truly had answered my questions. The enema expelled what WAS the very last of the tumor. Just five days before, when I'd had such gut pain that I'd almost passed out due to the grabbing sensation so deep inside of me, that WAS the epicenter of the tumor, the RBs, detaching and then "dying-off". The die off DID bring out the tumorous epicenter. And yes, it was a 3-foot-long rope biofilm, that I was foretold about in a dream. How do I know? We measured it because both my mom and I needed to see this as factual evidence. The RB epicenter had finally worked its way through my digestive system as the days passed since the grabbing sensation, just like in all other episodes of toxic pathogenic die-off, so that I was able to expel the epicenter of the tumor. It was going to be only a matter of time, soon to come, for my digestive tract to fully and fluently start working on its own again!

At that point in time, I was still doing my daily enema routine. I wasn't "at ease" as I usually was while doing my daily routine, however. I was starting to feel a noticeable shift. I listened, tuning-in to what my body was telling me.

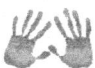

August 24th, 2016. I cut back from doing two, to doing only one enema a day. It wasn't easy. My lower abdomen became hard and uncomfortable. As a day progressed to evening, my entire abdomen would begin to hurt. Still, I wouldn't give in to doing an extra enema. I wanted, and needed, to see if my body could have a bowel movement on its own, just like Dr. North had recommended.

In the course of the last many weeks, I was having only a few RBs staggered here and there, and then the biggest portions of the tumor had been eliminated. Besides those big RBs, the epicenter of the tumor, it was mostly all intestinal lining coming out during the enemas now. Dr. North was right about shedding intestinal lining—it was now happening.

The same time that I had cut back to one enema/day, I'd decided to go off of all my supplements. I'd been getting a lot more gut and abdominal pain when taking the supplements. I thought this pain was due to my body reacting to the supplements. *Maybe it is time that I don't need to be taking these supplements anymore?* I thought to myself. I voiced my thoughts to Mom, telling her, "I'm thinking about going off of my supplements for a week and see how my body likes this change, or reacts to this change." Mom also thought this was a good idea. "I feel like the supplements aren't helping; like they are actually hindering the healing process more than helping right now, Mom," I'd said.

"You know your body best, Kelly. There is a difference between a helpful, healing hurt, and a hindering hurt. I think it's a good idea to try going off of all your supplements for a week. It will give you a good indication of the state of your gut health and how it's working on its own," she replied.

"I guess this would be the ideal timing, too, as I have a phone consult with Dr. North next week. I'd be able to hear what his advice is from that point," I thoughtfully commented.

"Go for it," Mom reassured me, smiling!

I didn't take any of Dr. North's supplements that day and I felt a lot better. Immensely better. In the next couple days, I was having a lot less symptoms and pain. I was still unable to have any bowel movements on my own, so I continued doing one enema a day, noticing that there was even less intestinal lining and only a few random RBs coming out.

As the week of taking no supplements ended, I had NO rope biofilms in my stools! At that same time, I woke up one morning and noticed another "shift". I'd just woke up and immediately felt the difference. I didn't say a word to anyone at the time, as I couldn't put my finger on what that shift--a noticeable difference, was. All I knew was that a healing shift had taken place! I also remembered saying aloud, "I thought I'd wake up one day and something would be different."

Was this heartfelt knowing I had real? Really happening, becoming reality just as the 3-foot-long rope biofilm had become reality? I thought. *Hmm?*

99

Dreams Become Reality

Kelly

I realize that writing my health journey for anyone to read can be interesting, but also weird in my sharing, especially about bowel movements and toxic pathogens coming out of me. However, bowel movements are important. If they weren't, then it would not be necessary for patients in hospitals to not be allowed to go home if they cannot have a bowel movement. During my journey of illness, normal bowel movements had become non-existent. Getting them back took a lot of time and patience, as one can see from my health journey story.

The morning of August 31st, 2016, I had my first NORMAL bowel movement all on my own! I had a feeling that I shouldn't do an enema that morning to see if I could go on my own. Mom confirmed my thoughts when I'd voiced them to her. Having a formed "normal" bowel movement was UNREAL! I couldn't remember the last time it was really "normal" LOOKING. I was SO excited! I was to have a phone consult with Dr. North later that morning. I was excited to tell him of the morning's event!

Later, my phone rang. Mom sat nearby as I put the phone on speaker. She had wanted to ask Dr. North a couple questions. "Hello Dr. North." I greeted him warmly.

"Hello, Kelly. I hope things have been going well this month." He inquired.

"My mom is sitting here. She wants to sit in on the consult, if you don't mind," I asked?

"Yes, that is perfectly fine. Hello, Amy!" Dr. North greeted Mom warmly.

I gave him an update about the progress I'd made over the past month, then said, "I still haven't done any coffee enemas! I've been doing lemon juice enemas. However, it wasn't until a week ago that I went down to one enema a day. I was still unable to go on my own until today!! I had my first normal bowel movement this morning without enemas, all on my own! I still feel like I need to go." I truthfully stated.

"Kelly! This is GREAT news" Dr. North exclaimed with pure joy in his voice!

"Yes, it is! Also, I need to tell you that when I went down to just the one enema a day, I discontinued taking all of my supplements. I was beginning to feel like they weren't helping me. Instead, they made me feel worse in a "not so good" kind of way. Upon discontinuing the supplements, my symptoms have improved and I feel better as a whole." I shared.

"I see no problem that you discontinued the supplements if you feel that your body is not getting the needed help from them. You can take a supplement here or there if you feel like your body needs it." He stated wisely.

I smiled, knowingly, at Mom. I'd already came to that conclusion before we'd started the phone consult! *You yourself are your own best doctor,* went flying through my head. I grinned at the thought. "Sounds good, Dr. North." I replied, smiling.

"Tell me the symptoms you currently have, Kelly." He requested.

"The symptoms only come when I need to have a bowel movement and am unable to actually have one. Then, I get bloated and have headaches. In addition, I get low-back pain. Sometimes there's a little left-side pain in the abdomen too. That left-side pain is usually very minimal. Other than that, that's about it for symptoms." I shared. As I finished speaking, the weight of my words hit me. *Wow!* I thought. *That's NOTHING if I had to compare them to the symptoms I 'd had a year ago, let alone a few months ago.* I looked out at the glistening water rippling on the lake, swallowing the lump that had formed in my throat.

"Dr. North, is it okay if I ask you a question?" Mom inquired.

"Why sure, go right ahead." He invited warmly.

Mom then gave him a very brief summary of when she and I were doing the on-line gut healing program together last spring, and how beneficial it was as part of my healing process. She shared a few more thoughts and commented about the Comprehensive Stool Analysis Test (CSAT) I'd done the previous fall, which had brought awareness to and confirmed the pancreatic cancer, candida overgrowth, the gut bacteria imbalances, and other important, valuable pieces of information. After, she asked, "Do you think Kelly could do that same CSAT again, in order to see what is going on inside of her gut now? I think it would help to provide information regarding her current health and if there are improvements that need to be made yet," Mom questioned, knowingly.

"Amy, you've brought up a very good point! I agree. I think a Comprehensive Stool Analysis Test is a VERY good idea. You're right, this test will give a lot of knowledge as to what is going on. I, too, think this would give a very helpful insight to see where Kelly's pancreas health is at. I'll send out the test." He stated.

"That would be great!" Mom and I both commented at the same time. We looked at each other, smiling at our choice of words. *The nut didn't fall from the tree,* I thought.

"Kelly, this month I'm not going to have you take any new supplements. Do as I told you earlier, take a supplement if you feel the need to. I also want to encourage you to continue to ease off the enemas so that you are doing only a couple each week. Eventually, I want you to be able to have bowel movements daily completely on your own without the help of an enema. I recommend that you don't do an enema today and wait it out, seeing if you can go on your own tonight or tomorrow." Dr. North encouraged me.

"Okay! Sounds good. Thank you," I said with a smile on my face. I looked out at the glistening lake again as the conversation continued, then we set up my next phone consult and said our good-byes.

Mom and I talked about some details of the phone consult afterwards. "Kelly, I would like to reaffirm, you should really try to wait until tomorrow to do an enema," Mom said. "You might not go number-two again today, but maybe tomorrow morning you'll be able to." She offered thoughtfully.

"Yes. I agree. I need to deal with symptoms today and find out if my body can continue with bowel movements on its own. Thank you, Mom. I love you!" We embraced in a hug and I kissed her on her cheek saying, "I'm so glad you were a part of the phone consult today!"

Later that same day I had a small bowel movement! Two times in one day! I was ecstatic! As I went to bed that night, I felt bloated… like I needed to have another BM. I massaged my abdomen as I always did before falling asleep, then I turned out the light. I slept pretty well.

Immediately upon awakening the next morning, I massaged my abdomen before getting out of bed. I still felt bloated, just like when I'd gone to bed. Not long after the abdominal massage, I felt the need to have a bowel movement. I got out of bed, unsure of what would happen, just as I did most mornings without results. I walked into the bathroom with an open mind, not thinking about *making* myself have a bowel movement. Surprise! I had a normal, healthy, bowel movement! "I did it," I laughed happily! I had a couple more bowel movements the same day! Needless to say, I didn't do an enema that day! The only symptoms I was having were bloating, some gas, and headaches; all of which were when I needed to actually have a BM.

Those subtle shifts that I'd been feeling lately had really been happening. I was healing! And the dream I'd had about waking up one day and feeling a shift, and then shorty after having BMs on my own? Well, that dream was now a reality too!

The next day, the Friday of Labor Day weekend, I had more bowel movements. I actually lost track of how many bowel movements I had that day! *It's REALLY happening,* I thought to myself, feeling utterly thank-ful. The dreams are truly becoming my reality! *THANK YOU, Papa!*

100

Gifts of Pain

Kelly
The end of August 2016 marked the start of year number six of my journey towards healing. The days of August brought a lot of memories that I reflected on at this time, days of this long, healing journey. At times, my heart was so overcome with thankfulness that tears of joy pooled in my eyes and ran down my face. Remembering all of those days that were so hard, yet, here I was! All the healing that had happened, was happening, was overwhelming to think about without having an emotional response!

"Thank you, Lord, from the bottom of my heart. I trust You, Papa. I love You! Please continue to heal me and use me for Your glory and honor. My life is in Your hands and always has been." I spoke softly to Papa God.

JE September 2nd, 2016
I am all better! I feel it! I believe it! And, I KNOW IT!!! Papa, thank You! MY heart, my whole being is full of pure joy, love, and thankfulness. Utter thankfulness! Feeling blessed beyond measure. And, I know that the healing will only continue!

Dad had asked me at supper, "How do you want to celebrate your healing you've had going on lately?" The family joked, forming and voicing their thoughts as to how I would respond while I ate my supper. As I was chewing and absorbing the meal, I listened to them chatter, marveling at the playfulness that flowed between them, how the atmosphere was so uplifting and fresh.
Tonight, I played cards, the game "500", with my parents and brother. I truly don't like playing that game anymore, but I agreed without hesitation to play as a way to celebrate. Doing something you don't like as a way of celebrating sure sounds backwards, but it's really not. It's a form of love, a willingness to

do something others will enjoy, a way to diversify and not stay stuck in my own ways. Thank you, Papa God, for answering prayers and doing so in YOUR perfect timing. Thank You for never leaving me or forsaking me.

My heart was joyful and at peace, knowing what we'd accomplished in the last six years. Yes, it was WE... me doing the bulk of the work, but all the health professionals that had helped in their own unique ways, my mom, my family, and my small tribe of people. It was such a rewarding feeling in my heart to know that I'd overcome pancreatic cancer and reversed other gut issues. As well.

I had to do my CSAT yet to see if the results were going to show my "heart's knowing" of being all well. Time would tell... and with that, I would soon start sharing my health story, and good news with other friends and relatives as the days continued, to those whom didn't know what I'd been going through these past six years.

Throughout my health journey thus far, I'd learned a lot about myself physically, mentally, emotionally, and spiritually--the four aspects of a whole human being. If I wanted to be healthy and well, I needed to address each area for healing to happen. This wasn't just a "one time" addressing of any one of the four areas. Sometimes it was a process, like layers of an onion, as I've stated before. The pain inflicted in our lives, in all of these four areas, impact us whether we know it or not.

When I think of pain, the first things that come to mind are: comparison, gnarly, trauma, a chance to overcome, forgiveness, darkness vs. light, and character growth opportunities. Maybe these words throw some people for a loop, and maybe they don't. What words come to your mind when you think about pain? Bully? Mean words? Abuse? Physical pain? Anger? Bitterness? Everyone's pain, their view of pain, and the way they handle pain, are different. I'm not going to say the way you or I handle pain is right or wrong, but I will say that I've learned a great deal from pain, not just from the course of where I'm at in my health journey, but in my entire life journey. I'd like to share some of the gifts of pain has brought to my life.

Wisdom. In complete vulnerability, and humbleness, I can truly say that some wisdom has been gained. I have a deep respect for pain in whatever of the four aspects it takes place: physical, emotional, mental, and spiritual. During my seven years of dis-ease to ease in health, wisdom was gained through firsthand experiences with a lot of pain. It wasn't easy, as you've read. Most of the time it was difficult. But I learned to embrace the pain as best I could, rather than become angry and bitter. I wanted to become a better person, a better version of myself, a healthier person, a more loving individual, and I wanted to understand how to better embrace life's continuous roller coaster that will always be a part of our lives. Pain IS painful, but that doesn't mean it has to define you, me, or the next person. We each have the choice to choose how pain affects us.

I've been told that painful experiences may help to handle pain in other circumstances not only in my life but in other's lives too. I've found this to be true. Having gained some wisdom from painful life experiences can be beneficial in helping others on their journey as well, in difficult times.

Expanded tolerance to and compassion for others. I'm a "Massage Therapist". I'm not lying when I say I have a big heart and LOVE for people. My compassion for others is sometimes earth shaking, as some have said. But my compassion isn't just in my job (which yes, I'm very passionate about my work, having compassion for people in pain), it's in all of daily life.

I used to be an introvert, as I've talked about on this journey. Long story short, I've changed from the person I once was. I've grown to have a respect and expanded tolerance for all people, no matter where we stand in a conversation about our beliefs, our life views, etc. I was NOT always like this. It used to be if it wasn't my way in my much younger years, then you can certainly hit the highway. And if you didn't want to, well, I was done with the conversation and the atmosphere was thick with tension. I'm guessing you probably know what I'm talking about as you've lived your life with other people. As I have changed, no matter our difference of beliefs, I now choose to tolerate and respect others. My compassion for others has also grown, probably ten-fold to be honest. It's a process, one that is seemingly never ending.

Self-Love. This is something that I've always had. In my younger years I was the odd person out. Oops, I guess I still am! I stayed true to who I was as an individual, staying true to my beliefs. I wasn't one to "go along to get along". That just wasn't who I was. However, this being said, I've also matured in the sense that self-love is more than what my narrow-minded beliefs were, to in my later years really stepping back and looking at myself and my life from outside the box, asking myself why do I do what I do? Is this really helping me?

Selflove isn't just about taking care of our bodies, such as exercise and feeding and fueling our bodies right. It's also about thinking right--positively, but yet realistically and responsibly, and taking time for self. Yes, I need to take care of me because I can't expect anyone else to take care of me or know me better than I know myself and what I need. Selflove isn't JUST a few aspects, it's a lot more! With time, practice, and maturing, selflove can grow, blossoming us to be more the person we were meant to be and become.

Claiming my power and living in my time essence. Okay, I actually don't like the word "power". In many peoples' eyes, power gets perceived as "more powerful" or "reigning over", or to put it bluntly, "I'm more powerful than you". I'm not a fan of any of those. My thinking about power is, "our power is our essence". Our power is the person that we are, the person we are becoming. This power is powerful, but NOT more powerful than any other person's power. We are ALL equal. No one is better than another. When we are living in the beautiful essence of the uniquely beautiful person THAT we are, then THAT IS our power. The way that we share our power is by sharing our lives with others. It's by living our lives in our own awestruck beauty, in our own skin, that we are being vulnerable with others in sharing who we are.

Our time here on earth is precious. We don't know the number of days that we have. Our lives, our time here, is ours to claim. Claiming it doesn't have to be big and bold. Claiming our power can be quiet and sweet. But by claiming it, we are living for such a time as this, to live our lives in our own essence. Our lives are continually changing. That means our essence is continually changing. Staying true to ourselves and embracing that power IS our power.

Wisdom, expanded tolerance to and compassion for others, self-love, and claiming my power, living in my time essence…these are all gifts I gained from pain that have helped change me to become more of the person I was meant to be. I am thankful for these gifts pain has bestowed on me.

101

Set Free

Kelly

The gifts of pain are numerous, truly. As I've stated, pain can happen in four aspects of our life: physically, emotionally, mentally, or spiritually. Also, as I've stated before pain is stored in our bodies: our muscles, our hearts, and our entire being, whether we are aware of it or not. Let me share an example.

It was nearly two years ago when I had a craniosacral massage appointment with the two therapists, Cathy and Donna. During that particular appointment, the therapists found trauma deeply stuck within my body, in my muscles and in my core being, all of which were unknown to me. Different areas of my body were indicating to them that there was "stored trauma". They asked what traumatic things had happened to me in my life. I shared about the time I physically went down hard on ice-packed snow, really fast, while alpine ski racing… and also shared another similar incident. Besides those, I was pretty "clueless". As they worked, they asked specific questions about my history, and I answered as best I could. And then they asked about my heritage. *My heritage?* I thought, *I wonder what they want to know?* They asked what nationality I was. I'd answered, "Jewish, and German, mostly." One therapist nodded her head up and down and said, "That's it. That's what this is, deeply embedded in your being, in your muscles. You have ancestral trauma stuck inside of you."

As I lay on the table, my mind was blown wide open. *What?* I thought. This was a trauma of wars involving hatred, antisemitism, evils being done against specific races of humanity, leaving the casualties of these crimes against humanity full of bitterness and unforgiveness EVEN through the generations

393

of unhealed people. "What do you know about the Jewish bloodline in you?" One of the therapists inquired. I answered the best I could. But honestly, I didn't know much about the history other than my dad had found out about his being Jewish when he was about 27 years old. Prior to that, my dad hadn't known his Jewish ancestry. It was a secret that was finally brought into the open shortly after he and my mom were married. Nothing else had ever been said to him about it before in his whole life.

With the help of the craniosacral therapists, through prayer and our combined efforts, we were able to pull out the ancestral trauma that was stuck inside of me, stemming from BOTH nationalities—German and Jewish. The Jews experienced rejection, betrayal, and terrible crimes against humanity. The bloodline carried thousands of years of wars, tribulations, and continuous persecutions. My mind was ALMOST blown away. How were they able to find this inside of ME? I mean, it wasn't written in plain writing to see. But, as I learned, it WAS written within my DNA.

God brings people into our lives for reasons. Thankfully, both of the craniosacral therapists were able to take all of this ugly history and extract it out of me, with each of their combined efforts and my willingness to let it go out of me as well. As I got off the table that day, something in me was lighter… I'd been set free. The ancestral bondage, the chains, were being taken away, setting me free at a whole new level.

This example of chains "as bondage", a depiction of a history of ancestral pain and trauma, really CAN continue through the blood of generations in humans. The bondage hadn't been addressed in past generations, but it now had with me, and the roots had been cut with an axe to the root, with the work done in our craniosacral therapy session that day. Our bloodlines do carry a lot of much information! This small-framed, olive-skinned, brown-eyed girl, with natural red highlights in her curly brown hair, are actually all Jewish embedded features in my DNA. Ha, I even got the nickname--with NO disrespect or pun intended, as I do NOT like racial jokes, "The little Jew" in our household. It was a nickname that I loved and embraced because the meaning behind it wasn't just my lineage, it was because I was cautious with money, a suggested Jewish trait, and of course I look the nationality. The nickname really does fit still to this day.

Through the years, I've wondered about our family history. I utilized google searches and ancestral resources to find out what I could. With all my efforts, I hadn't come up with much. I finally came to the point where I had to accept the reality that I may never know more about my Jewish family history. I needed to face this reality, accepting it.

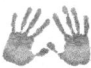

Fast Forward: During the year of 2019--which is well forward in my health journey story here, while working with Dr. North to tweak some VERY minor health maintenance issues and to get me on a more specific maintenance supplement plan, he suggested I have an ancestry test done. Why? In doing so, we could utilize the raw data to know what supplements are ones that my body is more apt to be in need of. *Cool! I've always been intrigued with these tests but had never done one!* I thought. So, I agreed to do an ancestry test.

The test arrived and I spit in the provided test tube, boxed up my bottled saliva, and whoosh, out in the mail it went. What I didn't realize in fullness at the time of doing this test was that I might get REAL answers to my ancestor's origins, some real family history. After nearly three weeks the results landed in my email inbox. I opened the mail while on vacation in Key West, FL that late winter, and was speechless. My history. My origins. Insights into our Jewish family heritage. All of this was in front of me and more. Tears pooled in my eyes as my heart raced with excitement.

I learned a lot from those results. Did those results tell me everything I wanted to know? Of course not, but I got a broad picture and was able to connect some dots, making some sense of things I had wondered about, and I better understand my heritage. Also, some aspects of myself that stemmed from my heritage were confirmed. I was seeing my GENETIC lineage!

I believe it's good to know our family history and health history. All those genes, DNA, going through the generations actually DO hold valuable information. In my opinion, that doesn't mean we are going to have those same genetic issues or that those genetics define us, so that we can't reverse them… because we CAN reverse some of our genetic dysfunctions! It IS possible! Do an internet search on "epigenetics" to learn more about how environments and nutrients play a huge role in who we become concerning our DNA.

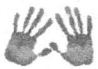

In general, I think we as human beings aren't aware of historical pain or trauma, or other "holdings" we have inside of us, whether it be in our muscles, heart, mind, gut, or being, unless someone brings it to our attention. At least that was my experience. Pain and trauma are unique to each human being, and needs to be addressed in its own unique way--on the surface level, and those deeper levels we may not even be aware of, not being exposed until the timing is right, then they come to the surface, like layers of an onion being peeled away. And that is what I've learned through layer after layer being peeled away in my healing journey, it's a process. Which, ultimately, has led me to truly believing after so many years that the journey IS truly the reward. So, enjoying the process of life, the pain it brings and embracing it as best we can, is an "important" part to our daily lives and the healing process.

Pain isn't always visible physically, or always understandable in our self-knowledge, like the pain carried in my body from history wasn't visible or even noticeable to me. It was inside of me as the craniosacral therapists had found it. It was truly unknown to me before this. Despite knowing of my heritage--family lineage, I had questions that I would have liked answers to, but I'd already grown up to a level where I accepted the reality of the situation of my not ever knowing my history at all. Was that the reason this "miracle" happened, why I got to learn some of my genetic history just recently? I don't know. I don't have all the answers, and I don't need to have all the answers. All I know for sure is that this all was revealed when the timing was right. As I always say, "In Papa God's perfect timing."

102

A Weekend to Remember

Kelly

On Labor Day weekend, 2016, Tiffany (who'd shared her "GOOP" recipe with us which aided in quickening the last of my heavy detoxification process-- unknown by us it would have that effect) and her husband were coming to spend the weekend with our family. We were looking forward to their visit!

Our family friends arrived on Saturday and were welcomed warmly. The day was filled with laughter, conversations, games, peace, and leisurely walks. After a late breakfast on Sunday, Tiffany and Junior, her husband, and I drove to town where my business is located. On the drive, Tiffany asked. "Kelly, how have you been feeling lately? I know last time I saw your mom and brother you weren't doing too well."

I glanced at her and then looked back at the road with a smile on my face. I took a breath before I answered. The emotion of the last few healing days was still so fresh. I swallowed then stated, "It's over. It's truly over." I felt a lump form in my throat. She glanced sideways at me, obviously trying to decipher what I'd just said. "It's really over," I restated, swallowing hard "I'm doing REALLY well. I feel the best I've ever felt in my entire life. In the last few days so much has changed, shifts for the better." I paused, looking at her.

Behind sunglasses, while focusing on her driving, she was trying to process the depth of what I had just shared. Junior sat in the back seat quietly listening. "In the last few days, I've started to have bowel movements completely on my own. I haven't done an enema since Wednesday. I have virtually no symptoms or any pain. My energy has greatly improved. Overall, I feel healthy and well! I talked to Dr. North on Wednesday. We are going to do a new CSAT and then we will see from the test results how my pancreas is functioning. It's the same test that I'd done last fall that detected the pancreatic cancer, the bacteria imbalances, yada, yada, yada. But, based on how I feel, I already know the results will come back good for my pancreas! The cancer is gone. I KNOW that. However, it will still be good to SEE the results on paper." I excitedly said! Deep in the inner most part of my heart, I knew it to be true, that the worst was over, the cancer was GONE. Continued healing was to happen, but I was over the worst of it.

"When you said, 'It's over. It's truly over', Kelly, I had to look at you to see exactly what you meant by that statement. Wow!" She exclaimed. Then paused before saying, "You've been at this such a long time. Many years. For someone your age to do this and stay that dedicated says a lot," she spoke openly. "So, what are you going to do now that you're healthy and have more free time" she inquired?

I chuckled as she asked a loaded question. "Well, I've had a dream, or a goal, for many years," I started to explain with a smile still plastered on my face! "For years I've dreamed of having a wellness center..." and I continued to share my heart.

Before that day in their car, I hadn't verbally told anyone my good news except for Mom, Dad, and Troy. It had only been a couple days since this big shift. Mom had shared the good news with her mom, "Grandma" to me, and another elderly woman who is very close to our family and lives close to my business in Ortonville, the elderly woman who would bring me flowers at work and check-in on me during my worst-of-worst years of illness. I shared with Hallie via a text message. But to speak the words out loud, "It's over. It's truly over. I'm doing really well!", that took on a whole new depth of conquering what many believe is the unconquerable. Talking and sharing with the couple in their car that Labor Day Sunday seemed natural... it felt so good.

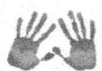

The thing was, and what I didn't see in fullness at that time of talking in Tiffany's car while driving to town, is I was already in the process of my dream, having a wellness center at my current business. Massage therapy, and the additional services that have been added since the initial grand opening in June of 2013, have broadened our wellness center, being diversified for various healing. It's interesting, looking back, that I didn't quite see this in fullness, that the wellness center was already in process and would take time for it to grow and diversify further.

Having a wellness center was actually a dream or goal that I'd had since starting my training at massage therapy school in 2012, and I was so very blessed to be able to follow my dreams with the help of my family, especially my parents, who helped it become a reality.

Today, I'm still so VERY humbled and thankful to be doing something that I absolutely love and am passionate about. It's such a blessing to be able to walk alongside of people on their health journey.

JE September 5th, 2016
I told Mom tonight, "This was the best weekend I've had in well over a year." It's the honest truth, regarding my health. This weekend was the first weekend that I've gotten to live, laugh, and love freely for days without pain or symptoms. I felt awesome ALL weekend and didn't get sick from different (healthy, organic) foods I wouldn't normally eat, or eat such a variety of in a short period of time. I ate grilled steak--grass-fed beef with no added hormones. I haven't had "grilled" meat in years! Absolutely NO symptoms! It's been a JOY getting to spend this treasured weekend with people I love. Papa God, You are so very special. And Your timing is so perfect! What a blessing.

It was absolutely marvelous to spend my first weekend, in YEARS, symptom free! To this very day, now years later in sharing my health story, it's hard to even express in fullness the reality of feeling well and healthy. In those years of being ill, having company wasn't something that happened very often, due to never knowing how I would be feeling physically.

Labor Day weekend 2016 was different. It was special because my health had turned around for the better. I remember a few times throughout the weekend, chills ran down my arms and back because the reality of this health change was hitting me in fullness--it WAS happening. Happy tears also crept in a few times without any forewarning. I didn't fight them.

JE September 6th, 2016

Thank You for continued healing, Papa. I'm eternally grateful! Wow, Papa, what peace I have. I feel like I am a brand-new person with a whole new life, a whole new start. I'm SO thankful and so ready for it to begin. WAIT, it has begun and I'm LOVING IT!!!

103

Real Sharing

Kelly

JE September 8th, 2016

Day #8 of AMAZINGNESS! To have virtually no symptoms, WOW! What a blessing to live, laugh, and love! Thank You, Papa!

Fall of 2016. Each day here-on after Labor Day weekend, the healing process continued. Having bowel movements on my own continued too! I'd spoken from the inner depths of my soul, tears spilling down my face, untouched, one evening, *"Thank You, Papa. I'm eternally grateful for the continued healing You are doing in and through me. I love You and trust You,"*

The Comprehensive Stool Analysis Test (CSAT) arrived by mail. I completed it with an easily offered specimen, then sent it to the lab for testing! I had no doubt in my mind that my pancreas was functioning well and that the cancer was truly eradicated. I had only a few symptoms, randomly. Overall, I was feeling the best that I had felt in years, maybe even the best I'd ever felt in my whole life! The smile on my face was back, without being forced, and it felt REALLY good!

Being these wonderful changes were still so fresh, it felt surreal to have bowel movements on my own. In addition, I had so much energy at times that I wanted to run around like young children do during school recess! I'd go through an entire day feeling well! This made work days easier too! I really loved the work I do. I'm glad I continued to work while battling my health ordeal. A friend had stated to me once, "All of the healing that you do for yourself every single day, despite not feeling well... then with the work you do, you are forced (actually it's my choice) to help people regardless of how you feel."

I remember smiling, thinking, and gently saying, "Some days my clients were one of the only things that kept me going." She and I had held our gaze, looking deep into each other's eyes while happy tears formed. When I had texted that same special friend, Hallie, telling her the good news that had happened in the last many days saying, "It's over. It's truly over!" Her response was immediate!

"KELLY! Words can't express the happiness, joy, and RELIEF I feel for you! That's so incredible! You are incredible. Thank you for sharing you, all of it, with me!" she had texted back. Hallie is one of my tribe sisters who knew all of what I'd gone through. Her love, concern, care, kindness, support, and encouragement never stopped.

As my health took this huge turn for the better, there were times when tears would spring forth from my eyes, coming straight from my heart. These were thankful tears of healing, and would pour out at any given time. I didn't fight the tears when they would come, but freely let them flow--a BIG change from not so many years ago.

After Labor Day weekend, Mom shared with family and friends the huge progress my health had made within the last week-and-a-half. She didn't go into great detail, but instead said, "Kelly is doing much better! Her digestive system is working. She is much improved!"

I shared the good news with my chiropractor, who knew the truth about my health situation and had played a role in directing me toward health professionals that aided in my healing during this health journey. His response was, "PRAISE THE LORD! That is wonderful news and it reflects the strength and commitment you made to yourself! You have an incredible story to share... and when you are ready it will have a kingdom impact here on earth. Kelly, you should be very proud of yourself. You've done what most (people) would think is impossible and would plain refuse to do. Wow! Praise God, and fantastic job, Kelly!"

Humbled. Blessed. Overwhelmed. Joyfully. Thankful. All of these were emotions that I felt. But mostly, I felt humbled and thankful, with my heart blown wide open.

JE September 11th, 2016

It seems like I'm living a dream as I'm learning to live life and function "normally" again. What a pure blessing! I feel truly WELL overall, needing less sleep, and having no abdominal or back pain. Thank You, Papa! It's been a long and hard journey, but oh so rewarding! I wouldn't trade it for anything! Thank You for this whole journey so far! I want You to ALWAYS be the center of my life, Papa. Help me to stay focused on You. I love and trust You!

On September 14th, 2016, I'd sent a text message to Mom. It read, "I've been thinking, seeing lately just how much this healing journey has God's hand ALL over it. The point in my saying this is Papa God makes beauty out of ashes, even the nastiest, most horrible, ugliest hardships and trying circumstances. This healing journey is a beautiful portrayal of Papa doing just that! Papa God wants me to share my story with people. It's time!"

Mom's text reply said, "Smiling BIG!"

Telling the truth about my health journey? Was I ready? I knew what Papa God wanted me to do, and I trusted that. In due time sharing my story WOULD HAPPEN. The reason I share this particular snippet of info is because I struggled in my mind, going back and forth, with if I should REALLY share my story with people. Yes, I knew in my heart of hearts Papa God was calling me to, but yet I still struggled.

If you've followed my story thus far, you well know my story is raw and personal. I'm completely vulnerable in sharing the fine details of my journey, being REAL transparent with nothing to hide. It has humbled me greatly to allow people to judge my choices. I, again, just want to thank you for having any interest at all in reading my story. I really and truly hope that you have been blessed. If you wouldn't mind, please do tell others and share the book with them.

104

Suspense

Kelly

It'd only been a week since I'd sent in my CSAT stool samples. The suspense was starting to get to me, making me a tad bit anxious. Normally, suspense didn't affect me. But this time was different.

"I sure hope the test results come in this week." I'd said to Mom. Only a day later, on September 16, 2016, I got my CSAT results via email. I'd just finished with my last client, and glancing at my cell phone screen I saw the email notice which read, "Enclosed is a copy of your CSAT results."

"MOM!" I exclaimed happily while trying to be quiet, as my client was still in the nearby therapy room.

"You got your test results?" She'd assumed wisely.

"YES" I replied, giddy with excitement.

"Don't read them yet! Let's look at them together." Mom squealed quietly.

"Okay!" I'd agreed. "I'm going to print them though." While the file of the test results was printing, Mom assisted my client with her payment and shortly thereafter it was just the two of us in office. I said, "Are you ready, Mom?"

"Yes." She'd replied.

"It looks like I still have some bacteria that aren't right in my gut. But overall, the results have drastically improved regarding the numbers compared to last year's test." I stated. "My pancreas numbers are good! They're NORMAL!" I stated happily.

"Your pancreas results were the first and only results that I saw!" Mom said and then laughed, smiling big. Mom's relief was evident on her face.

"Mom, I'm so glad that you were here to go over the results with me."

"Me too, Kelly. Me too." She'd replied with happy tears filling her eyes. We shared a long, warm hug, and I swallowed the lump that'd formed in my throat. Then both of our tears spilled freely, at ease. "You're my living miracle, Kelly." I truly AM my mom's living miracle. I'm in no way, shape, or form bragging, but actually quite the opposite. I'm humbled to know that I brushed death's door, enduring a hellish nightmare, and came out the other side of it alive and thankful FOR the experience and for the RBs. I'm truly humbled, thankful, and blessed beyond anything words can express.

I got home from work that night and sat down for supper with my parents and brother. As we talked and ate, I mostly listened to their conversation. It felt good just to sit and listen to them talking, catching up with one another's week. Turning to me, Mom inquired. "Are you going to tell them your test results, Kelly?"

"I got my CSAT results back today. The results detected how my pancreas is working along with many other vital insights." Dad looked at me waiting to hear what I'd say next. The words bubbled out of me, "The results showed that my pancreas is back to functioning as it should!" It was nice to see the joy and happiness in my dad's eyes. It was similar to Mom's when she read the test results just hours earlier. Their deep love and concern for me was always evident throughout this entire journey. To see the relief in their eyes and in their whole beings was a pure blessing, along with my brother's relief and caring concern for me. I continued, "There are still some bacteria in my gut that aren't balanced as optimally as they should be. This means my gut microbiome (my gut flora) isn't as balanced as it should be. But with the right supplements and with Dr. North's help, they should be balanced in due time. Healing takes time and doesn't happen overnight," I'd commented wisely, knowing healing DOES TAKE TIME and doesn't happen overnight!

"The other concern is that my immune system is very upregulated; hyper-active. These numbers are higher than they've ever been. My immune system is still attacking AND reacting to what it comes into contact with... which is literally everything. It's reacting this way because it's trying to understand the difference between good and bad. It makes perfect sense though, given what my body has been going through for so long. Why WOULDN'T it react to anything, given my immune system still views the cells, the bacteria, and food as the enemy? In time, my immune system will start to depict the difference to operate more accurately, eventually calming down. It's going to take some time though." I stated, knowingly. "I haven't talked with Dr. North about the results yet. I will in our next phone consult at the end of the month. Then, I'll hear what insights he has for what's left to balance." I told my family.

"Kelly, this is great news! The pancreas was the main focus though, right?" Dad asked.

"Yes. That was the main reason for the test; seeing how my pancreas was working and what has changed in my gut health. Also, checking to see that other organs are back working together as they were designed to work. This is HUGE!" I stated. "This test holds a lot of other very helpful information for Dr. North, giving him direction in the next step of healing."

"That's great, Kelly!" Dad voiced again, "I'm happy for you. You've really been a trooper!"

"Thank you." I smiled.

"I'm glad you're feeling better." Troy said. And he was truly thankful.

"You've still been able to have bowel movements on your own?" Dad inquired.

"Yes, I'm going on my own." I smiled again.

"You say that as if it's 'normal'." Mom said to me, chuckling.

"Ha! That's funny, Mom!" I said while turning to look at Dad. "Yes, I'm going on my own. I've not done ANY enemas to induce a bowel movement! Getting the last of the tumor, the rope biofilms, out was key. It was then that I could go on my own; my body started working as it was designed to. Pretty amazing."

I then swallowed the lump that had formed in my throat. My parents and brother started talking among themselves while I was engaged in my own thoughts, overcome with a vast array of emotions concerning the last six-plus years. *"Thank You, Papa. I'm so overcome with utter thankfulness. I trust You, Papa, for whatever You have in store for me. This hasn't been easy, but You have paved the way for me and I can never say 'thank You' enough. I love You. Please continue to heal me, using me for Your glory and honor."* I prayed inwardly.

All the memories of the endless days and nights of pain, being unable to laugh or cry because it made the physical abdominal and back pain that much worse. The diligence it took. Giving up things I loved to do and used to love to eat, trusting that my Papa was in control; making good of whatever was to happen. Thoughts of my loved ones and other well-meaning people that came alongside of me and our family to help. Mom choosing to do the on-line gut healing program with me. My pets and the roles they played in my healing. All the amazing healers that helped in so many ways. *"Papa,"* I prayed silently again with tears in my eyes, *"I'm left utterly speechless with the beauty that You have made of this entire process in these last six-plus years. Despite everything, it has truly been REWARDING! I wouldn't trade ANY of this for anything. Thank You for giving me a second chance at life. Lead me, direct me, and guide me."* Swallowing, and blinking while tears teased, then spilled over, all seemed well. My heart was at peace.

The next day, I saw Hallie for my monthly massage in the city. She enveloped me in a big hug upon hearing my test results. After the appointment, she said, "Your body seems really strong. It has surprised me throughout this whole process how strong it is, but today it is stronger and 'different'."

I smiled. My body was stronger. It was different. And I was different.

105

CSAT Results Revealed

Kelly

On September 28th, 2016, I was giddy with anticipation for my phone consult with Dr. North. I stood outside on a crisp fall Minnesota morning.

"Good morning, Kelly. I hope you are doing well?" Dr. North inquired.

"Hello! I am doing REALLY well!" I chuckled.

"GOOD! Tell me about how well you are doing." He said lightly.

"Well…" I said in my midwestern drawl, "I haven't done any enemas since I last talked to you! I've had bowel movements completely on my own. I've had virtually NO symptoms besides a few headaches which stem from smells like chemicals (petroleum and cleaning products), perfumes, and other toxins flying around in the air--such as burning garbage, particles from grains being harvested on farm fields locally around us, or fumes from gas- or diesel-powered trucks and equipment. Also, I've had a little gas and bloating. Those aren't daily occurrences though. That's it, as far as symptoms go, though!" I stepped back inside the house.

"Oh!" I stated before he had a chance to speak, "Another HUGE positive change started three days ago. I can now fall asleep faster and easier at night. Before it most often took 1-2 hours to fall asleep. Now, it's taking only 10-30 minutes. With that, I've found that I sleep deeper and am less restless. I don't feel the need to sleep as many hours in a night as I used to, and I still have plenty of energy," I shared excitedly!

"Kelly, this is all wonderful news! I'm SO glad to hear this!" responded Dr. North, his joy flowing through his voice. "Did you receive a copy of your test results via email?"

"Yes, I did. I have them in front of me." I stated. My heart, my mind, and my whole being were ready to hear what he had to say. I had anticipated this moment of time... and now it was FINALLY here!

"You have a couple strains of bacteria that still aren't quite balanced. One of them I'm wondering if you're taking in supplement form?" Dr. North named the bacteria and I listened to what information he had to share about it.

"No, I'm not taking any supplement that has that particular bacteria strain. The only other probiotic foods and beverages I'm taking include sauerkraut, coconut water kefir, and kombucha." I shared.

"Okay. The kombucha can get bacteria imbalances in it at times. Have you gotten a new mother scobi recently?" He asked.

"Interesting you mention that, because as of recently we've been having issues with our kombucha. It has a distinct taste to it that isn't quite right..." My voice trailed off as I'd walked into the kitchen where Mom was.

"That's a sign you should start the process over. There's probably a bacteria imbalance." He stated, then explained about what precautions should be used in order to maintain a stable bacterial environment. I listened intently and smiled at Mom, whom was listening to our conversation. I had Dr. Jack on speaker phone. Mom and I'd both had the thought that maybe the kombucha was aiding in my bacteria imbalance.

Dr. North then moved forward with the CSAT results saying, "The other bacteria imbalance we'll be able to eradicate through supplementation. Kelly, this month will be a purging month. We need to get rid of these remaining bad bacteria. Also, we'll need to get a few new bacteria in your body that you don't have. These are important to have." He stated knowingly.

"Okay." I replied, while stepping outside again, onto the deck.

"Overall, your pancreas and other organs are working well! The only other aspect we are looking at right now is your immune system. The test shows your immune system is currently VERY hyperactive. This is due to the bacteria imbalances. Once we correct these imbalances, your immune system should calm down." Dr. North informed me.

"So, in other words," I said, "my immune system is both attacking and reacting to anything and everything, due to the fact it's trying to decipher what is good and bad? And that is why I'm still having some symptoms?"

"Exactly." He confirmed. My face broke into a huge grin. The brisk fall air was chilly. I was starting to get cold. *Should have left my jacket on.* "Kelly, one more month of purging and you will be able to start maintaining good health." He said. "It will take another year of working together to get your GI track back to healthy and well. That being said, you're WELL on your way, and this month will be the last 'hard core' month. After that, you won't have to take all the supplements you've been taking. Instead, you will be using only food as medicine, and practicing preventative maintenance!" Dr. North chuckled deep down from his innermost being. His huge chuckle of joy caused me to break into a bigger, wider grin. "You'll just continue to feel better and better from this point on."

One more year. This feels surreal. Is this REALLY happening Papa God! My grin grew even bigger. I was about to finish a VERY long and drawn-out last step in the healing process! I was at the threshold of embarking on the homestretch. One more month of "hard core" supplementation and then it would be time to take the supplementation down to a subtler degree for the next year with food as my medicine, and to allow my body to start to fight bacteria on its own again! HUGE deal! *One more month!* Just one more month!

106

Special Memories

Kelly

Dr. North and I were both silent for a brief time, as if soaking in the depth of all this past year had encompassed... and for me, the many past years to getting to this point. I'd gone through the hard work of detoxifying my body, giving it what was needed to fight this long battle. Various organ's health was reversed by detoxification. I'd truly conquered pancreatic cancer, the deadliest cancer, with MANY helps!

Conquering cancer via alternative forms of healing are often looked down on by Western medical communities, and at times by the general public, disregarded as quackery and scoffed at as impossible. Like my chiropractor had put so clearly, "You've done what most people would think is impossible, or would plain refuse to do."

Thoughts continued racing through my mind of the last six years, while on the phone with Dr. North that crisp fall Minnesota morning. I broke our silence, saying, "Thank you, Dr. North," trying to refocus on our conversation, having just drifted off in my own thoughts. I looked up into the clouds and whispered in the inner most depths of my heart, *"Thank You, Papa."*

"You're welcome, Kelly. I'm going to finish working on your protocol for this month and we'll get the supplements sent out to you ASAP." He said warmly.

We scheduled another appointment, then Dr. North said, "Kelly, you've done such a good job! You have gone through A LOT of hard work. You have made so much progress and I'm so very happy for you!"

My throat felt thick. My eyes were filled with tears. I gently blinked, the tears falling down my face and said, my voice lurking through the thickness, "Dr. North, thank you so much for all of your help." My voice cracked. My words seemed so small compared to how thankful I truly was for his help.

"Oh Kelly, you are so welcome. You continue to be well and we'll talk again in a month. Bye-bye." Dr. North's famous "Bye-bye" always made me smile. He ALWAYS ended our phone consults this way

My heart felt like it was going to burst from the joy as I gently wiped the tears from my eyes. I turned and opened the screen door, stepping into the house again. Returning to the kitchen, Mom looked deep into my eyes. Tears had filled in her eyes, too, and without hesitation I reached out and we engulfed each other in a deep embrace, taking in another very special moment. "It's okay Mama. I'm all better." I choked out as tears and relief of "the worst being over" erupted from both of us in happy sobs. These words, "I'm all better" were the words any mama would love to hear after this journey. For years I'd wondered what this moment would be like. Now, finally it had happened, coming to fruition, on the morning of September 28, 2016 at 9:30a.m. I didn't know what to think or really how to feel. The one thing I did know was God had truly made a way for me to live and kept me in the palm of His hand every single step of the way. *Thank You, Papa. I'm eternally grateful. I love You and trust You.*

Dr. North had said it would take "one more year" to get me back to optimal health. I was eager to continue feeling better and better. Truthfully, I didn't even know what feeling better all encompassed, but I was ready for more healing to take place!

During the month of September 2016, I experienced "normal life" in many senses. Not only having bowel movements on my own, but being able to do activities with friends. I tried a few new foods. I was lighter in heart and more at ease than ever. I laughed. Papa had not only healed me physically, He'd healed me mentally, emotionally, and spiritually too throughout that whole health journey, and was continuing to do so. *My life is in Your hands,* I prayed in my heart.

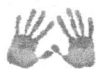

JE October 6th, 2016

Times are changing. I feel the change. Not just in my health, but for the future plans You have in store for me. I have NO doubt(s) in my mind about the future and all You have in store for me. I know You are in control; everything happens in Your perfect timing. I trust You, Papa God. My life is in Your hands. Continue to give me peace, patience, joy, love, healing, guidance, and direction. I know You are doing these things and I am at total peace. Papa, You are so good, ALL the time. You are beyond amazing.

As you well know from reading thus far, my mom was with me every step of the way on this healing journey. It wasn't easy for either of us, as I've talked about before. But in the moment when I said the words, "It's okay, Mama. I'm all better!" the full reality of all those years of complete vulnerability shared together were raw with emotion. To this day, it still brings happy tears to my eyes and a chill down my spine when I remember that day.

Looking back, today as I write, I won't lie--I'm still in awe of how God made absolute beauty out of ashes in my health. What some people could view as terrible, horrendous, and hellish, I literally choose not to LOOK at it that way. There's something to be said about looking at the reality of our lives and our situations, positively or negatively. I looked at it positively, as the years expanded. There's something to be said about positive thinking. I'm not saying being optimistic is going to fix a situation, but it helps to bring a different perspective and a lightness of heart... and for me, to be grateful all the more for anything and everything. No matter how awful or well I felt during my journey, I tried to not only stay positive, but most importantly for me, to be in constant communication with my Papa God.

My Papa God is my very best friend, as I've stated often here in sharing my journey. There's NO way I could have gone through this journey without Him in my life. I'm not trying to convince you to believe what I believe, pushing my faith on you. I'm simply sharing the truth of my reality. My Papa God was and is my CONSTANT solid rock. Truthfully, my Papa God blows my mind with His undying love for each and every one of us. No matter what we've done in our lives, no matter the choices we've made, will make in the future, no matter what place we are at in our lives, He NEVER leaves us or forsakes us. We can ALWAYS turn to Him. Papa delights in our constant relationship with Him, and speaking for myself, I do delight in the constant relationship with Him too. This not to say at times I don't get frustrated and want answers NOW. Interestingly, those moments of the unknowns while putting my trust in Him, were where our relationship blossomed ten-fold. Maybe you've experienced this too?

Again, I'm not trying to push my faith on you. The point is, Papa God delights in EACH and EVERY one of us. I truly want you to know that He delights IN YOU.

107

FULL CIRCLE!

Kelly

And so it was, one more month of hardcore supplements. After, I was taking very few supplements and focusing more on food as medicine. I continued to learn SO much from Dr. North, in his explaining the WHYs of intrinsic bodily functioning health details to help me be able to better help myself. He was teaching me so in a year's time I could be my own best doctor at a deeper level.

Truthfully, it was humbling to me that Dr. North would take the time to really hear me and answer my questions. He wasn't prideful or arrogant in his answers or the knowledge he shared. He always just laid what he knew out in the open, sharing it and letting me absorb the information. He reminded me a lot of Dr. Ann because she, also, took the time to talk with and educate her patients. It's refreshing to see there are still health professionals taking the time to educate their patients.

Throughout the next year, the few symptoms lingering at times disappeared, mostly bloating and gas, especially when introducing new foods. It was a slow process to implement new foods back into my diet, always starting in small quantities and working my way up to larger amounts as my body received the vital nutrients. I was becoming even more in-tune with my body, something I (we) should never stop listening to.

In a years' time I had so many noticeable shifts in my health. My energy was better than ever. My state of mind and overall health was the best it'd ever been. I was more vulnerable and more real with people than I'd ever been thus far in life. And I was humbler. There wasn't a day that I wasn't thankful to feel good, to have BMs on my own, and to be symptom free. Dr. North had said in the year to come this would happen, that I would feel better and better, and it WAS happening. I was in total awe that I continued to feel better and better. It was surreal to me, honestly.

Just shy of the one-year mark Dr. North had told me I would be well, he was right--my body felt totally WELL. This was in the fall of 2017. There was a "knowing" deep inside of me the timing was right, and it was time for me to take care of my own health. Shortly after sensing this "knowing", Dr. North and I had our last phone consult.

"It's time for you to implement all that you've learned into your lifestyle, Kelly." We were both silent for a few moments. We'd both been knowing this time would come. "Kelly, there were times in this journey…" in his genuine kind voice, "I really didn't know if you were going to make it. But you did. You're my miracle story!" Tears sprang out from my eyes, literally streaming endlessly down my cheeks. "You've reversed your health completely. I'm so proud of you and all your hard work."

I couldn't even say anything as the lump in my throat prevented me from even speaking. But when I could, my voice was thick and trembling, "Thank you, Dr. North. Thank you. You helped make it possible. I couldn't have done it without you." We each absorbed the short silence before we both knew that it was time to say our final "bye-bye", until we would again consult in a years' time the following October of 2018.

I can't even begin to describe all the feelings and emotions that were present in that split second, but here's a few of the biggest: gratitude, awestruck wonder, pure thankfulness, humbleness, peace, and a heart and mind that were both blown wide open.

Throughout my illness to wellness journey, it had been a desire of my heart to be able to meet Dr. North in person, to personally thank him for all his help. During my chronic state of health, it wasn't going to happen. But in my heart, I fully believed one day I would be able to meet him in person. I'd voiced this to Mom a few times during the next year after getting my clean bill of health, telling her, "I want to meet Dr. North and thank him personally for all his help. The timing isn't right, but at some point, it will be." Mom had smiled, nodding her head in agreement.

Since 2013 and beyond, my mom and I have done a "Girls Get-Away" on her birthday weekend, mid-October. The "Girls Get-Away" was something that we needed to plan ahead for, if others were going to be a part of it. **Fast-forward** to August, 2018. This year's "Girls Get-Away" 2018, I had an idea in mind that I thought she might enjoy. I attempted to present it to her by first asking, "Mom, what do you want to do for your birthday this year?" Yes, I DID ask her this before I even told her about my idea.

Mom thought for a little while. Then her eyes lit up, like a child's eyes do when they get a gift they really like! She squealed, "Wouldn't it be AWESOME to go down south to meet Dr. North in person!" She was giddy with anticipation of my response! My jaw literally dropped, giving her the "deer in the headlight look". *Does she SERIOUSLY live in my head or what?*

I shook my head in utter dismay, while chuckling responding, "How in the world did you know? That's EXACTLY what I was going to suggest to you!" We both erupted into a series of hoots and laughter. When we got ahold of ourselves, I elaborated. "I was thinking that since your birthday is on a Friday, MAYBE we could fly in the day before, IF he's available since he travels all over the world for speaking engagements, teaching, etc. And if so, see if he'd be willing to meet us in person for my yearly consult."

It was settled. I was to inquire of Dr. North, from the south, to see if he had time in his busy schedule to meet us in person to have my yearly consult with him.

Fast-forward AGAIN a few more months, to October 19th, 2018--Mom's birthday. As Mom, I, and my auntie Lori (Mom's sister) drove through the hills of the south, minutes away from meeting Dr. North! Auntie Lori asked me from the back seat, "Kelly, what are you thinking and feeling right now?"

I had to think for a little while before responding. "Truthfully, if I pick one word to sum it up, it would be 'surreal'." And it was exactly that, surreal, as we pulled into his driveway. Dr. North and his wife are in their 70's. They had invited us to their home for lunch, a gesture many doctors would never make with their clients. He and I had worked on my chronic health condition together always via phone consults, so we'd never actually met in person before this time. It was a very special time for all of us to finally meet face-to-face!

Our time together was nothing shy of memorable. Hugs were shared as we walked through the door. Mom was able to video our meeting for the first time. We also took a few pictures together before lunch. It was so nice to put names and faces together of his wife and an assistant, as I'd communicated to each of them over the span of two years of monthly consults, both in lining up appointments via phone and completing follow-ups via emails.

Dr. North's wife made the lunch, and then we were served while light chatter interwove before and throughout the meal. It was a really nice time enjoying one another's company. Truthfully, I mostly sat back and absorbed the conversations.

Afterwards, Dr. North took Mom and me back to his office to go over my yearly CSAT results. I'd asked him if I could do an annual CSAT prior to our meeting, (which he'd sent out to me, I'd completed my specimens, and test results were sent back to us both) so today we'd planned to go over the test results. The CSAT was done for purpose of "a map" for my routine maintenance. Together, the three of us talked, going over the test results-- which were all good! No issues were found.

Mom thought this was the best birthday present she could ever receive, meeting Dr. North with me and thanking him in person, AND my good test results!

As we walked out of his house into the mid-fall afternoon, he showed us his beautiful garden of fresh herbs out front in the landscaped yard, picking some for us to taste. I couldn't help but smile as he walked us to our vehicle. At the vehicle, he carefully tucked us inside while saying his final "bye-bye" whiling shut my car door. What a gentleman. Inevitably, my eyes got a bit misty.

Meeting Dr. North was something I felt the need to do since he was the person who played the most intricate role in reversing my health. If it wasn't for Dr.

North's wisdom in detoxification, gut health, nutrition, and so much more in the all-natural aspects of healing, I wouldn't be here today--nor would I be sharing my story with you.

Since the fall of 2018, I've had seasons of continued monthly consults with Dr. North. Together we've been able to tweak little things that come up in my health. Furthermore, we've improved some things so there hopefully won't be opportunity for issues in the future.

So, you see, everything came full circle. Well, almost! There was only one thing left after meeting Dr. North, that I knew in my heart of hearts that my Papa God called me to do. And what was that? To share my personal health journey story with you. And, so the story has come to fruition in the telling. It has truly come FULL CIRCLE!

108

What's Next?

Kelly

What's next? In order to answer this question, I've got to go back to when I was battling for my life. It was only a couple years into my 7-year health journey that I became a massage therapist. I absolutely love my job and am very passionate about it. In saying this, as my health wasn't all that I desired for it to be, being so sick, I came to realize just how crucial "food as medicine" truly is. My life has changed upside-down and inside-out because of the entire ill health experience.

When I hit the point in my health where it was unknown to IF I would wake to see another day, I felt a tugging in my heart; both a knowing and a desire in my heart to learn for myself, and for others IF they wanted to, learn more about "food as medicine". Not long after having this tugging in my heart, I got an email that opened my eyes in surprise, presenting me with an opportunity to become a "health coach".

Laying on the floor in pain at the time, I read the email then clicked on the link provided to "Learn More". I read in depth the information on health coaching all while battling my physical pain. I saved the email, knowing at that point in time I'd need it, but right then I needed to focus on my getting better, to be well again, before I could embark on another fabulous health endeavor. Although I set aside the email, it was always in the back of my mind, not to mention buried at the bottom of my email-inbox when years later I looked for it.

Now I'm healthy and well. I still love, and am passionate about, being a massage therapist. My business is truly the wellness center that I talked about in "A Weekend to Remember". I am a self-employed business owner that offers a variety of services that can aid in a person's all-natural health journey. In the fall 2019, I embarked on a new health endeavor while still working and operating my business.

And then God answered; "Write this. Write what you see. Write it out in big block letters so that it can be read on the run. This vision-message is a witness pointing to what's coming. It aches for the coming – it can hardly wait! And it doesn't lie. If it seems slow in coming, wait. It's on its way. It will come right on time." -Habakkuk 2:2-3(MSG)

I attended school online at the "Institute for Integrative Nutrition", right from home. Health coaching training took a year's time, which allowed me to attend classes and study on my time-frame, daily.

It's my hearts' desire to serve people in an all-natural, healthy way. Yes, I did this in my business already, but this health "nerd" who is always wanting to learn more, asking WHY this, or HOW COME that, wanted to open up yet another avenue for healing to happen in an individual's life.

What is a health coach? A health coach is a wellness-authority figure and supportive mentor who helps their clients shift their behavior toward healthier habits. Whether the goal is losing weight, improving digestion, reducing stress, addressing mental and emotional behaviors, boosting energy, or just developing an overall healthier lifestyle, health coaches support their clients to develop sustainable lifestyle changes. By addressing all facets of wellness, in addition to diet, relationships, career, physical activity, and spirituality, a health coach takes a holistic approach to health, helping clients find the unique foods and lifestyle choices that make their clients feel their best.

In becoming a health coach, my desire to be able to help people that want to change their lives is open for the making of that to happen. By making small changes, with the help of a health coach, it can be easier for someone to become healthier with guidance and direction.

I chose the specific health coaching training because I wanted to be able to help myself become healthier and more whole, too. I want to know the WHYs and HOWs of nutrition, food, emotions, illness, food chemistry, brain patterns and functions, diseases, the problems stemming from GMOs and how processed foods impact our health and brain, food intolerances and sensitivities, emotional eating, nutritional health for children, food addiction, and so much more! I also wanted to understand people better. I want to understand why our thoughts, our thinking, is the way it is. What if I could understand myself better than I already do? What if you could understand yourself better with some guidance? I wanted to understand the impact food has on us, and what makes us the people we are. To be able to see how illness can be reversed with specific foods, spices, herbs, supplements, etc., is pretty fantastic. I knew this for a fact!

I don't know if you want to, but this health nerd wants to dig deeper into natural health and healing all the time! It's my joy to share things that I learn with clients and you, a reader of my health story, but I NEVER want anyone to feel like I shove my beliefs, thoughts, or interests at them. This being said, no matter where life takes each of us, I value you and your health. I hope and pray that you value your health too.

As you've read, my pets are a big part of my life. After I obtained my clean bill of health, our family lost a dear friend--my adventure partner, my cat Goofy. The year before we put her down, two little kittens became part our family. What an exciting season it was! If you'd like to hear these happenings-- how the kittens came into our lives, how Goofy acquired "cancer" from a routine vaccine, and about our newest pet, "Aggie", a puppy—then visit my business website at **yourlifeletthehealingbegin.com** and click on "blog" tab, then check out the blogs titled, "SURPRISE!", "MORE SURPRISES!", "What A Day", "Furry Friends", "Injected", and "Love at First Sight ". My blogs include health tips and life stories.

A final note. Life's a roller coaster. There are highs and lows in life. Always remember that there IS beauty that comes out from ashes. Let's all take a step back and look for the beauty in our ashen moments of life. May you find the beauty in every one of them. God bless!

Epilogue

Kelly

Dear Reader,

Life, what a blessing. Life, what an adventure! And life, what a rollercoaster--it's full of ups, downs, twists and turns. Without all of those, life wouldn't be an adventure, nor would we be who we are today. Isn't that pretty neat when you really think about it?

It is currently the year 2022 as I write this epilogue. I've continued to invest in my health as well. I've completed my health coaching training and integrated it into my business. I've been working and spending quality time with my family and my pets, and I've been doing all the outdoor activities that I've desired to do, mostly around the area that I live. I have routine in my life, and I feel light and free. I can sit back and relax and breathe deeply.

In the last two years, our world as we used to know it has changed drastically. I've realized at yet another level how important freedom, health, and peace are. Freedom of speech, freedom to choose what you want to do, freedom of health choices, etc.

Freedom of attaining my health choices, to me means the ability to eat organic, non-GMO food, and to consume good, quality, whole foods that nourish my mind and my body. It's an absolute freedom I've come to greatly appreciate. And then there's freedom to attain peace. As you've read in my health story, my Papa God is the one that ultimately gives me life, breath, peace, and love. Without my Papa I wouldn't be here today, nor would I be who I am right now, or actually BE right now! I have peace because of my Papa God. No one can ever take Him away from me.

It is my ultimate hope and prayer you have, or soon find freedom, health, and peace in ways that are right for YOU. These are not the same for everyone, so please, find what's right for you as an individual and stick to it. You are loved, you are worthy, and you can have freedom, good health, and peace in your life. Don't give up, it's a process. Every step makes a difference.

Life is nothing short of an incredible journey! I truly don't know what my future holds beyond today, but I do look forward to whatever it entails. For the time being, I'm enjoying having a "normal life", a "healthy routine", and "finding joy" in everyday life adventures. That's really what it's about, finding joy in ALL things. May you find peace, love, joy, health, and freedom in the days, months, and years to come. And never forget that it's a process. Again, don't give up!

Thank you for taking the time to read my health journey from dis-ease to ease. I hope and pray that you took some things away from my story which may have inspired you to become a better version of yourself.

Much love always,

Kelly Lang

Amy
A personal message to my daughter
Kelly, you've had so much healing take place in your young life, through your actions in caring for yourself, through caring for your clients and pets, through journaling, and in the space of time writing your story so candidly for others to read. Your commitment to follow through in caring for yourself in these multiple areas of healing from various traumas in living your life, and writing those experiences into this book, have blessed you and those of us around you. Thank you for speaking so much truth in the arena of "health", with such boldness and faith! ***"God love ya, girl!"*** *Thank you for being a warrior, a forerunner, a vessel for God to speak through, and a change-agent. I'm so happy in my heart you hung on for "one more month"!*

Dear Reader,
What may seem like a "healthy" life-style can become something other than "healthy" in a matter of a day's time, be it a short or long life. One day, symptoms appear. Then doctoring. Doctors diagnose. A life blows up instantly with stress, having to make major health decisions--choices. We all know people who've experienced this, even ourselves perhaps.

Kelly was making choices--doing many holistic practices to help her body digest properly during her many years of illness. When she started detoxing during the online gut healing program, the timing of that was impeccable--she was already almost five years into helping herself all-naturally via eating an all-natural organic diet—free of chemicals, dyes, hormones and other destructive additives which promote damage in human cells. She'd not been given a cancer diagnosis from any Western medical doctor, only an initial IBS (irritable bowel syndrome) diagnosis. The proof of the pancreatic cancer showed up on the Comprehensive Stool Analysis Test later while working with Dr. North. And thanks be to God, the timing of therapies and people to help her gain back her health all worked together to detox cancer from her pancreas! I'm ONE THANKFUL mama!

Naturally, I'm thrilled over the choices Kelly made to become whole and well in health. The choice of self-respect demonstrated, with discipline in the process of healing herself and patiently waiting for her body to heal itself, has made my heart so happy for the woman she is today. Her story matters for such a time as this.

We all go through seasons in our lives. Seasons of great joy. Seasons of loss. Seasons of learning. Seasons of love, and seasons of seemingly little love or patience. Seasons of unrest in the world, always, some seasons more than others. I love seasons, and what they teach me. I seek to find truth in this life. The "season of detoxing" for Kelly evolved into a few years, although she was sick for a longer season prior to detoxing--seven years total. It takes a long time to get really sick, and it takes a hard season, and a dedicated person to become well, as one can see as you've read Kelly's health journey in the over 400 pages here.

I believe God allows us "gifts of pain, situations in which pain is used to grow us. God had Kelly's health situation in the palm of His hands at all times. Kelly chose an all-natural approach to her healing. When you, the reader, read about that day on the bathroom floor in our home when Kelly was battling for her life while heavily detoxing, you'll recall God gave her a choice to let go, to die in her earthly existence, or for her to breathe again and continue to demolish the stronghold of illness in her young life. For me, I know to Whom I was praying to as she lay partially on my lap and on the floor during this time, having no idea of WHAT she was experiencing with her Papa God. One could assume I prayed for her to not have pain and to be made well. You're free to assume so. What I do recall is an "always prayer" that fills my mind so often for many people, including myself--"Not my will, or anyone else's will be done, but Thy will be done". All I can really say about her amazing experience on this particular day is, "THANK GOD".

I don't take my health, or anyone's health, for granted. Patients choose their path of healing, at least presently as this book is being completed. Which is just the point; we make choices. We have the freedom TO choose. This is what I love most about, **"Your Life Your Choice Let the Healing Begin…"**, all the talk about freedom of choice. What I also love about Kelly's life shared here and on her blog is her transparent love of Papa God that she so candidly shares with us.

But God! God is the answer to all the problems in our world and problems among human beings. God is the Healer of nations, the One who is with us at all times. God is waiting to hear from us individually and corporately. If you want to know Him, call out to Him. He hears you. Trust me on this one. He hears and sees everything every day, and still loves us unconditionally in this fallen cellular experience called a human life. Life here on earth is a short journey for us. This world is not our home. Eternity is forever. Evil cannot prevail. Love always wins. *This world has gotten quite crazy down here. Help us, dear God. How much longer? Amen.*

Do not be overcome by evil, but overcome evil with good. -Romans 12:21

May our lives, with all the seasons we go through, be filled with much learning in the experiences, much seeking of truth, and speaking out for such a time as this. Peace is a choice to enter into with God, only through His Son Jesus Christ, who paid the ultimate price for mankind to be made right with the Father, God. Knock and the door will be opened. Seek and you will find. Ask and you shall receive.

"As I look back, I realize the obvious. God never wastes a tear. He never squanders the significant lessons acquired through our suffering. He does not disconnect our present pain from our future growth and fruitfulness." -Daniel Henderson

Peace be with you,

Amy Lang

426